Current Updates in Total Ankle Arthroplasty

Editor

J. CHRIS COETZEE

FOOT AND ANKLE CLINICS

www.foot.theclinics.com

Consulting Editor
MARK S. MYERSON

June 2017 • Volume 22 • Number 2

ELSEVIER

1600 John F. Kennedy Boulevard • Suite 1800 • Philadelphia, Pennsylvania, 19103-2899

http://www.theclinics.com

FOOT AND ANKLE CLINICS Volume 22, Number 2
June 2017 ISSN 1083-7515, ISBN-13: 978-0-323-53007-1

Editor: Lauren Boyle
Developmental Editor: Meredith Madeira

Foot and Ankle Clinics (ISSN 1083-7515) is published quarterly by Elsevier, Inc., 360 Park Avenue South, New York, NY 10010-1710. Months of issue are March, June, September, and December. Periodicals postage paid at New York, NY, and additional mailing offices. Subscription price per year is $320.00 (US individuals), $489.00 (US institutions), $100.00 (US students), $360.00 (Canadian individuals), $588.00 (Canadian institutions), $215.00 (Canadian students), $460.00 (international individuals), $588.00 (international institutions), and $215.00 (international students). To receive student/resident rate, orders must be accompanied by name of affiliated institution, date of term, and the *signature* of program/residency coordinator on institution letterhead. Orders will be billed at individual rate until proof of status is received. Foreign air speed delivery is included in all *Clinics* subscription prices. All prices are subject to change without notice. **POSTMASTER:** Send address changes to *Foot and Ankle Clinics*, Elsevier Health Sciences Division, Subscription Customer Service, 3251 Riverport Lane, Maryland Heights, MO 63043. **Customer Service: 1-800-654-2452 (US and Canada). From outside of the United States and Canada, call 314-447-8871. Fax: 314-447-8029. E-mail: JournalsCustomerService-usa@ elsevier.com (for print support); JournalsOnlineSupport-usa@elsevier.com (for online support).**

Reprints. For copies of 100 or more, of articles in this publication, please contact the Commercial Reprints Department, Elsevier Inc., 360 Park Avenue South, New York, NY 10010-1710. Tel.: 212-633-3874; Fax: 212-633-3820; E-mail: reprints@elsevier.com.

Editorial Advisory Board

Contributors

CONSULTING EDITOR

MARK S. MYERSON, MD
Medical Director, The Foot and Ankle Association, Inc., Baltimore, Maryland

EDITOR

J. CHRIS COETZEE, MD
Orthopedic Foot and Ankle Surgeon, MOSMI and Twin Cities Orthopedics, Edina, Minnesota

AUTHORS

YOUSEF ALRASHIDI, MD, SB-Ortho
Assistant Professor, Orthopaedic Foot and Ankle Surgeon, Orthopaedic Department, College of Medicine, Taibah University, Almadinah Almunawwarah, Kingdom of Saudi Arabia

YASH J. AVASHIA, MD
Resident, Division of Plastic Surgery, Duke University, Durham, North Carolina

ALEXEJ BARG, MD
Assistant Professor, Department of Orthopaedics, University of Utah, Salt Lake City, Utah

GREGORY C. BERLET, MD
Orthopedic Foot and Ankle Center, Westerville, Ohio

MICHAEL M. BRAGE, MD
Associate Professor of Orthopaedic Surgery, Department of Orthopaedics and Sports Medicine, University of Washington and Harborview Medical Center, Seattle, Washington

JAMES W. BRODSKY, MD
Director, Foot and Ankle Surgery Fellowship Program, Baylor University Medical Center, Dallas, Texas; Clinical Professor of Orthopaedic Surgery, University of Texas, Southwestern Medical School; Professor of Surgery, Orthopedics, Texas A & M HSC College of Medicine, Medical Director, Human Motion and Performance Laboratory, Baylor University Medical Center, Dallas, Texas

SCOTT COLEMAN, MS, MBA
Baylor Human Motion and Performance Laboratory, Baylor University Medical Center, Dallas, Texas

TIMOTHY R. DANIELS, MD, FRCSC
Full Professor, Department of Surgery, St. Michael's Hospital, University of Toronto, Toronto, Ontario, Canada

ANDREW DODD, MD, FRCSC
Clinical Lecturer, Department of Surgery, University of Calgary, Calgary, Alberta, Canada

NORMAN ESPINOSA, MD
Institute for Foot and Ankle Reconstruction Zurich, Zurich, Switzerland

AHMED E. GALHOUM, MSc, MRCS (England)
Orthopaedic Surgeon, Nasser Institute for Research and Treatment, Cairo, Egypt; Fellow, Orthopaedic Surgery, Department of Orthopaedics and Traumatology, Swiss Ortho Center, Schmerzklinik Basel, Basel, Switzerland

TAGGART T. GAUVAIN, MD
Assistant Clinical Professor, Department of Orthopaedic Surgery, University of Texas Health Science Center-Houston, Houston, Texas

MARK GLAZEBROOK, MD, FRCS(C), MSc, PhD
Orthopedic Surgeon and Professor, Dalhousie University, QE2 Health Science Center, Halifax, Nova Scotia, Canada

MICHAEL A. HAMES, MD
Private Practice Orthopaedics, Wichita Falls, Texas

MARIO HERRERA-PÉREZ, MD
Head, Foot and Ankle Surgery, and Associate Professor, Orthopaedic Department, University Hospital of Canary Islands, La Laguna, Tenerife, Spain

BEAT HINTERMANN, MD
Associate Professor and Chairman, Orthopaedic Clinic, Kantonsspital Baselland, Liestal, Switzerland

RAYMOND Y. HSU, MD
Fellow, Foot and Ankle Surgery, Department of Orthopaedics, University of Utah, Salt Lake City, Utah

JUSTIN M. KANE, MD
Foot and Ankle Division, Orthopedic Surgeon, Orthopedic Associates of Dallas; Faculty, Foot and Ankle Surgery Fellowship Program, Baylor University Medical Center, Dallas, Texas

GEORG KLAMMER, MD
Institute for Foot and Ankle Reconstruction Zurich, Zurich, Switzerland

SHU-YUAN LI, MD, PhD
Administrative Coordinator, The Foot and Ankle Association, Inc., Baltimore, Maryland

CAMILLA MACCARIO, MD
C.A.S.C.O. Foot and Ankle Unit- IRCCS Galeazzi Milan, Milan, Italy; Universita' degli Studi di Milano, Milan, Italy

WILLIAM C. McGARVEY, MD
Associate Clinical Professor, Orthopaedic Surgery Residency Program Director, Foot and Ankle Fellowship Program Director, Department of Orthopaedic Surgery, University of Texas Health Science Center-Houston, Houston, Texas

SUHAIL K. MITHANI, MD
Assistant Professor, Division of Plastic Surgery; Assistant Professor, Department of Orthopaedic Surgery, Duke University, Durham, North Carolina

JOEL MORASH, MD, FRCS(C)
Orthopedic Surgeon and Assistant Professor, Dalhousie University, QE2 Health Science Center, Halifax, Nova Scotia, Canada

DAWSON MUIR, FRACS
Grace Orthopaedic Centre, Tauranga, New Zealand

MARK S. MYERSON, MD
Medical Director, The Foot and Ankle Association, Inc., Baltimore, Maryland

SELENE G. PAREKH, MD, MBA
Partner, North Carolina Orthopaedic Clinic; Professor, Department of Orthopaedic Surgery; Adjunct Faculty, Fuqua Business School, Duke University, Durham, North Carolina

MAJ UMA E. RAMADORAI, DO
Assistant Professor, Uniformed Services University of the Health Sciences, Department of Orthopaedic Surgery, San Antonio Military Medical Center, San Antonio, Texas

CHRISTOPHER W. REB, DO
Division of Foot and Ankle Surgery, Department of Orthopaedics and Rehabilitation, University of Florida College of Medicine, Gainesville, Florida

ROXA RUIZ, MD
Senior Attending Foot and Ankle Surgeon, Orthopaedic Clinic, Kantonsspital Baselland, Liestal, Switzerland

RONNIE L. SHAMMAS, BS
Research Fellow, Division of Plastic Surgery, Duke University, Durham, North Carolina

FEDERICO GIUSEPPE USUELLI, MD
C.A.S.C.O. Foot and Ankle Unit- IRCCS Galeazzi Milan, Milan, Italy

VICTOR VALDERRABANO, MD, PhD
Professor, Chairman, Orthopaedic Department, Swiss Ortho Center, Schmerzklinik Basel, Swiss Medical Network, Basel, Switzerland

ANDREA VELJKOVIC, MD, BComm, MPH, FRCSC
Assistant Clinical Professor, University of British Columbia, Vancouver, British Columbia, Canada

DAVID M. WALTON, MD
Beaumont Hospital, Michigan Orthopedic Institute, Southfield, Michigan

MARTIN WIEWIORSKI, MD
Head, Foot and Ankle Surgery, Orthopaedic and Trauma Department, Kantonsspital Winterthur, Winterthur, Switzerland

STEPHAN H. WIRTH, MD
Department of Orthopaedics, University of Zurich, Zurich, Switzerland

ALASTAIR YOUNGER, MB, ChB, ChM, MSc, FRCSC
Professor, Department of Orthopaedics, University of British Columbia, Vancouver, British Columbia, Canada

Contents

the pathophysiology. Surgeons managing these patients with total ankle arthroplasty need to be familiar with extra-articular and intra-articular surgical methods to correct pes planus and pes cavus deformities, including bony procedures and soft tissue procedures. Performing these procedures in 1 or 2 stages depends on surgeon preference and the severity of the deformities. This article recommends a two-staged reconstruction for more severely deformed feet.

Ankle replacement results may be compromised by malposition of the components. An anterior displacement can be measured on a lateral standing radiograph. The ankle may appear anteriorly translated because the ankle is overstuffed, the heel cord is tight, or the posterior capsule is tight. In ankle instability with degenerative arthritis, the talus may be anteriorly translated, internally rotated, and in varus. In an ankle replacement, this deformity may persist and will require correction. On occasion, the talus is inserted too anterior; revision to a flat cut talar component and posterior translation of the talar component will result in correction.

One of the main challenges in ankle replacement is correction of any deformities in the operative limb. Deformity can be found proximal and distal to the ankle joint as well as in the ankle joint. There are static and dynamic deformities that can create unbalanced ankle joints causing early and often catastrophic failure. Surgeons must recognize the deformities that are present and use sound judgment to balance the ankle joint with procedures before, during, or after total ankle implantation. This article helps clinicians to identify deformity and provides a basic template to consider how to address each challenge.

Total ankle arthroplasty has advanced rapidly in the last 20 years. Early agility implants enjoyed improved survivability compared with more archaic total ankle implants. When talar subsidence occurs, the revision options include a stemmed component to improve stability by spanning the subtalar joint. Removal and revision of these stemmed components can be difficult because of ingrowth and bone loss.

Component subsidence has been found to be the top complication that leads to failure of the total ankle arthroplasty (TAA). The cause of subsidence formation is unclear, and is multifactorial. Talar subsidence is more frequently met than tibial subsidence, and the subsequent big bone loss is demanding to handle. As a revision treatment option, neither a revision TAA nor a salvage ankle and/or hindfoot arthrodesis procedure is easy to perform or can obtain a definite outcome. The Salto XT can be used to treat most of the TAA systems available for use in the United States with acceptable short-term outcomes.

FDA-approved navigated TAR system with limited but encouraging outcomes data. Therefore, its value can be estimated only based on benefits other than a proven clinical outcomes improvement over conventional systems. These include unique preoperative planning through 3-dimensional templating and virtual surgery and the patient-specific cut guides, which also reduce overall instrumentation needed for the case. To better inform this conversation, well-observed longitudinal outcomes studies are warranted.

FOOT AND ANKLE CLINICS

RELATED INTEREST

Orthopedic Clinics of North America, January 2017 (Vol. 48, No. 1)
Controversies in Fracture Care
Frederick M. Azar, James H. Calandruccio, Benjamin J. Grear et al, *Editors*

THE CLINICS ARE NOW AVAILABLE ONLINE!
Access your subscription at:
www.theclinics.com

FOOT AND ANKLE CLINICS

Preface

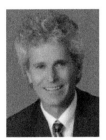

J. Chris Coetzee, MD
Editor

Over the past 15 years, since I was the Guest Editor for the 2002 issue *Foot and Ankle Clinics of North America* on Total Ankle Replacement (Volume 7, Issue 4), significant and positive steps have been taken in the field.

Total Ankle Arthroplasty (TAA) is not "experimental" any more and is an established option for certain patients with ankle arthritis. Multiple ankle replacement designs are now on the market, and there are more to come.

I believe the next 10 years will further clarify several points of concern and discussion. The purpose of this issue is to look into some of these issues. Several important topics about the indications for total ankle replacement versus arthrodesis are covered as well as the correction of complex deformities.

Another subject that will garner attention over the next decade is the controversy of fixed versus mobile bearing in TAA. The knee literature did not show a significant advantage of one over the other, but that has not been studied in the ankle yet. Hopefully that is a topic we could cover in the next issue on Total Ankle Arthroplasty.

Inevitable with any joint replacement are the unpleasant realities of complications and failures. There are several excellent articles in this issue dealing with some of the important questions.

This will be a very informative issue of the *Foot and Ankle Clinics of North America* with great contributions from some of the leaders in the field. I would like to personally thank all the contributors for spending the time to share their experience with everyone.

J. Chris Coetzee, MD
Orthopedic Foot and Ankle Surgeon
MOSMI and Twin Cities Orthopedics
4010 West 65th Street
Edina, MN 55435, USA

E-mail address:
jcc4bf@gmail.com
Website: http://www.tcomn.com

http://dx.doi.org/10.1016/j.fcl.2017.01.015
1083-7515/17/© 2017 Published by Elsevier Inc.

foot.theclinics.com

Kinematics and Function of Total Ankle Replacements Versus Normal Ankles

Justin M. Kane, MD[a,b], Scott Coleman, MS, MBA[c],
James W. Brodsky, MD[a,b,d,e,]*

KEYWORDS

- Total ankle arthroplasty • Gait • Kinematics • Biomechanics • Arthritis

KEY POINTS

- Patients with ankle arthritis have alterations in nearly all temporal-spatial, kinematic, and kinetic parameters of gait.
- Total ankle arthroplasty (TAA) significantly improves function, as meaured by multiple parameters of gait.
- TAA does not normalize gait function compared with healthy controls.

INTRODUCTION

A significant amount of disability is experienced by patients with end-stage ankle arthritis.[1–18] Numerous studies have equated the morbidity in patients with end-stage arthritis of the ankle to patients suffering from hip arthritis, end-stage renal disease, or congestive heart failure.[19,20] Numerous features differentiate patients with end-stage ankle arthritis from those with end-stage hip and knee arthritis. Post-traumatic arthritis is a common cause of end-stage ankle arthritis.[21] Because of the high degree of clinical success in total hip arthroplasty (THA) and total knee arthroplasty (TKA), total ankle arthroplasty (TAA) was first introduced in the 1970s. Although ankle arthrodesis had been used to successfully treat ankle arthritis in the past, the theoretic benefit of preserving motion at the tibiotalar joint was the primary motivator

The authors have nothing to disclose.
[a] Foot and Ankle Division, Orthopedic Associates of Dallas, Baylor University Medical Center, 3900 Junius Street, Suite 500, Dallas, TX 75246, USA; [b] Foot and Ankle Surgery Fellowship Program, Baylor University Medical Center, 3500 Gaston Avenue, Dallas, TX 75246, USA; [c] Human Motion and Performance Laboratory, Department of Orthopaedic Surgery, Baylor University Medical Center, 411 North Washington Avenue, Suite 2100, Dallas, TX 75246, USA; [d] Department of Orthopaedic Surgery, University of Texas Southwestern Medical School, Dallas, TX, USA; [e] Texas A & M HSC College of Medicine, BUMC Dallas Campus, 3500 Gaston Avenue, Dallas, TX 75246, USA
* Corresponding author. Foot and Ankle Division, Orthopedic Associates of Dallas, 3900 Junius Street, Suite 500, Dallas, TX 75246.
E-mail address: james.brodsky@baylorhealth.edu

along with the proven track record of hip and knee arthroplasty. Unfortunately, outcomes were disappointing for early implant designs and the procedure was largely abandoned given the success of ankle arthrodesis.[3–8]

Even though tibiotalar arthrodesis was more reliable than early arthroplasty designs, numerous limitations, including loss of motion and the development of adjacent joint arthritis,[22–26] along with a better understanding of ankle joint kinematics, spurred a renewed interest in ankle arthroplasty. TAA still lags behind THA AND TKA with respect to longevity and improvement in subjective and objective outcomes compared with hip and knee arthroplasty but there is a large body of evidence supporting the newer generations of implants. High levels of patient satisfaction, durable pain relief, and significant improvements in objective measures of function, along with midterm survivorship approaching 80% to 95%, have led to an enthusiastic opinion of ankle arthroplasty.[1,2]

Several objective outcome studies have evaluated postoperative function after TAA. Although arthroplasty does not restore gait to that of healthy controls, improvements across nearly all parameters of gait have been observed, with gait function approaching that of controls.[9–11] Perhaps more meaningful is the improvement demonstrated when patients undergoing TAA have their gait function compared with their preoperative function. TAA clearly demonstrates marked improvement compared with preoperative function.[11–17]

BIOMECHANICS AND ANATOMY

The talocrural joint is a highly constrained articulation composed of the interface between the tibia, fibula, and dorsal surface of the talus. In part, due to the poor understanding of its biomechanics, early TAA implant designs had an unacceptably high rate of early failure. A more thorough understanding of the anatomy and biomechanics has contributed to the vast improvement in newer implant designs.[27,28]

Because of the 3-dimensional anatomy of the talocrural joint, motion throughout the gait cycle is multiplanar. With dorsiflexion, there is concomitant external rotation and abduction. As the ankle plantarflexes, there is a component of internal rotation and adduction. The 3-dimensional osteology of the talar dome contributes to this multiplanar motion. There are 2 distinct domes to the dorsal surface of the talus. The medial dome has a smaller radius of curvature than the lateral dome. This size difference explains the secondary motion seen at the talocrural joint with dorsiflexion and plantarflexion.[29,30] In addition to the difference between the medial and lateral talar domes, the talus has an asymmetric width. The articular surface is wedge-shaped with the anterior portion wider than the posterior.[29,31]

As the talus plantarflexes under the tibial plafond, the axis of rotation shifts from anterior to posterior. The complete arc of sagittal motion of the talocrural joint is 70°.[32] However, in vivo studies have demonstrated the working range of motion of the talocrural joint to be 25° (15° of plantarflexion and 10° of dorsiflexion) for the gait cycle.[33]

During gait, greater than 5 times the bodyweight is transmitted vertically at the talocrural joint.[34] This is also experienced after TAA. Additionally, shear forces exceed 2 to 3 times the bodyweight during the gait cycle. The significant forces exerted across the talocrural joint, combined with the relatively small weightbearing surface (7 cm²), necessitate for careful design considerations for implant survivorship.[34,35]

CLINICAL OUTCOMES

As implant designs and technique have improved, patient-reported outcomes have been reported to be either good or excellent in nearly 80% of patients at greater than 2-year follow-up.[1] In a recent meta-analysis, Haddad and colleagues[1] reported a 10-year survival rate of 77%. Revision rates were only 7% during the same time period. Additionally, the average postoperative American Orthopedic Foot and Ankle Society (AOFAS) hind-foot score was 78.2.

The positive impact TAA had on patients with end-stage ankle arthritis was further demonstrated in a meta-analysis conducted by Zaidi and colleagues.[36] Survivorship at 10 years was found to be 89% in 7942 total ankle replacements. The mean AOFAS hind-foot score improved from 40 to 80. The investigators concluded that TAA "has a positive impact on patients' lives, with benefits lasting 10 years, as judged by improvement in pain and function, as well as improved gait and increased range of motion."

GAIT ANALYSIS

To effectively understand the disability end-stage ankle arthritis has on gait and the improvements achieved with TAA, a basic understanding of the parameters of gait is necessary. Three general categories are studied with respect to gait.

Temporal-spatial parameters (TSPs) are often referred to as the vital signs of gait.[37] TSPs measure the speed of walking, as well as the components contributing to walking speed, including support time for each limb. Walking speed is the product of step length and cadence (steps per minute). In the evaluation of TSPs, it is important to remember that factors such as pain and stiffness may influence function irrespective of the underlying ankle pathologic condition.[9,38–44]

Kinematic parameters are a measure of movement at the individual segments being analyzed. These are measured separate of the forces driving locomotion. The individual parameters measured include displacement (linear or angular), velocity, and acceleration.[37] Modern analyses of gait use motion capture devices to measure the specific angles and trajectories around the anatomic areas of interest. The newest models for gait analysis have evolved from treating the foot as a single segment to multisegment analyses that are capable of distinguishing motion between and among the different joints of the foot in the coronal, axial, and sagittal planes.[45,46]

Kinetic parameters of gait are the final component of a gait analysis. They measure the forces generated during gait. Kinetic parameters are expressed as power and moment (force plus direction). Ground reaction forces, joint moments, and joint mechanical power are all measured as part of a complete assessment of gait kinetics.[44]

Temporal Spatial Parameters of Gait

Cadence, walking speed, and single limb support time for the affected limb are all abnormal in patients with end-stage ankle arthritis.[9,34,47] Although the disease process itself contributes the abnormalities seen in gait analysis, protective measures to reduce load and, therefore, pain associated with the affected joint also play a role.[48]

In studies evaluating gait before and after TAA, improvements in TSPs have been consistently demonstrated. Valderrabano and colleagues[9] studied preoperative and postoperative gait after TAA with a 3-component implant. Stride length improved by 5 cm, cadence by 5.6 cm/s, walking speed by 12 cm/s, and support time by −0.04 seconds for the affected limb. For the unaffected limb, improvements were also noted. Stride length improved by 7 cm, cadence by 4.8 steps/min, walking speed by 12 cm/s, and support time by −0.07 seconds. Brodsky and colleagues[15] found similar outcomes with a different 3-component implant. Stride length increased by 17 cm, cadence by 12.9 steps/min, and walking speed by 25.6 cm/s. Although the improvements in these studies did not reach the values for healthy controls, the parameters measured were markedly improved approaching gait function in controls. Queen and colleagues[16] studied preoperative and postoperative gait after TAA with a 2-component implant. Stride length improved by 13.9 cm, walking speed by 31 cm/s, and double-limb support time by −6%. All improvements were clinically and statistically significant.

Equally important to evaluate are the improvements in gait comparing TAA with the alternative option of ankle arthrodesis. Flavin and colleagues[12] compared preoperative and postoperative gait of patients undergoing either TAA or ankle arthrodesis for end-stage ankle arthritis. Both groups exhibited significant improvements over their preoperative function. However, neither group reached the gait function seen in healthy controls. Additionally, TAA and ankle arthrodesis exhibited different levels of improvement across the multiple parameters of gait, with each having an advantage over the other in many individual measurements.

Kinematic Parameters of Gait

In patients with end-stage ankle arthritis, there is loss of motion through all 3 planes. The greatest reduction is seen in the sagittal plane (dorsiflexion or plantarflexion).[9,34,47]

The driving factor for any arthroplasty procedure is preserving joint motion while effectively reducing pain. Although TAA has not been able to restore sagittal plane motion to the level of healthy controls, significant and clinically important improvements are clear when comparing to preoperative range of motion. In the study of 3-component implants by Valderrabano and colleagues,[9] improvements were seen in numerous planes of motion. Ankle plantarflexion improved by 4.3°, inversion movement improved by 1.1°, and adduction movement improved by 1.6°. Brodsky and colleagues'[15] comparison of preoperative and postoperative gait analysis after a 3-component implant demonstrated an improvement of total sagittal range of motion about the ankle of 3.7°, knee of 6.6°, and hip of 4.9°. Choi and colleagues[49] studied a 2-component implant design and found that, in contrast to 3-component ankle arthroplasty designs, most sagittal plane motion improvement was in dorsiflexion.

In a multisegment 3-dimensional gait analysis comparing TAA with the unaffected limb, Brodsky and colleagues[50] noted less overall motion in the sagittal, coronal, and axial planes in the side that had an arthroplasty.

When comparing TAA and ankle arthrodesis, kinematic parameters demonstrate improvements after both procedures. Flavin and colleagues[12] reported a greater overall sagittal range of motion in patients who had undergone TAA. They further noted that coronal plane eversion motion was less after undergoing TAA compared with ankle arthrodesis. In a study comparing postoperative gait analyses in patients who had undergone either TAA or ankle arthrodesis with healthy controls, Singer and colleagues[11] similarly found greater sagittal plane range of motion in patients undergoing TAA (+4.4°). A greater improvement in coronal plane motion was also experienced in patients undergoing TAA (+2.5°). Neither of these improvements reached the values of healthy controls. Tibial rotation was greater in patients undergoing TAA (+1.4°) and this reached the values of healthy controls. In a comparison of patients undergoing TAA or ankle arthrodesis, Hahn and colleagues[51] reported an overall increase in sagittal range of motion for patients undergoing TAA (+3°), whereas patients who had undergone ankle arthrodesis experienced a decrease in sagittal range motion of (−3°).

Kinetic Parameters of Gait

Distinct patterns of kinetic abnormalities exist in end-stage ankle arthritis compared with hip and knee arthritis. Power is clearly diminished as a result of abnormal temporal-spatial and kinematic parameters of gait. In addition to a reduction in power, moment is also abnormal. The largest reduction in ankle moment is seen in the axial plane. In contrast, knee osteoarthritis results in the largest reduction in coronal plane moment.[52,53] Although it is unclear why these differences exist, they may be attributable to the different causes responsible for hip or knee arthritis and ankle arthritis. Most cases of end-stage ankle arthritis can be attributable to post-traumatic causes. In contrast, primary osteoarthritis is responsible for most cases of end-stage hip and knee arthritis. In patients who have experienced significant trauma resulting in arthritic changes around the ankle, associated muscle and soft-tissue compromise may be the cause of reduced function. Another possibility is due to the complex motion at the ankle joint and gait changes to reduce discomfort may have a role.

Valderrabano and colleagues[9] reported improvements in ankle power (0.75 W/kg), ankle plantarflexion moment (0.04 Nm/kg), and ankle inversion moment (0.03 Nm/kg) after undergoing TAA with a 3-component design. Brodsky and colleagues[15] reported similar improvements. Ankle power (0.31 W/kg), and ankle plantarflexion moment (0.21 Nm/kg) both improved after TAA with a different 3-component design. Although these improvements were noted to be statistically significant and clinically meaningful, they did not reach the values recorded in healthy controls. In a study of 2-component implants, Queen and colleagues[16] also reported improvements in kinetic parameters of gait. Peak anterior ground reaction force and posterior ground reaction force improved, as did ankle plantarflexion moment.

Flavin and colleagues[12] compared the improvements seen after TAA and ankle arthrodesis and noted a more symmetric vertical ground reactive force after arthroplasty, which produced a more symmetric pattern of gait closer to that seen in healthy controls. Singer and colleagues[11] noted that after TAA, gait more closely replicated that of healthy controls when compared with ankle arthrodesis patients with respect to ankle power (watts), ankle extension moment (Nm/kg), and ankle moment at heel rise (Nm/kg).

THE DEBATE: MOBILE-BEARING VERSUS FIXED-BEARING IMPLANTS

TAA has evolved significantly from early implant designs. First-generation designs were broadly categorized as either constrained or unconstrained. Neither afforded results that compared with ankle arthrodesis or to the results seen with total knee and total hip arthroplasty. Unconstrained designs had the advantage of increased mobility and decreased strain at the bone-implant interface. The tradeoff was a high degree of instability and unacceptable rate of wear on the polyethylene component, which resulted in a high rate of early and midterm failure. Constrained devices remedied the instability and polyethylene wear due to a more even force distribution on the polyethylene. However, motion was restricted to the sagittal plane and the high degree of constraint resulted in early loosening at the bone-implant interface.[3–7,53,54] The high rate of failure led to many abandoning TAA in favor of the more durable and reliable ankle arthrodesis.

Although there were problems with first generation designs for TAA, further understanding of the biomechanics of the ankle and advances in implant design has led to the creation of the current generation of implants used today.[55,56] The newest implants are categorized as either 2-component or 3-component designs. In 2-component designs, the polyethylene implant is seated on the tibial component and motion occurs solely between the polyethylene and the talar component. In 3-component designs, the polyethylene is not fixed to the tibial component. This allows for motion to occur between the interface at the tibial component and the polyethylene, as well as the talar component and the polyethylene. Theoretically, this results in an improvement in multiplanar motion. Despite these differences, limited data exist supporting the superiority of either implant design.

Queen and colleagues[13] compared the outcomes of 2-component and 3-component implants. The average improvement at 2 years was 32.9 to 65 for AOFAS hindfoot scores. Foot and Ankle Disability Index (FADI) scores improved from 60.0 to 17.4 at 1 year and improved further to 13.3 at 2 years. Two-component arthroplasties exhibited a greater overall improvement in SF-36 (SHORT FORM -36) scores, whereas patients with 3-component implants exhibited a greater reduction in visual analog scale pain scores. The study concluded that, although both designs resulted in dramatic improvements in patient function and outcomes, it was unclear which design was more efficacious in the treatment of end-stage ankle arthritis.

SUMMARY

The literature clearly demonstrates that TAA results in clinically and statistically significant improvements in gait compared with preoperative function. It's important to note that these improvements, although approaching the gait parameters, do not match the gait of healthy controls. Many of these studies also show heterogeneous improvements in gait when comparing TAA and ankle arthrodesis. Although many of the improvements are greater in patients undergoing TAA, some improvements were greater in patients undergoing ankle arthrodesis.

One of the limiting factors in the study of gait is differentiating improvements as a result of pain relief versus biomechanical changes at the joint. This gray area may be a contributing factor in the many similarities seen between TAA and ankle arthrodesis as it relates to improvement in gait function.

Going forward, more sophisticated models are needed to better understand the effects of TAA on the biomechanics of gait. This is especially true as it pertains to studying the effects of arthritis and surgery on not just the ankle but the adjacent hindfoot and midfoot articulations.

REFERENCES

1. Haddad SL, Coetzee JC, Estok R, et al. Intermediate and long-term outcomes of total ankle arthroplasty and arthrodesis: a systematic review of the literature. J Bone Joint Surg Am 2007;89:1899–905.
2. Gougoulias N, Khanna A, Maffulli N. How successful are current ankle replacements?: a systematic review of the literature. Clin Orthop 2010;468:199–208.
3. Bolton-Maggs BG, Sudlow RA, Freeman MA. Total ankle arthroplasty. A long-term review of the London Hospital experience. J Bone Joint Surg Br 1985;67:785–90.
4. Dini AA, Bassett FH. Evaluation of early results of Smith total ankle replacement. Clin Orthop 1980;146:228–30.
5. Kitaoka HB, Patzer GL. Clinical results of the Mayo total ankle arthroplasty. J Bone Joint Surg Am 1994;76:974–9.
6. Stauffer RN, Seagal NM. Total ankle arthroplasty. Four years experience. Clin Orthop 1981;160:217–21.
7. Kofoed H, Sorensen TS. Ankle arthroplasty for rheumatoid arthritis and osteoarthritis: prospective long-term study of cemented replacements. J Bone Joint Surg 1998;80B:328–32.
8. Demottaz JD, Mazur JM, Thomas WH, et al. Clinical study of total ankle replacement with gait analysis. A preliminary report. J Bone Joint Surg Am 1979;61(7):976–88.

9. Valderrabano V, Nigg BM, von Tscharner V, et al. Gait analysis in ankle osteoarthritis and total ankle replacement. Clin Biomech 2007;22:894–904.

10. Doets HC, van Middelkoop M, Houdijk H, et al. Gait analysis after successful mobile bearing total ankle replacement. Foot Ankle Int 2007;28(3):313–22.

11. Singer S, Klejman S, Pinsker E, et al. Ankle arthroplasty and ankle arthrodesis: gait analysis compared with normal controls. J Bone Joint Surg Am 2013; 95(e191):1–10.

12. Flavin R, Coleman SC, Tenenbaum S, et al. Comparison of gait after total ankle arthroplasty and ankle arthrodesis. Foot Ankle Int 2013;34(1):1340–8.

13. Queen RM, Sparling TL, Butler RJ, et al. Patient-reported outcomes, function, and gait mechanics after fixed and mobile-bearing total ankle replacement. J Bone Joint Surg Am 2014;96:987–93.

14. Piriou P, Culpan P, Mullins M, et al. Ankle replacement versus arthrodesis: a comparative gait analysis study. Foot Ankle Int 2008;29(1):3–9.

15. Brodsky JW, Polo FE, Coleman SC, et al. Changes in gait following the Scandinavian total ankle replacement. J Bone Joint Surg Am 2011;93:1890–6.

16. Queen RM, DeBiasio JC, Butler RJ, et al. Changes in pain, function, and gait mechanics two years following total ankle arthroplasty performed with two modern fixed-bearing prostheses. Foot Ankle Int 2012;33(7):535–42.

17. Queen RM, Butler RJ, Adams SB Jr, et al. Bilateral differences in gait mechanics following total ankle replacement: a two year longitudinal study. Clin Biomech 2014;29:418–22.

18. Kapandji JA. Physiologie articulaire, fasc II. 4th edition. Paris: Maloine SA; 1974. p. 140.

19. Glazebrook M, Daniels T, Younger A, et al. Comparison of health-related quality of life between patients with end-stage ankle and hip arthrosis. J Bone Joint Surg Am 2008;90(3):499–505.

20. Saltzman CL, Zimmerman MB, O'Rourke M, et al. Impact of comorbidities on the measurement of health in patients with ankle osteoarthritis. J Bone Joint Surg Am 2006;88(11):2366–72.

21. Saltzman CL, Salamon ML, Blanchard GM, et al. Epidemiology of ankle arthritis. Iowa Orthop J 2005;25:44–6.

22. Beischer AD, Brodsky JW, Pollo FE, et al. Functional outcome and gait analysis after triple or double arthrodesis. Foot Ankle Int 1999;20:545–53.

23. Buchner M, Sabo D. Ankle fusion attributable to posttraumatic arthrosis: a long-term followup of 48 patients. Clin Orthop Relat Res 2003;406:155–64.

24. Buck P, Morrey BF, Chao EY. The optimum position of arthrodesis of the ankle. A gait study of the knee and ankle. J Bone Joint Surg 1987;69A:1052–62.

25. Coester LM, Saltzman CL, Leupold J, et al. Long-term results following ankle arthrodesis for post-traumatic arthritis. J Bone Joint Surg 2001;83A:219–28.

26. Fuchs S, Sandmann C, Skwara A, et al. Quality of life 20 years after arthrodesis of the ankle. A study of adjacent joints. J Bone Joint Surg 2003;85B:994–8.

27. Deland JT, Morris GD, Sung IH. Biomechanics of the ankle joint. A perspective on total ankle replacement. Foot Ankle Clin 2000;5:747–59.

28. Gill LH. Principles of joint arthroplasty as applied to the ankle. American academy of orthopaedic surgeons. Rosemont (AAOS) Instructional course lectures. Rosemont (IL): American academy of orthopaedic surgeons; 2002. p. 117–28.

29. Barnett C, Napier JR. The axis of rotation at the ankle joint in man. Its influence upon the form of the talus and the mobility of the fibula. J Anat 1952;86:1–9.

30. Hicks JH. The mechanics of the foot I. The joints. J Anat 1953;87:345–57.

31. Inman VT. The joints of the ankle. In: Stiehl JB, editor. Biomechanics of the ankle joint. 2nd edition. Baltimore (MD): Williams & Wilkins; 1991. p. 31–74.
32. Tooms RE. Arthroplasty of ankle and knee. In: Crenshaw AH, editor. Campbell's operative orthopedics. St Louis (MO): C.V. Mosby Company; 1987. p. 1145–50.
33. Stauffer RN. Total joint arthroplasty. The ankle. Mayo Clin Proc 1979;54:570–5.
34. Stauffer RN, Chao EYS, Brewster RC. Force and motion analysis of the normal, diseased, and prosthetic ankle joint. Clin Orthop 1977;127:189–96.
35. Hintermann B. Total ankle arthroplasty: historical overview, current concepts, and future perspectives. New York: SpringerWien; 2005. p. 35–49.
36. Zaidi R, Cro S, Gurusamy N, et al. The outcome of total ankle replacement: a systematic review and meta-analysis. Bone Joint J 2013;95B:1500–7.
37. Kirtley C. Clinical gait analysis: theory and practice. New York: Elsevier; 2006.
38. Kawamura K, Tokuhiro A, Takechi H. Gait analysis of slope walking: a study on step length, stride width, time factors and deviation in the center of pressure. Acta Med Okayama 1991;45:179–84.
39. McIntosh AS, Beattyy KT, Dwan LN, et al. Gait dynamics on an inclined walkway. J Biomech 2006;39:2491–502.
40. Ilgin D, Ozalevli S, Kilinc O, et al. Gait speed as a functional capacity indicator in patients with chronic obstructive pulmonary disease. Ann Thorac Med 2011;6: 141–6.
41. Inam S, Vucic S, Brodaty NE, et al. The 10-metre gait speed as a functional biomarker in amyotrophic lateral sclerosis. Amyotroph Lateral Scler 2010;11: 558–61.
42. Ledoux WR, Rohr ES, Ching RP, et al. Effects of foot shape on the three-dimensional position of foot bones. J Orthop Res 2006;24:2176–86.
43. Potter JM, Evans AL, Duncan G. Gait speed and activities of daily living function in geriatric patients. Arch Phys Med Rehabil 1995;76:997–9.
44. Queen RM, Nunley JA. The effect of footwear on preoperative gait mechanics in a group of total ankle replacement patients. J Surg Orthop Adv 2010;19:170–3.
45. Mayich DJ, Novak A, Vena D, et al. Gait analysis in foot and ankle surgery – topical review, Part 1: principles and uses of gait analysis. Foot Ankle Int 2014; 35(1):80–90.
46. Novak AC, Mayich DJ, Perry SD, et al. Gait analysis for foot and ankle surgeons – topical review, part 2: approaches to multisegment modeling of the foot. Foot Ankle Int 2014;35(2):178–91.
47. Khazzam M, Long JT, Marks RM, et al. Preoperative gait characterization of patients with ankle arthrosis. Gait Posture 2006;24:85–93.
48. Lewis G. The ankle joint prosthetic replacement: clinical performance and research challenges. Foot Ankle Int 1994;15(9):471–6.
49. Choi JH, Coleman SC, Tenenbaum S, et al. Prospective study of the effect on gait of a two-component total ankle replacement. Foot Ankle Int 2013;34(11):1472–8.
50. Brodsky JW, Coleman SC, Smith S, et al. Hindfoot motion following STAR total ankle arthroplasty: a multisegment foot model gait study. Foot Ankle Int 2013; 34(11):1479–85.
51. Hahn ME, Wright ES, Segal AD, et al. Comparative gait analysis of ankle arthrodesis and arthroplasty: initial findings of a prospective study. Foot Ankle Int 2012; 33(4):282–9.
52. Hurwitz DE, Ryals AB, Case JP, et al. The knee adduction moment during gait in subjects with knee osteoarthritis is more closely correlated with static alignment than radiographic disease severity, toe out angle and pain. J Orthop Res 2002; 20:101–7.

53. Mundermann A, Dyrby CO, Hurwitz DE, et al. Potential strategies to reduce medial compartment loading in patients with knee osteoarthritis of varying severity: reduced walking speed. Arthritis Rheum 2004;50:1172–8.
54. Kakkar R, Siddique MS. Stresses in the ankle joint and total ankle replacement design. Foot Ankle Surg 2011;17(2):58–63.
55. Reggiani B, Leardini A, Corazza F, et al. Finite element analysis of a total ankle replacement during the stance phase of gait. J Biomech 2006;39(8):1435–43.
56. Espinoza N, Walti M, Favre P, et al. Misalignment of total ankle components can induce high joint contact pressures. J Bone Joint Surg Am 2010;92(5):1179–87.

Ankle Arthrodesis Versus Total Ankle Arthroplasty

Joel Morash, MD, FRCS(C)[a],*, David M. Walton, MD[b],
Mark Glazebrook, MD, FRCS(C), MSc, PhD[a]

KEYWORDS

- Ankle arthroplasty • Ankle replacement • Ankle arthrodesis • Ankle fusion

KEY POINTS

- Reoperation rates are higher in total ankle arthroplasties (TAAs) compared with ankle arthrodesis. Infection rates for primary TAAs are 1.4% to 2.4%.
- The survival rate of TAA is approximately 75% to 90% at 10 years.
- Arc of motion is maintained with TAAs compared with ankle arthrodesis. Ankle arthrodesis increases arc of motion through the talonavicular joint, which is a cause for concern for adjacent joint disease in the future.
- Several factors are strong reasons to favor ankle fusion rather than TAA; patients without protective sensation or clear neuropathy should not undergo TAA.
- TAA and ankle arthrodesis both are effective treatments of end-stage ankle arthritis but the choice must be tailored to individual patients.

INTRODUCTION

End-stage ankle arthritis is a debilitating condition that affects the lives of patients to the same magnitude physically as end-stage kidney disease, congestive heart failure, and end-stage hip arthritis.[1,2]

The ankle joint is subject to more pressure and is more commonly injured than any other joint in the body. Although the rate of osteoarthritis of the ankle is not as high as for osteoarthritis of the hip and knee, the frequency of traumatic events to the ankle predisposes the joint to late arthritis.[3] The gold standard surgical treatment of end-stage ankle arthritis has been arthrodesis of the tibiotalar joint.

Because total ankle arthroplasty (TAA) has reestablished its superiority as the gold standard of treatment, ankle arthrodesis is in debate. Although abundant ongoing research and comparative trials are attempting to discern which treatment

---

Disclosure: The authors have nothing to disclose.
[a] QE2 Health Science Center, Halifax Infirmary (Room 4867), 1796 Summer Street, Halifax, Nova Scotia B3H 3A7, Canada; [b] Beaumont Orthopedics, Michigan Orthopedic Institute, Royal Oak, MI 21601, USA
* Corresponding author.
E-mail address: joel.morash@dal.ca

Foot Ankle Clin N Am 22 (2017) 251–266
http://dx.doi.org/10.1016/j.fcl.2017.01.013
1083-7515/17/© 2017 Elsevier Inc. All rights reserved.
foot.theclinics.com

option is superior, decisions must currently be made with the existing understanding. There are several causes for end-stage disease of the ankle joint. The most common are inflammatory and posttraumatic arthropathies.[4] In these conditions it is important to assess the entire hindfoot and midfoot to confirm that symptoms are isolated to the tibiotalar joint. Chronic ankle instability has become more appreciated as a common cause of isolated tibiotalar degeneration. Charcot arthropathy of the ankle is frequently seen in patients with diabetic neuropathy or other neurosensory derangements. Failed total ankle replacements (TARs) and avascular necrosis of the talus often necessitate ankle fusion. In addition, stage IV posterior tibial tendon dysfunction or other severe deformities of the ankle, which are not amenable to periarticular osteotomies, can be successfully treated with ankle fusion.[3,5]

The Canadian Orthopedic Foot and Ankle Society (COFAS) ankle arthritis classification (**Table 1**) is useful to guide treatment. Type 1 is isolated ankle arthritis and may be treated with isolated ankle fusion or TAA. Type 2 refers to ankle arthritis with intra-articular coronal plane abnormality, ankle instability, or tight heel cord. These ankles may require a second incision for ankle arthrodesis or may require ligament balancing, reconstruction, and possible midfoot or forefoot correction for TAA. Type 3 ankle arthritis is defined in conjunction with hindfoot deformity, tibial malunion, midfoot deformity, or plantar-flexed first ray. Treatment may include tibial, fibular, or calcaneal osteotomy or midfoot arthrodesis for ankle arthrodesis or TAA. In addition, any previously mentioned ankle arthritis with ipsilateral hindfoot degeneration (type 4) may be best treated with TAA because ankle arthrodesis is likely to transfer motion lost in the ankle to the already arthritic ipsilateral periarticular joints.[6]

ANKLE ARTHRODESIS

At present, the most accepted surgical treatment of end-stage ankle arthritis is ankle arthrodesis. The procedure is straightforward and is suitable for surgical treatment of almost all types of ankle arthritis. There exists ample evidence in the literature ranging from level I to IV studies to support a grade A recommendation (good evidence with consistent findings from level I studies) or at least a grade B recommendation (fair evidence with consistent level II or III studies) for the use of ankle arthrodesis in treatment of end-stage ankle arthritis.

Contraindications

Arthrodesis of the ankle is a reliable and highly effective treatment of end-stage ankle disease in most patients. The contraindications are similar to those of any definitive orthopedic procedure: active infection, insufficient vascular supply, and inadequate soft tissue envelope. The last contraindication can be ameliorated by the various approaches to the ankle. Some investigators suggest that contralateral ankle fusion is a mild contraindication for ankle arthrodesis if the patient is a candidate for ankle arthroplasty.[7] Also, careful consideration should be given to avoid ankle arthrodesis in patients afflicted with COFAS type 4 ankle arthritis if a TAA is not contraindicated.

Technique

There are numerous approaches and fixation techniques commonly done for ankle arthrodesis. The surgical approach is dictated by surgeon comfort, previous hardware, and condition of the soft tissue envelope. Often in posttraumatic ankle arthritis

Table 1
The Canadian Orthopedic Foot and Ankle Society preoperative and postoperative classification system for end-stage ankle arthritis

	Type 1	Type 2	Type 3	Type 4
Preoperative classification	Isolated ankle arthritis	Ankle arthritis with intra-articular varus or valgus deformity, ankle instability, and/or a tight heel cord	Ankle arthritis with hindfoot deformity, tibial malunion, midfoot abductus or adductus, supinated midfoot, plantar-flexed first ray, and so forth	Types 1–3 plus subtalar, calcaneocuboid, or talonavicular arthritis
Postoperative classification	AA or TAR with no procedure requiring a second incision except syndesmosis fusion	AA or TAR with a soft tissue procedure requiring a separate incision	AA or TAR with an additional osteotomy including midfoot arthrodesis	AA or TAR with an additional hindfoot arthrodesis
Concurrent procedures	None, hardware removal	Deltoid ligament release, ligament reconstruction, tendo Achilles lengthening, gastrocnemius recession, tendon transfer, capsule release, forefoot reconstruction, metatarsal osteotomy, dissection of neurovascular structures, plantar fascia release, syndesmosis reconstruction	Fibular osteotomy, calcaneal osteotomy, tibial osteotomy, midtarsal arthrodesis	Arthrodesis: triple, subtalar, talonavicular, calcaneocuboid

Abbreviation: AA, ankle arthrodesis.
From Krause FG, Di Silvestro M, Penner MJ, et al. The postoperative COFAS end-stage ankle arthritis classification system. Foot Ankle Spec 2012;5(1):32; with permission.

a previous incision is used to protect the skin flaps as well as to ease the hardware removal. The location of the prior incision can limit access to the joint, requiring additional incisions and occasionally staging of the fusion. Alternatively, if the anterior soft tissue envelope is poor, a posterior approach can be used to avoid a high-risk wound.

Classically, access to the tibiotalar joint through a lateral incision has been advantageous because it is the familiar approach for ankle fractures, it avoids neurovascular structures, it permits easy correction of varus deformity, and it allows for morselized fibula to be used as autograft. If a lateral approach is used, care should be taken to ensure appropriate coronal alignment and stability because the fibula serves as inherent resistance to lateral subluxation of the talus as well as valgus deformity. In addition, a fibular-sparing approach should be used, which preserves the ankle mortise.[8] This technique allows later conversion to ankle arthroplasty, which has shown pain relief and improved function in patients who did not tolerate their ankle fusions (**Fig. 1**).[9,10]

More recently, arthroscopic arthrodesis has been performed successfully in an attempt to reduce morbidity. In a recent comparative case series, arthroscopic ankle arthrodesis outperformed traditional open arthrodesis by Ankle Osteoarthritis Scale (AOS) scores at 1 and 2 years as well as duration of hospital stay. Although equivalent pain relief and return of function have been shown, most investigators recommend this as an advanced technique by experienced surgeons operating on ankles with minimal deformity.

In addition, as the anterior approach has been more widely implemented during the advancement of TAA, more surgeons have chosen to perform arthrodesis through this exposure as well. This choice offers the advantage of supine positioning and convenient clinical and radiographic assessment of anatomic structures and alignment. The anterior approach requires exposure of the neurovascular bundle and is often less familiar than the lateral approach. There is also concern for higher wound complications.

Fixation strategies are chosen on a case-by-case basis. With soft tissue compromise, external fixation with compression has been shown to be successful with outcomes similar to those of internal fixation. This technique can be achieved by both static and dynamic methods, the latter being technically more difficult but allowing deformity correction more slowly as well as late postoperative adjustments. Ringed external fixation can provide compression at the same level as plate and screw fixation.[11]

Transarticular screw fixation has had good outcomes over several decades. Holt and colleagues[12] reported their series in 1991 with a fusion rate of 93% using a 3-screw technique with an emphasis on the importance of the posterior-to-anterior screw, which is the technique of choice in conjunction with arthroscopic joint debridement, minimizing the exposure required for the fixation.

Plate fixation is a comfortable and reliable approach to achieving stability of the arthrodesis site, and can be applied from any of the formal approaches. Kestner and colleagues[13] showed that dual anterior plating is the most biomechanically stable choice. Many surgeons choose to use a combination of strategies, using compression screws and a plating system of choice to neutralize rotational forces, enhancing stability.

Regardless of the approach and the fixation technique, it is generally accepted that the most important aspects of the arthrodesis surgery are the basic tenets of fusion: joint preparation, opposition and compression of joint surfaces in an appropriate position, and stable fixation.

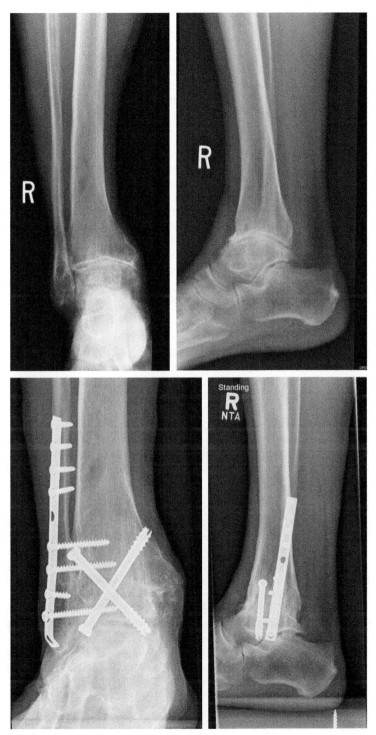

Fig. 1. A 74-year-old man 9 years after from ankle arthrodesis using the fibular osteotomy ankle arthrodesis technique.

Outcomes

Pain relief

After successful ankle fusion, patients typically have excellent pain relief and minimal physical limitations with return to activities as tolerated.[14–17] Arthrodesis of the ankle is a definitive treatment of end-stage disease and therefore the durability and longevity are unmatched with respect to alternative treatment. Common complications include nonunion, malunion, infection, hardware irritation, persistent pain, and progressive hindfoot or midfoot degeneration.

Union rates

Union rates vary from 60% to 100%, with larger studies consistently showing 90% to 95% union rates.[14,18,19] In a series of 215 cases of uncomplicated ankle arthrodesis reported by Chalayan and colleagues[14], there was a union rate of 91% at 6 months. They observed a 3 times higher increase in nonunions in patients who had previous subtalar fusion, and nonunions were twice as likely in patients with preoperative varus deformity. In a series of 121 ankles that were followed for 9 years, there was a union rate of 91%.[18] A recent review by O'Connor and colleagues[20] suggested that many of the risk factors for nonunion are difficult to absolutely conclude based on small samples and heterogeneous populations; however, there is fair evidence that smoking and diabetes are patient-specific risk factors for nonunion.

Gait biomechanics

Investigations into gait biomechanics after ankle arthrodesis have aided understanding of the optimal neutral sagittal plane position for fusion.[21,22] Other studies have shown a clear disturbance of gait after ankle arthrodesis.[23] The clinical impact has not been fully elucidated. There is no evidence of a negative impact on the knee; however, there is a suggestion that ankle arthrodesis can accelerate the hindfoot and midfoot degeneration.[23–26]

Singer and colleagues[27] in 2013 compared gait analyses in 17 patients who underwent TAR, 17 patients who underwent ankle arthrodesis, and 10 patients in a control group. The TAR group's gait pattern more closely resembled that of the control group. However, within this study there were no self-reported differences in clinical outcome.

Periarticular degeneration

Treatment with ankle arthrodesis improves gait relative to the preoperative state, likely because of pain relief as well as compensatory motion through the adjacent joints.[25,28,29] In the first year an average of 11° of increased motion was seen in the subtalar joint. In a prospective analysis of sagittal plane hindfoot motion after ankle arthrodesis, Sealey and colleagues[30] noted statistically significant early increase in both subtalar and talonavicular motion compared with the preoperative state. This increase was positively associated with quality-of-life scores.

This increased motion was seen specifically at the posterior facet of the subtalar joint and was hypothesized to be a cause of early progression of subtalar degeneration.[30] Long-term studies of ankle arthrodesis have suggested accelerated peritalar degeneration but no definite causation has been established.[18,31–34] Other investigators have noted less compelling evidence that the arthrodesis has a contribution and that the root cause centers on the indication for the initial arthrodesis (**Box 1**).[35–37]

ANKLE ARTHROPLASTY

Ankle arthroplasty is growing in popularity for the treatment of end-stage ankle arthritis. As surgical techniques and implants improve, the clinical results of ankle

---

Box 1
Take-home points for ankle arthrodesis

Ankle arthrodesis is a definitive, safe, and reliable procedure to relieve pain and improve function.

Ankle arthrodesis can be performed using a variety of techniques and approaches, allowing flexible surgical planning.

There are no definite activity restrictions after ankle fusion.

Approach and fixation strategy should be decided on a case-by-case basis.

COFAS type IV and ipsilateral midfoot and hindfoot fusion have a negative effect on union rates.

There is a compensatory increase in hindfoot and midfoot motion after ankle arthrodesis.

Some literature suggests that ankle arthrodesis can accelerate the progression of hindfoot and midfoot degeneration.

---

arthroplasty do so as well. Note that it is still a very technical operation and surgeons' experience has been shown to influence complication rates.

Indications and Contraindications

As surgical techniques and prosthesis improve, indications and contraindication for TAA continue to change. Every patient should be treated as an individual case and it is difficult to come up with concrete parameters on how to treat all ankle arthritis. The American Orthopaedic Foot & Ankle Society (AOFAS) issued a position statement in 2014 stating that, "Before considering total ankle replacement, patients should have exhausted or failed conservative treatment, should have satisfactory vascular perfusion in the involved extremity, and appropriate current or planned soft-tissue coverage about the ankle that affords a safe surgical approach to total ankle replacement."

Survivorship

Basques and colleagues[38] in 2016 reviewed 4800 TAAs and compared complications rates between surgeons with a volume in the 90th percentile and those below the 90th percentile. They identified that surgeons must complete 21 TAAs a year to be in the 90th percentile. This group had a significantly lower rate of overall complications, medial malleolus fractures, and decreased length of hospital stay.

One of the most important questions for patients is the expected survival rate of the implant. This question is clearly a concern for patients wishing to minimize the number of surgeries in their lifetimes when trying to choose between ankle arthrodesis and arthroplasty. With the increasing number of TAAs now in their 10th to 15th year of survival it is possible to make some generalized statements about survival rates, but it must be stressed to the patients that these are estimations and are patient specific. Without a standardized system for terminology of reporting complications of TAA, the published results have a high variability.[39]

Daniels and colleagues[15] in 2014 studied 388 ankles using the COFAS Prospective Ankle Reconstruction Database records from 2001 to 2007. They were able to follow 321 ankles (83%; 232 ankle replacements and 89 arthrodeses) for a mean follow-up of 5.5 ± 1.2 years. Seven (7%) of the arthrodeses and 48 (17%) of the ankle replacements underwent revision. The major complications rate was 7% for arthrodesis and 19% for ankle replacement (**Fig. 2**).

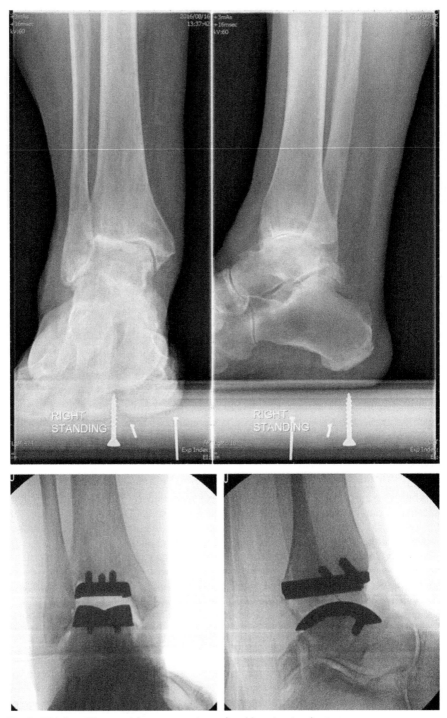

Fig. 2. TAA in a 72-year-old woman, using a fixed-bearing implant.

Registries from Europe, New Zealand, and Australia have been reported for short-term to medium-term survival. They report failure rates from 7.1% to 19% at 5 years and 24% to 31% at 10 years.[17,40–44] This finding is similar to the 13.8% failure rate found from 1997 to 2010 using the Statewide Planning and Research Cooperative System database.[45] These numbers differ from a meta-analysis using methodology of the Cochrane collaborations, reviewing 7942 TAAs, which found that the overall survivorship was 89% at 10 years with an annual failure rate of 1.2%.[46] This finding is consistent with a few multicenter studies showing survivorship rates of 96% at 5 years and 90% at 10 years.[47] It is important to note that comparisons of international registries are difficult to do because many of the implants differ from country to country.

Comorbidities

Expected rates must take into consideration patients' comorbidities and any social habits that may increase failure rates.

LaMothe and colleagues[48] in 2016 studied the survivorship of 1593 TAAs in 6 states between 2005 and 2009 and found an overall survivorship of 90.1%. Patients with rheumatoid arthritis or who were readmitted to hospital within 90 days had a significantly higher risk of failure, which was defined as revision, arthrodesis, amputation, or implant removal.[48] Other studies have shown no difference between rheumatoid patients and patients undergoing TAA for posttraumatic or primary arthritis.[15]

Body mass index (BMI) did not show any significant difference in complication, infection, or failure rates in a prospective study by Gross and colleagues[49] in 2016 comparing 455 primary TAAs in patients who were divided into 3 groups: BMI less than 30, BMI 30 to 35, and BMI greater than 35. Similarly, diabetes did not show any significant difference in complication or infection rate in a retrospective series of 813 primary TAAs.[50]

Smoking

There are few articles that directly compare patients' smoking status with outcome and complication rates. Lampley and colleagues[51] in 2016 reviewed 642 patients between 2007 and 2014, showing that active cigarette smokers had a significantly higher risk of wound complications and worse outcome scores compared with nonsmokers and former smokers.

Clinical Outcomes

Saltzman and colleagues[17] in 2009 compared clinical outcome between 465 TAAs (all STAR prosthesis) and 47 ankle arthrodeses. They found a significant higher reported Buechel-Pappas function score in the TAA group and an equivalent Buechel-Pappas pain score at 24 months' postoperative follow-up.

Daniels and colleagues[15] in 2014 used the COFAS Prospective Ankle Reconstruction Database at 4 centers between 2001 and 2007 and found TAAs to have more than double (19%) the rate of major complications compared with arthrodesis (7%). This study included 281 TAAs (Agility, STAR, Mobility, HINTEGRA) and 107 arthrodesis. There was no difference in AOS and Short Form 36 (SF-36) scores between the two groups.

In an 11-year study from 2004 to 2015, Popelka and colleagues[52] in 2016 followed 132 TAAs. TAA outcomes were poorer in patients with posttraumatic arthritis than in those with rheumatoid arthritis or primary arthritis. In patients with posttraumatic arthritis, the average AOFAS score increased to 78.6 because of restricted motion of the ankle, and some patients continued to have pain when walking. The average

AOFAS score in a total of 49 patients who had rheumatoid arthritis or primary arthritis reached a value of 86.4.

Infections

Minimizing the risk of infection is always of top priority when performing a TAA and/or ankle arthrodesis. It is often difficult to quantify overall infection rates with TAA because there is not a true registry. Also the description of an infection may differ depending on the surgeon and the clinical presentation. In a retrospective review of 966 TAAs at one institution from 1995 to 2012, they had 29 cases that were infected (3.2%). This incidence was lower in the primary TAAs (2.4%) and higher in the revision TAAs (4%). There was no difference in infection rates with respect to age, smoking, BMI, and operative time.[53]

Younger and colleagues[54] in 2016 prospectively followed 213 ankle arthrodeses and 474 TAAs from 2002 to 2010. There was a 0.9% infection rate in the arthrodesis group compared with a 2.3% infection rate in the TAA group. These infections required revision surgery. This study was also successful in creating a coding system to more reliably track complications for ankle arthrodesis and TAAs. The new coding system may provide a more standardized, clinically useful framework for assessing reoperation rates and resource use than prior complication and diagnosis-based classification systems. Analyzing reoperations at the primary site may enable a better understanding of reasons for failure, and may therefore improve the outcomes of surgery in the future.

Oliver and colleagues[55] in 2014 reported a lower infection rate (1.4%) when they completed a retrospective review of 300 consecutive patients (321 TAAs) at 1 institution with a minimum of 2 years' follow-up.

Postoperative Range of Motion

One of the main reasons for patients to choose arthroplasty rather than arthrodesis is to maintain motion. Pedowitz and colleagues[56] in 2016 were able to quantify this in a recent report comparing arc of motion in 41 patients who received a TAA and 27 patients who received an ankle arthrodesis. They showed a significantly higher arc of motion in the TAA group and a significantly higher arc of motion at the talonavicular joint in the arthrodesis group. They also found an increase in pain relief and better patient-perceived outcomes in the TAA group (**Box 2, Fig. 3**).

SUMMARY

TAA has reemerged as a viable and often preferable option to ankle arthrodesis for patients with end-stage ankle disease so it is vital to understand how patients should be counseled. The decision between ankle arthroplasty and arthrodesis should be made on a case-by-case basis. There are no consensus guidelines, but a recent decision analysis using a Markov model suggested that TAR was a superior option.[57] However, this model does not account for patient-specific risk factors.

There are several patient-specific situations in which an ankle arthrodesis could be deemed a better choice than TAA. Patients with a contralateral ankle arthrodesis are a clear indication for a TAA because the gait disturbance from a second ankle arthrodesis is more significant, including increasing difficulty with stairs and difficult terrain.[58]

For patients with ipsilateral hindfoot disease, many surgeons offer an ankle replacement more readily than an arthrodesis. Limiting the ankle motion causes added stress across the hindfoot, which could accelerate the disease but will certainly exacerbate symptoms.[25,30,31] In addition the rates of nonunion of the subtalar joint after ipsilateral ankle arthrodesis have been shown be much higher. In one cohort, nonunion rate was

---

Box 2
Take-home points for TAA

Survival rate is approximately 75% to 90% at 10 years.

No differences in complication or infection rates in obese patients or patients with diabetes.

Differing results reported increased complication rates in patients with rheumatoid arthritis.

Ensuring that patients with rheumatoid arthritis are followed by a rheumatologist so that appropriate medications are held preoperatively and postoperatively helps to decrease complication rates, especially wound healing complications.

Arc of motion is maintained with TAA compared with ankle arthrodesis.

Ankle arthrodesis increases arc of motion through the talonavicular joint, which is a cause for concern for adjacent joint disease in the future.

TAA gait pattern more closely resembles that of a control group.

Reoperation rates are higher in TAAs compared with ankle arthrodesis.

Arthroplasty clinical outcomes were poorer in patients with posttraumatic arthritis than in those with rheumatoid arthritis or primary arthritis.

Young, active, high-demand patients with ankle arthritis may be better candidates for arthrodesis than for TAA.

Infection rates for primary TAAs are 1.4% to 2.4%.

It is hoped that recent coding systems will help standardize reoperation and complication rates to enable a better understanding of reasons for failure, and may therefore improve the outcomes of surgery in the future.

38% compared with 8% without ipsilateral fusion.[59] The converse is also true, there is up to a 3 times risk increase for ankle arthrodesis nonunion in patients with ipsilateral subtalar fusion.[14]

Several factors are strong reasons to favor ankle fusion rather than TAA. Patients without protective sensation or clear neuropathy should not undergo TAA. These patients lack the proprioceptive ability to protect the joint and are at high risk for developing pressure ulcers, which can lead to severe septic arthritis. In addition, the authors recommend against TAA in patients with diabetes, because there is a high likelihood that they will develop distal extremity neuropathy.

Young active patients and patients who are laborers are traditionally recommended to undergo ankle arthrodesis, which causes minimal limitations and activity restrictions. However, biological age should be taken into account. For example, a patient severely afflicted by rheumatoid arthritis may be as low demand as an octogenarian and ankle arthroplasty could be considered.

Smoking is a modifiable risk factor and patients should be counseled to quit regardless of the surgical procedure that is planned. Lampley and colleagues[51] showed a significantly increased risk of wound complications in patients who smoke and undergo TAA. Smoking also increases the risk for nonunion and wound complications for ankle arthrodesis, but these risks can be mitigated by surgical approach and grafting options.[60,61]

Soft tissue envelope can dictate which procedure should be performed. Poor blood supply or previous surgical procedures may preclude TAA. The approaches for TAA are limited to anterior and lateral. If a posterior approach is required, ankle arthrodesis is recommended.

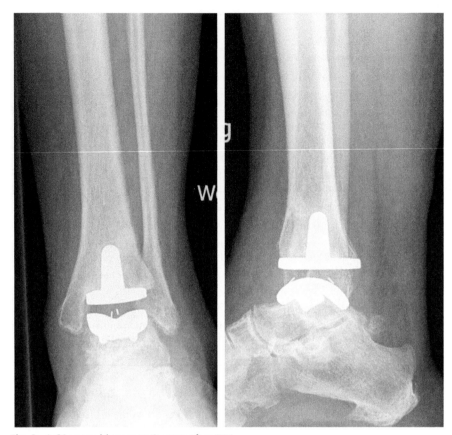

Fig. 3. A 66-year-old woman 9 years after TAA.

The degree of deformity is a moderate decision-making tool. More experienced arthroplasty surgeons may choose to perform TAA in severe cases; however, deformity greater than 15° to 20° in the coronal plane should be approached with caution.

Other patient characteristics have an unknown effect on surgical preference. Obesity, osteoporosis, alcohol use, and need for early weight bearing are all factors that need more study to determine their impact on the decision between ankle arthroplasty and arthrodesis.

Cost is an important consideration in the current health care setting. Younger and colleagues[62] in 2014 investigated the initial hospital-related cost associated with ankle arthroplasty and arthrodesis. In their analysis it was noted that ankle arthroplasty has costs similar to those of total knee and hip arthroplasty, all of which are more than twice the expense of ankle fusion. This difference is important to consider when making administrative decisions. Ankle arthroplasty should not be refused on a cost basis given its hip and knee counterparts; however, more global health care impacts should be studied with regard to long-term ankle fusion and replacement.

Patient expectation is an important factor that must be addressed, but this is not easily accounted for in functional outcome scoring. Younger and colleagues[63] investigated this using expectation and satisfaction scores. They reported that patients who undergo TAA have higher expectation scores and higher satisfaction scores after surgery than patients who undergo ankle fusion; however, both cohorts have the same expectation scores. There was no difference in other clinical preoperative or postoperative scores. The investigators concluded that accurate preoperative education to ameliorate misconceptions is critical in setting appropriate patient expectations and thus is critical to satisfaction with the procedures.[63]

In conclusion, TAA and ankle arthrodesis both are effective treatments of end-stage ankle arthritis but the choice must be tailored to individual patients. More studies are needed to better define when TAA and ankle arthrodesis are best applied to the surgical treatment of end-stage ankle arthritis.

REFERENCES

1. Glazebrook M. Comparison of health-related quality of life between patients with end-stage ankle and hip arthrosis. J Bone Joint Surg Am 2008;90(3):499–505.
2. Saltzman CL, Zimmerman MB, O'Rourke M, et al. Impact of comorbidities on the measurement of health in patients with ankle osteoarthritis. J Bone Joint Surg Am 2006;88(11):2366–72.
3. Thomas RH, Daniels TR. Ankle arthritis. J Bone Joint Surg Am 2003;85A(5): 923–36.
4. Pedersen E, Pinsker E, Younger ASE, et al. Outcome of total ankle arthroplasty in patients with rheumatoid arthritis and noninflammatory arthritis: a multicenter cohort study comparing clinical outcome and safety. J Bone Joint Surg Am 2014;96(21):1768–75.
5. Mann RA, Rongstad KM. Arthrodesis of the ankle: a critical analysis. Foot Ankle Int 1998;19(1):3–9.
6. Krause FG, Di Silvestro M, Penner MJ, et al. The postoperative COFAS end-stage ankle arthritis classification system: interobserver and intraobserver reliability. Foot Ankle Spec 2012;5(1):31–6.
7. Cottino U, Collo G, Morino L, et al. Arthroscopic ankle arthrodesis: a review. Curr Rev Musculoskelet Med 2012;5(2):151–5.
8. Glazebrook MA, Holden D, Mayich J, et al. Fibular sparing z-osteotomy technique for ankle arthrodesis. Tech Foot Ankle Surg 2009;8(1):34–7.
9. Huntington WP, Davis WH, Anderson R. Total ankle arthroplasty for the treatment of symptomatic nonunion following tibiotalar fusion. Foot Ankle Spec 2016;9(4): 330–5.
10. Pellegrini MJ, Schiff AP, Adams SB, et al. Conversion of tibiotalar arthrodesis to total ankle arthroplasty. J Bone Joint Surg Am 2015;97(24):2004–13.
11. Ogut T, Glisson RR, Chuckpaiwong B, et al. External ring fixation versus screw fixation for ankle arthrodesis: a biomechanical comparison. Foot Ankle Int 2009;30(4):353–60.
12. Holt ES, Hansen ST, Mayo KA, et al. Ankle arthrodesis using internal screw fixation. Clin Orthop Relat Res 1991;268:21–8.
13. Kestner CJ, Glisson RR, Nunley JA. A biomechanical analysis of two anterior ankle arthrodesis systems. Foot Ankle Int 2013;34(7):1006–11.
14. Chalayon O, Wang B, Blankenhorn B, et al. Factors affecting the outcomes of uncomplicated primary open ankle arthrodesis. Foot Ankle Int 2015;36(10):1170–9.
15. Daniels TR, Younger ASE, Penner M, et al. Intermediate-term results of total ankle replacement and ankle arthrodesis: a COFAS multicenter study. J Bone Joint Surg Am 2014;96(2):135–42.

16. Haddad SL. Intermediate and long-term outcomes of total ankle arthroplasty and ankle arthrodesis. A systematic review of the literature. J Bone Joint Surg Am 2007;89(9):1899–905.

17. Saltzman CL, Mann RA, Ahrens JE, et al. Prospective controlled trial of STAR total ankle replacement versus ankle fusion: initial results. Foot Ankle Int 2009;30(7):579–96.

18. Hendrickx RPM, Stufkens SAS, de Bruijn EE, et al. Medium- to long-term outcome of ankle arthrodesis. Foot Ankle Int 2011;32(10):940–7.

19. Maurer RC, Cimino WR, Cox CV, et al. Transarticular cross-screw fixation. A technique of ankle arthrodesis. Clin Orthop Relat Res 1991;268:56–64.

20. O'Connor KM, Johnson JE, McCormick JJ, et al. Clinical and operative factors related to successful revision arthrodesis in the foot and ankle. Foot Ankle Int 2016. http://dx.doi.org/10.1177/1071100716642845.

21. Buck P, Morrey BF, Chao EY. The optimum position of arthrodesis of the ankle. A gait study of the knee and ankle. J Bone Joint Surg Am 1987;69(7):1052–62.

22. King HA, Watkins TB, Samuelson KM. Analysis of foot position in ankle arthrodesis and its influence on gait. Foot Ankle Int 1980;1(1):44–9.

23. Thomas R, Daniels TR, Parker K. Gait analysis and functional outcomes following ankle arthrodesis for isolated ankle arthritis. J Bone Joint Surg Am 2006;88(3):526–35.

24. Flavin R, Coleman SC, Tenenbaum S, et al. Comparison of gait after total ankle arthroplasty and ankle arthrodesis. Foot Ankle Int 2013;34(10):1340–8.

25. Fuentes-Sanz A, Moya-Angeler J, Lopez-Oliva F, et al. Clinical outcome and gait analysis of ankle arthrodesis. Foot Ankle Int 2012;33(10):819–27.

26. Rouhani H, Favre J, Aminian K, et al. Multi-segment foot kinematics after total ankle replacement and ankle arthrodesis during relatively long-distance gait. Gait Posture 2012;36(3):561–6.

27. Singer S, Klejman S, Pinsker E, et al. Ankle arthroplasty and ankle arthrodesis: gait analysis compared with normal controls. J Bone Joint Surg Am 2013;95(24). e191(1–10).

28. Kozanek M, Rubash HE, Li G, et al. Effect of post-traumatic tibiotalar osteoarthritis on kinematics of the ankle joint complex. Foot Ankle Int 2009;30(8):734–40.

29. Wang Y, Li Z, Wong DW-C, et al. Effects of ankle arthrodesis on biomechanical performance of the entire foot. PLoS One 2015;10(7):e0134340.

30. Sealey RJ, Myerson MS, Molloy A, et al. Sagittal plane motion of the hindfoot following ankle arthrodesis: a prospective analysis. Foot Ankle Int 2009;30(03):187–96.

31. Coester LM, Saltzman CL, Leupold J, et al. Long-term results following ankle arthrodesis for post-traumatic arthritis. J Bone Joint Surg Am 2001;83A(2):219–28.

32. Conti RJ, Walter JHJ. Effects of ankle arthrodesis on the subtalar and midtarsal joints. J Foot Surg 1990;29(4):334–6.

33. Muir DC, Amendola A, Saltzman CL. Long-term outcome of ankle arthrodesis. Foot Ankle Clin N Am 2002;7(4):703–8.

34. Trouillier H, Hansel L, Schaff P, et al. Long-term results after ankle arthrodesis: clinical, radiological, gait analytical aspects. Foot Ankle Int 2002;23(12):1081–90.

35. Ling JS, Smyth NA, Fraser EJ, et al. Investigating the relationship between ankle arthrodesis and adjacent-joint arthritis in the hindfoot: a systematic review. J Bone Joint Surg Am 2015;97(6):513–9.

36. Sheridan BD, Robinson DE, Hubble MJW, et al. Ankle arthrodesis and its relationship to ipsilateral arthritis of the hind- and mid-foot. J Bone Joint Surg Br 2006; 88(2):206–7.
37. van der Plaat LW, van Engelen SJPM, Wajer QE, et al. Hind- and midfoot motion after ankle arthrodesis. Foot Ankle Int 2015;36(12):1430–7.
38. Basques BA, Bitterman A, Campbell KJ, et al. Influence of surgeon volume on inpatient complications, cost, and length of stay following total ankle arthroplasty. Foot Ankle Int 2016. http://dx.doi.org/10.1177/1071100716664871.
39. Mercer J, Penner M, Wing K, et al. Inconsistency in the reporting of adverse events in total ankle arthroplasty: a systematic review of the literature. Foot Ankle Int 2016;37(2):127–36.
40. Easley ME, Adams SB, Hembree WC, et al. Results of total ankle arthroplasty. J Bone Joint Surg Am 2011;93(15):1455–68.
41. Goldberg AJ, Sharp RJ, Cooke P. Ankle replacement: current practice of foot & ankle surgeons in the United Kingdom. Foot Ankle Int 2009;30(10):950–4.
42. Labek G, Todorov S, Iovanescu L, et al. Outcome after total ankle arthroplasty–results and findings from worldwide arthroplasty registers. Int Orthop 2013;37(9): 1677–82.
43. Skyttä ET, Koivu H, Eskelinen A, et al. Total ankle replacement: a population-based study of 515 cases from the Finnish Arthroplasty Register. Acta Orthop 2010;81(1):114–8.
44. van den Heuvel A, Van Bouwel S, Dereymaeker G. Total ankle replacement. Design evolution and results. Acta Orthop Belg 2010;76(2):150–61.
45. Seaworth CM, Do HT, Vulcano E, et al. Epidemiology of total ankle arthroplasty: trends in New York State. Orthopedics 2016;39(3):170–6.
46. Zaidi R, Cro S, Gurusamy K, et al. The outcome of total ankle replacement: a systematic review and meta-analysis. Bone Joint J 2013;95B(11):1500–7.
47. Mann JA, Mann RA, Horton E. STAR™ ankle: long-term results. Foot Ankle Int 2011;32(05):473–84.
48. LaMothe J, Seaworth CM, Do HT, et al. Analysis of total ankle arthroplasty survival in the United States using multiple state databases. Foot Ankle Spec 2016;9(4): 336–41.
49. Gross CE, Lampley A, Green CL, et al. The effect of obesity on functional outcomes and complications in total ankle arthroplasty. Foot Ankle Int 2016;37(2): 137–41.
50. Gross CE, Green CL, DeOrio JK, et al. Impact of diabetes on outcome of total ankle replacement. Foot Ankle Int 2015;36(10):1144–9.
51. Lampley A, Gross CE, Green CL, et al. Association of cigarette use and complication rates and outcomes following total ankle arthroplasty. Foot Ankle Int 2016. http://dx.doi.org/10.1177/1071100716655435.
52. Popelka S, Sosna A, Vavřík P, et al. Eleven-year experience with total ankle arthroplasty. Acta Chir Orthop Traumatol Cech 2016;83(2):74–83 [in Czech].
53. Patton D, Kiewiet N, Brage M. Infected total ankle arthroplasty: risk factors and treatment options. Foot Ankle Int 2015;36(6):626–34.
54. Younger ASE, Glazebrook M, Veljkovic A, et al. A coding system for reoperations following total ankle replacement and ankle arthrodesis. Foot Ankle Int 2016. http://dx.doi.org/10.1177/1071100716659037.
55. Oliver SM, Coetzee JC, Nilsson LJ, et al. Early patient satisfaction results on a modern generation fixed-bearing total ankle arthroplasty. Foot Ankle Int 2016. http://dx.doi.org/10.1177/1071100716648736.

56. Pedowitz DI, Kane JM, Smith GM, et al. Total ankle arthroplasty versus ankle arthrodesis: a comparative analysis of arc of movement and functional outcomes. Bone Joint J 2016;98B(5):634–40.
57. Kwon DG, Chung CY, Park MS, et al. Arthroplasty versus arthrodesis for end-stage ankle arthritis: decision analysis using Markov model. Int Orthop 2011; 35(11):1647–53.
58. Fuchs S, Sandmann C, Skwara A, et al. Quality of life 20 years after arthrodesis of the ankle. J Bone Joint Surg Am 2003;85(7):994–8.
59. Zanolli DH, Nunley JA, Easley ME. Subtalar fusion rate in patients with previous ipsilateral ankle arthrodesis. Foot Ankle Int 2015;36(9):1025–8.
60. DiGiovanni CW, Baumhauer J, Lin SS, et al. Prospective, randomized, multi-center feasibility trial of rhPDGF-BB versus autologous bone graft in a foot and ankle fusion model. Foot Ankle Int 2011;32(4):344–54.
61. Scranton PE. Comparison of open isolated subtalar arthrodesis with autogenous bone graft versus outpatient arthroscopic subtalar arthrodesis using injectable bone morphogenic protein-enhanced graft. Foot Ankle Int 1999;20(3):162–5.
62. Younger ASE, MacLean S, Daniels TR, et al. Initial hospital-related cost comparison of total ankle replacement and ankle fusion with hip and knee joint replacement. Foot Ankle Int 2015;36(3):253–7.
63. Younger ASE, Wing KJ, Glazebrook M, et al. Patient expectation and satisfaction as measures of operative outcome in end-stage ankle arthritis: a prospective cohort study of total ankle replacement versus ankle fusion. Foot Ankle Int 2015;36(2):123–34.

Osteolysis in Total Ankle Replacement

How Does It Work?

Norman Espinosa, MD[a],*, Georg Klammer, MD[a],
Stephan H. Wirth, MD[b]

KEYWORDS

- Total • Ankle • Replacement • Arthroplasty • Periprosthetic • Osteolysis
- Mechanisms • Pathophysiology

KEY POINTS

- Aseptic loosening of total ankle replacement remains enigmatic regarding its underlying mechanisms.
- Although great scientific efforts have been made to explain the mechanisms, it remains poorly understood, complex and multi factorial.
- Many factors, including age, body weight, activity lesions, implant designs, fixation methods, material properties, immunologic responses and biomechanical adaptations to total ankle replacement all contribute to the development of perioprosthetic osteolysis.

INTRODUCTION

The first observations and reports on periprosthetic osteolysis date back to the 1970's and were followed by scientific works to investigate the pathophysiology and clinical impact on patients, mainly focusing on total hip and knee arthroplasty.

However, only sparse literature exists regarding periprosthetic osteolysis in total ankle replacement (TAR). The first report on periprosthetic osteolysis in TAR was published in 2004 by Knecht and colleagues.[1] Similar to total hip and total knee arthroplasty, periprosthetic osteolysis has been seen as a risk factor for TAR failure and revision surgery.

Disclosure: The authors have nothing to disclose.
[a] Institute for Foot and Ankle Reconstruction Zurich, Kappelistrasse 7, Zurich 8002, Switzerland; [b] Department of Orthopaedics, University of Zurich, Forchstrasse 340, Zurich 8008, Switzerland
* Corresponding author.
E-mail address: espinosa@fussinstitut.ch

Foot Ankle Clin N Am 22 (2017) 267–275
http://dx.doi.org/10.1016/j.fcl.2017.01.001
1083-7515/17/© 2017 Elsevier Inc. All rights reserved.

CONTEMPORARY TOTAL ANKLE REPLACEMENT DESIGNS

Anatomic designs and improved biomechanical properties of contemporary TAR improved the survivorship of implants.[2,3] As a result TAR regained interest among the orthopedic foot and ankle community and patients. The more TARs are implanted, the greater the potential for complications after the procedures. The mean revision rate per 100 observed component years was 3.29 for TAR compared with 1.29 and 1.26 for total hip and total knee arthroplasty.[4]

OSTEOLYSIS IN TOTAL ANKLE REPLACEMENT

Adverse responses in periprosthetic bone and soft tissues to implant-derived material components of wear debris have been recognized as relevant factors inducing aseptic implant failure.[5] Recent works by Yoon and colleagues,[6] Kohonen and colleagues,[7] and Koivu and colleagues[8] showed that the presence of periprosthetic osteolysis in TAR ranged between 35% and 37% 3 to 4 years postoperatively. Scientific publications have linked TAR failure to periprosthetic osteolysis.[6,8–12] In the publication by Yoon and colleagues,[6] osteolysis associated with TAR was a common phenomenon in the postoperative period. Most of the osteolytic lesions observed were quiescent, but the investigators pointed out that these lesions raise concerns in contemporary TAR because of their incidence rate and the potential for later mechanical failure compared with arthrodesis. Yoon and colleagues[6] recommended early diagnosis and careful evaluation of osteolysis in order to detect those lesions as early as possible and reduce revision surgery and failure rates of TAR.

QUESTIONING POLYETHYLENE DEBRIS–INDUCED PERIPROSTHETIC OSTEOLYSIS

In total hip and total knee arthroplasty it is widely accepted that polyethylene wear leads to osteolysis and thus to aseptic loosening and failure of the implant components.[13] The question is whether polyethylene wear could also be found in TARs with periprosthetic osteolysis and whether this is associated with failure of the TAR. Dalat and colleagues[14] showed extremely high percentages of polyethylene debris in the osteolytic areas of examined TAR. In addition, Vaupel and colleagues[15] were able to show macroscopic and microscopic wear patterns of the polyethylene inserts in 8 failed Agility TAR systems, concluding that polyethylene wear results in component loosening and failure of the implants.

In an early study performed by Kobayashi and colleagues,[16] the shape, size, and concentration of polyethylene particles in the synovial fluid of 15 Scandinavian TARs and 11 posterior-stabilized total knee arthroplasties were investigated. The particles in both groups were similar in shape, size, and concentration. Based on the conclusion that periprosthetic osteolysis in TAR is associated with polyethylene debris, the investigators assumed that the long-term results of second-generation TAR should be comparable with posterior-stabilized total knee arthroplasties. However, this has not been the case. The data from the Norwegian Joint Registry reported a survivorship of only 75% at 10 years for the scandinavian total ankle replaement system (STAR) arthroplasty compared with 95% survivorship at 15 years for the posterior-stabilized total knee arthroplasty.[17,18] This finding questions the sole assumption of polyethylene debris–induced periprosthetic osteolysis in TAR. Certain mechanisms other than polyethylene wear alone may be responsible for or promote development of osteolysis. This statement might be supported by the fact that not all patients with periprosthetic osteolysis reveal polyethylene debris in the histopathologic analysis. Koivu and colleagues[19,20] were able to show that early osteolysis is caused by Receptor Activator of NF-κB

Ligand (RANKL)-driven foreign body inflammation directed against necrotic tissues of the patients but not against the TAR-derived particles.

van Wijngaarden and colleagues[11] concluded that polyethylene particles are not the primary cause of osteolytic cyst formation but a secondary contributing factor that might accelerate the process of osteolysis. The investigators postulated that "implant design, biomechanical factors and local anatomical-physiological factors play an important role."[11]

THEORIES TO EXPLAIN PERIPROSTHETIC OSTEOLYSIS

In order to understand osteolysis it is necessary to realize how this process is induced. Insertion of an implant into bone results in localized, adjacent tissue necrosis. This necrosis is caused by the approach, preparation of surfaces, and local effect of the implant on tissues. The response to this step is the formation of reparative granulomatous tissue creating a natural envelope to enclose the implant components. The thickness of this envelope may vary from start of implantation throughout further evolution of the TAR. Loose implants have shown thicker reparative tissue coats than stable implants. Those thick tissue envelopes, also called pseudomembranes, include large amounts of foreign body macrophage and giant-cell responses to wear material with variable amounts of lymphocyte reactions.[5] Macrophages become activated in an inflammatorylike cascade, which activates osteoclasts or they become osteoclasts themselves while initiating bone resorption.[21] Polyethylene particles become phagocytosed by macrophages. As a result, cytokines are released, which modulate osteoblast and osteoclast activity stimulating further osteolysis. As already mentioned, macrophages differentiate into osteoclasts as a result of polyethylene particle stimulation.[5] This stimulation has been attributed to the submicrometer-sized particles.[22] With regard to current polyethylene materials used in orthopedic practice, Brulefert and colleagues[23] were able to confirm that nano-sized wear particles promote osteoclast differentiation without alteration of bone resorptive activity of mature osteoclasts. The investigators concluded that the nano-sized wear particles could be considered as important factors in periprosthetic osteolysis of the newest generation of polymer bearing surfaces. More recently, Jonitz-Heincke and colleagues[24] showed that human osteoblasts were directly involved in the proinflammatory cascade of bone matrix degradation. The simultaneous activation and recruitment of monocytes/macrophages boosted osteolytic processes in the periprosthetic tissue. By the downregulation of tissue inhibitors of matrix metalloproteinases and the concomitant upregulation of matrix metalloproteinases as a response to particle exposure, bone formation around implants may be suppressed, resulting in implant failure.[24]

The Role of Polyethylene Wear

The first and central theory related to cemented total hip implant loosening caused by periprosthetic osteolysis is that of so-called particle disease. As a consequence, uncemented implants were developed to avoid that disorder but with no superior outcome compared with cemented ones.

Modern TAR designs include ultrahigh-molecular-weight polyethylene (UHMWPE) with yield stresses ranging between 18 and 20 MPa. Above a pressure level of 23 MPa the polyethylene material undergoes either permanent deformation or macroscopic damage. However, delamination of UHMWPE occurs at 10 MPa.[3] It is therefore a prerequisite to protect the polyethylene from early degradation and wear, which means that material properties should be optimized and that the design of the implant must respect the interface in a manner that avoids damage to the polyethylene. Highly cross-linked polyethylene reduces the risk of periprosthetic osteolysis caused by wear particles.[25]

Polyethylene ages by oxidative degradation resulting in increased density, less molecular weight, and increased crystallinity and elastic modulus. To reduce oxidative degeneration, smooth surfaces are necessary in order to provide optimal material properties and to reduce friction.[26,27] The higher the friction between the interfaces, the greater the probability of polyethylene damage with consequent dispersion of wear particles around the implant.

Repetitive UHMWPE particle injections into rabbit knees with weight-bearing articulating osseointegrated prosthetic joints did not show any radiographic, histologic, or biomechanical difference compared with the healthy contralateral sides.[22] The investigators concluded that polyethylene wear alone might not be responsible for the loosening process and that it may be initiated by additional factors. The pathways of cell activation in particle disease are complex and difficult. However, although not yet known in detail, an imbalance of bone-resorbing cytokines and bone-forming cytokines plays an important role in osteolysis.

Rate of Wear and Joint Size

The rate of wear is important. Annual wear (these data are derived from hip studies) greater than 0.2 mm resulted in impaired implant survivorship.[28] Wear rate depends on TAR design and material properties.

In addition, the size of affected joint seems to be important: large joints are less quickly affected by this process than small joints. The ankle joint is a small joint compared with the hip and knee joints, and significant forces are transmitted through this articular complex.[29] Therefore, it could be speculated that, in the ankle joint, lytic processes might develop earlier than in the knee where, because of its large size, a long time is needed to reach a critical dose of particles.

The Role of Micromotion

Micromotion at the bone-implant interface might promote the development of periprosthetic osteolysis.[30] The initial stability and alignment achieved during surgery is vital to reduce micromotion and therefore to avoid any premature loosening (**Figs. 1** and **2**). The process is analogous to fracture healing: Stability ensures proper fracture healing and mechanical strength. However, it is difficult to assess micromotion at the interfaces in the early phase after implantation of a TAR. Bone deformation caused by bone compression and soft tissue deformation in the fibrous capsule around the implants have been considered to cause micromotion. Micromotion cannot be accurately detected by conventional imaging techniques. Nowadays, computed tomography (CT) or single-photon emission CT (SPECT)–CT (**Fig. 3**) can help to evaluate possible metabolic alterations at the interface but it is unlikely that, in the early phase (ie, within 6–12 months postoperatively), an accurate conclusion could be drawn because in the initial postoperative period many adaptive biological processes dominate, masking the true value of that imaging technique and resulting in false interpretation of the data.[7]

Based on studies regarding knee and hip arthroplasty, migration of implants may take up to 3 years.[31] No exact data exist in the literature regarding TAR. The material properties of TAR play a role in the ingrowth of the implant components and reduction of micromotion. Espinosa and colleagues[3] investigated the influence of TAR design and malpositioning and found that a more congruent TAR yielded more evenly distributed and lower-magnitude joint contact pressures compared with a less congruent TAR design. Proper TAR positioning has been found to be an important requirement

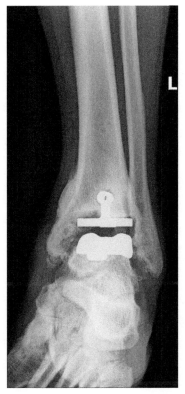

Fig. 1. An anteroposterior standing and weight-bearing radiography of a left ankle 2 years after implantation of a Salto total ankle replacement. There are cysts around the tibial component (medially) and medial malleolus that are easily visible.

to protect the components from premature failure. Based on those data it seems likely that micromotion affects implant stability and that it may promote joint fluid and polyethylene wear particle intrusion into the implant interfaces. As a result, inflammatory cascades are initiated that lead to weakening of the bone plate and loosening of the implant.

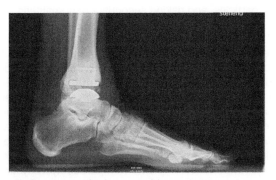

Fig. 2. Anteroposterior extension tibial cysts and loosening.

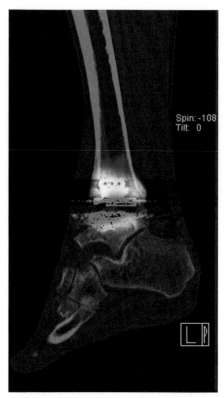

Fig. 3. SPECT-CT of the same ankle as shown in **Figs. 1** and **2**. The metabolic uptake is remarkable around the tibial and talar component. In addition, a large talar cyst can be identified, which is located in the talar neck and underneath the talar component stem.

The design of an implant can promote biomechanical alterations at the bone-implant interface, which in turn may have detrimental effects.[32,33] The phenomenon is called stress shielding and is the result of new loading conditions imposed by the implant.[26,34] It may play an important role in deciding what type of tibial and talar fixation should be used and whether the polyethylene insert is mobile or fixed. Areas around an implant that are not loaded reveal local bone loss. Stress shielding may create bone loss caused by remodeling but with the risk of opening the interface to joint fluid and wear particles, and risking secondary periprosthetic osteolysis.

The Role of Fluids

High fluid pressure has also been identified as a possible causative factor regarding the development of periprosthetic osteolysis.[35–38] Experimental studies were able to show osteocyte death and osteolysis as a result of oscillating fluid pressure.[39] In degenerative joint disease the intra-articular fluid pressure is greater than in normal joints.[40,41] Because of the accompanying inflammation, fluid production is accelerated and therefore the pressure increases to pathologic levels. As a consequence, the bone undergoes a washout or geyser effect, resulting in bone resorption and osteolysis. A similar effect could also be present in TAR. Therefore, the sealing of an implant is of major importance. Implants with porous hydroxyapatite-coated surfaces were less affected by UHMWPE particles at the interface.[22,42] In contrast, Singh and colleagues[9] showed that hydroxyapatite-coated TARs were prone to cyst formation and had a higher risk of undergoing revision surgery. Nevertheless, if an implant does not provide a proper sealing of the bone-implant interface, this will result in dispersion of wear particles into the joint fluid, which are then forced along the bone-implant interface.

Individual Factors: Genetics

Besides pure mechanical causes, it has been suggested that genetics are involved in the process of periprosthetic osteolysis formation. It has been postulated that the individual variation between patients regarding polyethylene wear might be associated not only with age, activity level, or body weight but also with aberrant cellular responses.[43] This sensitivity of some patients to polyethylene wear particles has led to the term implant looseners.[44,45] However, although it might sound logical that all individuals would react in different ways through variable immunologic pathways and that those mechanisms could ultimately lead to implant loosening through osteolysis, the correlation between sensitivity to wear particles and implant failure still needs further scientific clarification.

SUMMARY

Aseptic loosening of implants remains the most common reason for revision surgery for hip, knee, or ankle prostheses. Although a great scientific effort has been made to explain the underlying mechanisms it remains poorly understood, complex, and multifactorial. Many factors, including age, body weight, activity lesions, implant design, fixation methods, material proprieties, immunologic responses, and biomechanical adaptations to TAR all contribute to the development of periprosthetic osteolysis.

REFERENCES

1. Knecht SI, Estin M, Callaghan JJ, et al. The Agility total ankle arthroplasty. Seven to sixteen-year follow-up. J Bone Joint Surg Am 2004;86-A(6):1161–71.
2. Espinosa N, Wirth SH. Revision of the aseptic and septic total ankle replacement. Clin Podiatr Med Surg 2013;30(2):171–85.
3. Espinosa N, Walti M, Favre P, et al. Misalignment of total ankle components can induce high joint contact pressures. J Bone Joint Surg Am 2010;92(5):1179–87.
4. Labek G, Thaler M, Janda W, et al. Revision rates after total joint replacement: cumulative results from worldwide joint register datasets. J Bone Joint Surg Br 2011; 93(3):293–7.
5. Athanasou NA. The pathobiology and pathology of aseptic implant failure. Bone Joint Res 2016;5(5):162–8.
6. Yoon HS, Lee J, Choi WJ, et al. Periprosthetic osteolysis after total ankle arthroplasty. Foot Ankle Int 2014;35(1):14–21.
7. Kohonen I, Koivu H, Pudas T, et al. Does computed tomography add information on radiographic analysis in detecting periprosthetic osteolysis after total ankle arthroplasty? Foot Ankle Int 2013;34(2):180–8.
8. Koivu H, Kohonen I, Sipola E, et al. Severe periprosthetic osteolytic lesions after the Ankle Evolutive System total ankle replacement. J Bone Joint Surg Br 2009; 91(7):907–14.
9. Singh G, Reichard T, Hameister R, et al. Ballooning osteolysis in 71 failed total ankle arthroplasties. Acta Orthop 2016;87(4):401–5.

10. Cottrino S, Fabrègue D, Cowie AP, et al. Wear study of total ankle replacement explants by microstructural analysis. J Mech Behav Biomed Mater 2016;61:1–11.
11. van Wijngaarden R, van der Plaat L, Nieuwe Weme RA, et al. Etiopathogenesis of osteolytic cysts associated with total ankle arthroplasty, a histological study. Foot Ankle Surg 2015;21(2):132–6.
12. Kokkonen A, Ikävalko M, Tiihonen R, et al. High rate of osteolytic lesions in medium-term followup after the AES total ankle replacement. Foot Ankle Int 2011;32(2):168–75.
13. Sukur E, Akman YE, Ozturkmen Y, et al. Particle disease: a current review of the biological mechanisms in periprosthetic osteolysis after hip arthroplasty. Open Orthop J 2016;10:241–51.
14. Dalat F, Barnoud R, Fessy MH, et al. Histologic study of periprosthetic osteolytic lesions after AES total ankle replacement. A 22 case series. Orthop Traumatol Surg Res 2013;99(6 Suppl):S285–95.
15. Vaupel Z, Baker EA, Baker KC, et al. Analysis of retrieved agility total ankle arthroplasty systems. Foot Ankle Int 2009;30(9):815–23.
16. Kobayashi A, Minoda Y, Kadoya Y, et al. Ankle arthroplasties generate wear particles similar to knee arthroplasties. Clin Orthop Relat Res 2004;(424):69–72.
17. Fevang BT, Lie SA, Havelin LI, et al. 257 ankle arthroplasties performed in Norway between 1994 and 2005. Acta Orthop 2007;78(5):575–83.
18. Espehaug B, Furnes O, Havelin LI, et al. Registration completeness in the Norwegian Arthroplasty register. Acta Orthop 2006;77(1):49–56.
19. Koivu H, Takakubo Y, Mackiewicz Z, et al. Autoinflammation around AES total ankle replacement implants. Foot Ankle Int 2015;36(12):1455–62.
20. Koivu H, Mackiewicz Z, Takakubo Y, et al. RANKL in the osteolysis of AES total ankle replacement implants. Bone 2012;51(3):546–52.
21. Archibeck MJ, Jacobs JJ, Roebuck KA, et al. The basic science of periprosthetic osteolysis. Instr Course Lect 2001;50:185–95.
22. Sundfeldt M, Widmark M, Johansson CB, et al. Effect of submicron polyethylene particles on an osseointegrated implant: an experimental study with a rabbit patello-femoral prosthesis. Acta Orthop Scand 2002;73(4):416–24.
23. Brulefert K, Córdova LA, Brulin B, et al. Pro-osteoclastic in vitro effect of polyethylene-like nanoparticles: involvement in the pathogenesis of implant aseptic loosening. J Biomed Mater Res A 2016;104(11):2649–57.
24. Jonitz-Heincke A, Lochner K, Schulze C, et al. Contribution of human osteoblasts and macrophages to bone matrix degradation and proinflammatory cytokine release after exposure to abrasive endoprosthetic wear particles. Mol Med Rep 2016;14(2):1491–500.
25. Lachiewicz PF, Soileau ES. Highly cross-linked polyethylene provides decreased osteolysis and reoperation at minimum 10-year follow-up. J Arthroplasty 2016; 31(9):1959–62.
26. Sundfeldt M, Carlsson LV, Johansson CB, et al. Aseptic loosening, not only a question of wear: a review of different theories. Acta Orthop 2006;77(2):177–97.
27. Wennergren D, Ekholm C, Sundfeldt M, et al. High reliability in classification of tibia fractures in the Swedish Fracture register. Injury 2016;47(2):478–82.
28. Sochart DH. Relationship of acetabular wear to osteolysis and loosening in total hip arthroplasty. Clin Orthop Relat Res 1999;(363):135–50.
29. Snedeker JG, Wirth SH, Espinosa N. Biomechanics of the normal and arthritic ankle joint. Foot Ankle Clin 2012;17(4):517–28.
30. Goodman SB, Huie P, Song Y, et al. Loosening and osteolysis of cemented joint arthroplasties. A biologic spectrum. Clin Orthop Relat Res 1997;(337):149–63.

31. Ryd L, Linder L. On the correlation between micromotion and histology of the bone-cement interface. Report of three cases of knee arthroplasty followed by roentgen stereophotogrammetric analysis. J Arthroplasty 1989;4(4):303–9.
32. Affatato S, Taddei P, Leardini A, et al. Wear behaviour in total ankle replacement: a comparison between an in vitro simulation and retrieved prostheses. Clin Biomech (Bristol, Avon) 2009;24(8):661–9.
33. Schmalzried TP, Guttmann D, Grecula M, et al. The relationship between the design, position, and articular wear of acetabular components inserted without cement and the development of pelvic osteolysis. J Bone Joint Surg Am 1994; 76(5):677–88.
34. Oh I, Harris WH. Proximal strain distribution in the loaded femur. An in vitro comparison of the distributions in the intact femur and after insertion of different hip-replacement femoral components. J Bone Joint Surg Am 1978;60(1):75–85.
35. Linder L. Implant stability, histology, RSA and wear–more critical questions are needed. A view point. Acta Orthop Scand 1994;65(6):654–8.
36. Alidousti H, Taylor M, Bressloff NW. Periprosthetic wear particle migration and distribution modelling and the implication for osteolysis in cementless total hip replacement. J Mech Behav Biomed Mater 2014;32:225–44.
37. Catelas I, Jacobs JJ. Biologic activity of wear particles. Instr Course Lect 2010; 59:3–16.
38. Skripitz R, Aspenberg P. Pressure-induced periprosthetic osteolysis: a rat model. J Orthop Res 2000;18(3):481–4.
39. Aspenberg P, van der Vis H. Fluid pressure may cause periprosthetic osteolysis. Particles are not the only thing. Acta Orthop Scand 1998;69(1):1–4.
40. Schmalzried TP, Campbell P, Schmitt AK, et al. Shapes and dimensional characteristics of polyethylene wear particles generated in vivo by total knee replacements compared to total hip replacements. J Biomed Mater Res 1997;38(3): 203–10.
41. Schmalzried TP, Akizuki KH, Fedenko AN, et al. The role of access of joint fluid to bone in periarticular osteolysis. A report of four cases. J Bone Joint Surg Am 1997;79(3):447–52.
42. Reikeras O, Johansson CB, Sundfeldt M. Bone ingrowths to press-fit and loose-fit implants: comparisons between titanium and hydroxyapatite. J Long Term Eff Med Implants 2006;16(2):157–64.
43. Jasty MJ, Floyd WE 3rd, Schiller AL, et al. Localized osteolysis in stable, non-septic total hip replacement. J Bone Joint Surg Am 1986;68(6):912–9.
44. Matthews JB, Mitchell W, Stone MH, et al. A novel three-dimensional tissue equivalent model to study the combined effects of cyclic mechanical strain and wear particles on the osteolytic potential of primary human macrophages in vitro. Proc Inst Mech Eng H 2001;215(5):479–86.
45. Matthews JB, Green TR, Stone MH, et al. Comparison of the response of three human monocytic cell lines to challenge with polyethylene particles of known size and dose. J Mater Sci Mater Med 2001;12(3):249–58.

Total Ankle Replacement in the Presence of Talar Varus or Valgus Deformities

Andrew Dodd, MD, FRCSC[a],*, Timothy R. Daniels, MD, FRCSC[b]

KEYWORDS

- Ankle arthritis • Varus talus • Valgus talus • Total ankle replacement

KEY POINTS

- Ankle replacement in moderate or severe talar valgus or varus deformity as a 1-stage or 2-stage procedure is becoming a more reliable treatment option for patients.
- Orthopedic surgeons managing ankle arthritis with talar valgus or varus deformities need to be familiar with surgical reconstruction of pes planus or pes cavus deformities.
- Talar valgus deformities can be associated with a pes planus or pes cavus deformity, surgeons need to understand the clinical differences because this will influence the surgical reconstruction required.
- The hindfoot alignment radiographic view should be considered a part of the standard radiographic assessment of patient with end-stage ankle arthritis.

INTRODUCTION

End-stage ankle arthritis (ESAA) is a debilitating condition that often requires surgical management. More than 50% of patients with ESAA present with significant intra-articular and/or extra-articular deformities that can involve multiple anatomic areas, including from the knee to the midfoot.[1–6] These deformities, if not understood and addressed appropriately, will result in early failure of the total ankle replacement (TAR).[4,5,7–9]

The goal of TAR is to provide long-term improvement in pain and function for patients suffering from ESAA. For any total joint arthroplasty, implant alignment has an impact on loading patterns and subsequent polyethylene wear rates; TAR is no

Disclosure Statement: Dr T.R. Daniels is a consultant for Integra, Design team of Cadence Ankle (Intergra). Dr A. Dodd has nothing to disclose.
[a] Department of Surgery, University of Calgary, Bone & Joint Clinic, South Health Campus, 4448 Front Street Southeast, Calgary, Alberta, T3M 1M4, Canada; [b] Department of Surgery, St. Michael's Hospital, University of Toronto, Suite 800, 55 Queen Street East, Toronto, Ontario M5C-1R6, Canada
* Corresponding author.
E-mail address: andrewedodd@gmail.com

Foot Ankle Clin N Am 22 (2017) 277–300
http://dx.doi.org/10.1016/j.fcl.2017.01.002
1083-7515/17/© 2017 Elsevier Inc. All rights reserved.

exception. Malalignment of TAR components increases edge-loading and can lead to early failure.[4,5,7-9] The goal in TAR is to place the components perpendicular to the weightbearing (mechanical) axis of the lower extremity.[5,10] Normal ankle alignment, based on the lateral distal tibial angle, is 89° plus or minus 3°.[11] The anatomic and mechanical axes of the tibia are parallel, therefore placement of the TAR components perpendicular to the anatomic axis of the tibia is recommended.[1,12]

Post-traumatic arthritis is the most common cause of ESAA, and residual deformity is common.[13] Significant talar varus or valgus deformities of greater than 10° is common and increases the difficulty of reconstructive efforts. Previous investigators have advocated against TAR in patients with significant coronal plane deformity and arbitrary cutoffs of 15° to 20° have been recommended.[3,4,7,14,15] However, the evidence for these cutoffs is based on case-series. Given that deformity of greater than 10° is present in 10% to 40% of patients with ESAA,[1-6] a substantial portion of patients would not be candidates for TAR if these recommendations were followed. Recently, several clinical publications have demonstrated that TAR can be performed safely and effectively in talar deformities of up to 30°.[3,5,16] The type of ancillary procedures required to balance the foot and ankle is better understood and becoming a part of mainstream thinking. Up to 75% of patients with preoperative deformity will require ancillary procedures to properly balance the foot and ankle.[9]

No evidence-based guidelines are available to help with preoperative and intraoperative decision-making when performing TAR in the setting of significant deformity. This article describes the preoperative assessment and surgical techniques used by the senior author to obtain a stable, well-aligned TAR in patients presenting with coronal plane malalignment.

CLASSIFICATION OF DEFORMITY

When considering malalignment about the foot and ankle, it is important to differentiate between intra-articular and extra-articular sites of deformity. Extra-articular sites of deformity may be adjacent to the tibiotalar joint, or remote. It is useful to categorize deformity as extra-articular remote, extra-articular local, and intra-articular (**Table 1**).

Extra-articular remote deformities are important to recognize because they may need to be corrected before TAR if they have a substantial impact on ankle and hindfoot alignment. Decision-making becomes difficult when, in the rare situation, a patient presents with significant proximal deformity that is asymptomatic. An example of this is varus or valgus osteoarthritis of the knee that is not yet symptomatic enough to consider total knee arthroplasty (**Fig. 1**A–C). These situations require thorough discussion with an orthopedic knee reconstruction specialist and patient education. The author's practice is to address any proximal deformity that significantly affects ankle alignment (causing 10° or more of varus or valgus deformity) before undertaking

Table 1 Categorizing deformity	
Deformity Location	**Examples**
Extra-articular remote	Femoral deformity or malunion, varus or valgus knee deformity, proximal tibia deformity or malunion
Extra-articular local	Distal tibia deformity or malunion, hindfoot varus or valgus, foot cavus or planus
Intra-articular	Post-traumatic deformity, bone erosion, malleolar dysplasia

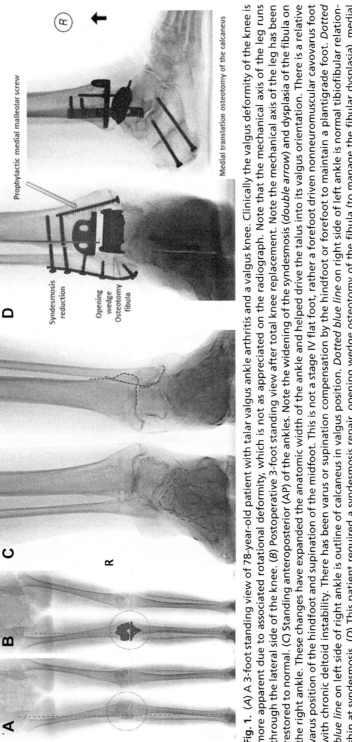

Fig. 1. (*A*) A 3-foot standing view of 78-year-old patient with talar valgus ankle arthritis and a valgus knee. Clinically the valgus deformity of the knee is more apparent due to associated rotational deformity, which is not as appreciated on the radiograph. Note that the mechanical axis of the leg runs through the lateral side of the knee. (*B*) Postoperative 3-foot standing view after total knee replacement. Note the mechanical axis of the leg has been restored to normal. (*C*) Standing anteroposterior (AP) of the ankles. Note the widening of the syndesmosis (*double arrow*) and dysplasia of the fibula on the right ankle. These changes have expanded the anatomic width of the ankle and helped drive the talus into its valgus orientation. There is a relative varus position of the hindfoot and supination of the midfoot. This is not a stage IV flat foot, rather a forefoot driven nonneuromuscular cavovarus foot with chronic deltoid instability. There has been varus or supination compensation by the hindfoot or forefoot to maintain a plantigrade foot. *Dotted blue line* on left side of right ankle is outline of calcaneus in valgus position. *Dotted blue line* on right side of left ankle is normal tibiofibular relationship at syndesmosis. (*D*) This patient required a syndesmosis repair, opening wedge osteotomy of the fibula (to manage the fibular dysplasia), medial translation osteotomy of the calcaneus and deltoid ligament imbrication to properly balance the ankle arthroplasty. This alignment correction (*arrow*) could not have been achieved without addressing the multidirectional valgus deformity of the knee first.

TAR, regardless of symptomatology. We are less aggressive with lesser degrees of deformity; however, there is little literature to guide these decisions.

Extra-articular local deformities and intra-articular deformities are common and can be addressed at the time of TAR or in a staged fashion. A thorough discussion of these deformities and their management follows.

PREOPERATIVE ASSESSMENT
History and Physical Examination

Assessment always begins with a thorough history and physical examination. In addition to a general medical and surgical history, a focused history on the affected ankle is important. This includes a pain history, elucidation of potential causes (eg, inflammatory, post-traumatic), any prior treatments whether successful or not, prior surgical interventions on the foot or ankle, and an assessment of the level of disability caused by the ankle arthritis. Pertinent information surrounding previous trauma and/or surgery is listed in **Table 2**.

Important comorbidities and key information regarding comorbidities are listed in **Table 3**.

Physical examination begins with a standing examination of alignment. The entire lower extremity is examined for areas of deformity. Ankle and hindfoot alignment should be observed from anterior and posterior, and the degree of varus or valgus deformity of the ankle or hindfoot complex is assessed. The examiner must gain an understanding of the relative contributions of the tibiotalar joint, hindfoot, midfoot, and forefoot to the deformity. Determining the relative degree of deformity in the ankle and subtalar joint (STJ) is clinically challenging and radiographs are necessary to confirm clinical assessment. Midfoot alignment includes assessment of planus, cavus, adduction, and abduction deformities. Forefoot deformities presence and severity should be noted (see **Fig. 1C**).

Following standing examination, sitting examination begins with inspection. The lower extremities are examined for deformity, swelling, surgical scars, muscle bulk, and skin or soft tissue health. Boney prominences are carefully inspected for calluses and ulcerations. A thorough neurovascular examination is performed to ensure normal sensation in the peripheral nerves and palpable dorsalis pedis and posterior tibial pulses. Signs of vascular insufficiency (arterial and venous, **Table 4**) should not be overlooked.[17,18]

Table 2 Information regarding previous trauma and/or surgery	
Trauma	Mechanism of injury (high or low energy)
	Specific type of injury to ankle
	Other lower injuries to lower extremities
	Open fractures
	Neurovascular compromise
	Treatments
Surgery	Type of surgery
	Location of surgery (to obtain records)
	Outcomes
	Complications
	Infection
	Neurovascular injury
	Chronic regional pain syndrome
	Nonunion

Table 3
Comorbidities and key information

Comorbidity	Important Information
Diabetes mellitus	Duration of disease Hemoglobin A1C levels Presence of neuropathy, retinopathy, nephropathy History of ulcerations plus Charcot arthropathy Medications
Obesity	Body mass index
Vascular disease	Coronary events Ischemic events in extremities Interventions or surgeries Medications (anticoagulants)
Smoking	Pack-year history
Inflammatory arthropathy	Type Duration of disease Severity of disease Previous surgeries Medications (immune-suppressants)

Following inspection, palpation for areas of tenderness is performed. Patients with ESAA often have degenerative changes in multiple adjacent joints. Not all joints with degenerative changes on radiographs are symptomatic, thus clinical examination must determine which joints are painful.

Range-of-motion (ROM) assessment is very important. Ankle ROM in plantarflexion and dorsiflexion is assessed. Preoperative ROM largely influences postoperative ROM[19]; therefore, patients with extremely stiff ankles will tend to remain stiff postoperatively unless an aggressive posterior debridement is performed through a separate posterior-lateral incision. The tendoachilles should be examined for contracture, including the Silfverskiöld test. Assessment of the hindfoot complex is also vital. For both varus and valgus hindfoot deformities, the examiner must determine the remaining arc of motion of the hindfoot complex, including subtalar, talonavicular, and calcaneocuboid joints (CTJs). This can be classified as a rigid deformity, correction to neutral, or correction beyond neutral, because this will influence surgical planning (**Table 5**). It is important to determine the arc of inversion or eversion. If a patient

Table 4
Signs of vascular insufficiency

Vascular Insufficiency	Physical Examination Findings
Arterial	Pallor Decreased or absent pulses Ankle-brachial index <0.9 Ulceration (toes, boney prominences)
Venous	Telangiectasis Varicose veins Edema Skin color changes (hemosiderin) Skin fibrosis Ulceration (malleolar regions)

Table 5
Assessment of hindfoot deformity correction (varus or valgus)

Correction of Hindfoot	Surgical Considerations
Correction past neutral	No correction necessary
Correction to neutral	Calcaneal osteotomy 1st metatarsal osteotomy Cuneiform osteotomy Soft tissue releases Tendon transfers
No correction; rigid deformity	Hindfoot arthrodesis (+/− above)

with a talar varus deformity has lost the arc of eversion, an aggressive release of the posterior tibial tendon (PTT), talonavicular capsule, and spring ligament is required to correct the talar varus. Too much emphasis is placed on deltoid ligament release in these scenarios. It is important to understand that in the severe talar varus deformities the medial malleolus is often bare because the deep fibers of the deltoid ligament have been worn off by the bone-on-bone articulation with the underlying talus and calcaneus (**Fig. 5A and 9B**). The senior author often does a 2-stage procedure on the severe talar varus deformities (**Fig. 2**). In severe talar valgus deformities and stage IV flat foot, if the arc of inversion has been lost, a 2-stage reconstruction is often required with aggressive correction of the pes planus deformity performed first, including deltoid reconstruction with allograft. After which, the TAR is performed at 6 to 12 weeks after pes planus.

Contribution of the midfoot and forefoot to the hindfoot deformity should also be considered at this point. Midfoot collapse may be present in planovalgus deformities. Although the area of collapse is difficult to pinpoint on clinical examination, severity can be assessed. Excessive plantarflexion of the first ray causing a forefoot-driven hindfoot varus should also be gauged. The Coleman block test can be used to assess the contribution of the first ray to hindfoot varus; however, the senior author has found that seated examination of the posture of the first ray and ability to passively correct the hindfoot varus is equally effective.

Diagnostic Imaging

Diagnostic imaging plays a vital role in the preoperative workup of the ESAA patient. Each patient should have standing foot and ankle radiograph series of the affected ankle. The authors also recommend a standing hindfoot alignment view (HAV) be performed on each patient (**Fig. 3**).[20] Bilateral radiographs are useful for comparison purposes. Radiographs are examined to identify the degree of degenerative changes; presence of osteophytes; bone stock; and presence, location, and severity of deformities. The distal tibia should be assessed for extra-articular deformity and the center of rotation of angulation (CORA) should be located (**Fig. 4**).[11] Intra-articular deformities include talar tilt, erosive changes of the tibial plafond, and malleolar dysplasia (**Fig. 5**). The foot radiographs are inspected for degenerative changes in the hindfoot complex, planus and cavus deformity, and abduction or adduction deformities.

The HAV is essential for gauging the degree of varus and valgus contributed by the ankle and hindfoot, respectively. Varus and valgus deformity can be isolated to the ankle joint, or the patient may have double varus or double valgus (stage IV flat foot deformity), with deformity at both the ankle and SJ (**Fig. 6**). Less commonly, the ankle and SJ assume opposing deformities as the SJ attempts to compensate for the ankle

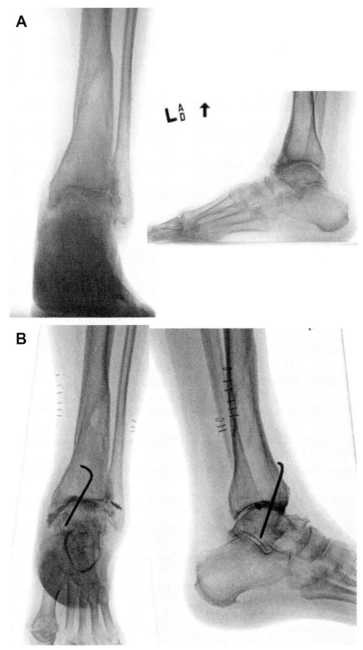

Fig. 2. (*A*) A 72-year-old woman with a history of a distal tibial fracture treated nonoperatively 45 years previous. She has developed an incongruent talar varus deformity with ESAA. The tibial deformity is minimal, the ankle varus deformity is intra-articular. (*B*) First stage of a 2-staged procedure. The patient has undergone a medial release of the foot, including transfer of the PTT to the peroneus brevis, combined with a talonavicular and spring ligament release. The ankle osteophytes have been debrided and the lateral ankle ligaments reconstructed. The talar varus deformity has been corrected and held with cement and an intra-articular K-wire. The patient will be weightbearing in a cast after 2 weeks and return to the OR for an ankle arthroplasty at 8 weeks postoperatively.

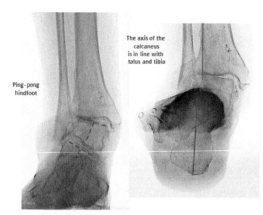

The axis of the
calcaneus
is in line with
talus and tibia

Ping-pong
hindfoot

Fig. 3. Patient with talar valgus and compensatory hindfoot varus (ping-pong hindfoot). This can be best appreciated with a HAV in which it becomes evident that the calcaneus is not in the same degree of valgus as the talus. The HAV clearly demonstrates that the axis of the calcaneus is parallel to the axis of the tibia. This can create a paradoxic situation in which, after the ankle joint is packed with a total ankle arthroplasty, the remainder of the foot behaves as a cavovarus deformity, even though it started with a talar valgus deformity. In these scenarios, the senior author has had to release or perform a posterior tibial to peroneus brevis tendon transfer. Each case is different and needs to be managed accordingly.

deformity (see **Fig. 3**). The senior author has termed this the ping-pong effect. These situations warrant special attention (see later discussion).

Computed tomography (CT) scans, including 3-dimensional reconstructions, are essential for preoperative planning by allowing for a detailed understanding of bone erosions or cysts, osteophytes, degenerative changes, and planes of deformity (**Fig. 7**A). Special attention should be paid to large anteromedial and inferolateral talar osteophytes that can prevent reduction of the talus into the ankle mortise. These osteophytes can form a ring around the talar neck and have previously been dubbed the horseshoe osteophyte by the senior author.[9] There are often large anterior fibular osteophytes that also require resection. The CT scan also helps define the presence and degree of malleolar dysplasia, which may need to be addressed surgically. The hindfoot complex and midfoot should be assessed for degenerative changes. The presence of degenerative changes may influence the decision to proceed with arthrodesis procedures rather than osteotomies to correct deformity. The benefit of weightbearing CT scans is increasingly being reported in the literature. These scans may improve the understanding of deformity preoperatively. Their role in TAR is still under investigation.

VARUS DEFORMITY
Medial Release

Before performing the anterior approach for TAR, a decision is made regarding the need for a medial release. A medial release is performed on patients whose hindfoot deformity can be corrected to neutral but not beyond.

An incision is placed directly medially over the talonavicular joint (TNJ). Dissection down to the joint capsule is performed. The tibialis posterior (TP) tendon is released from the navicular, and a TNJ arthrotomy is performed. The TNJ capsule is elevated slightly from the talus and navicular in a plantar and dorsal direction. The dorsal capsule is left intact to preserve blood supply to the talar head.

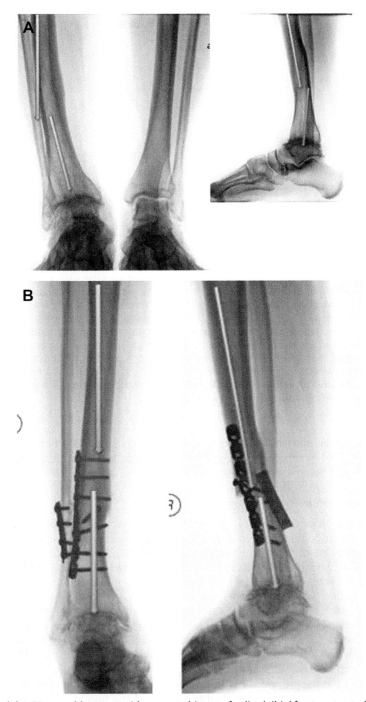

Fig. 4. (*A*) A 74-year-old woman with a remote history of a distal tibial fracture treated nonoperatively. The tibial deformity measures 12° of varus on the standing AP view and 10° of recurvatum on the lateral radiograph. A CT scanogram measured 17° of external rotation. (*B*) In this case, the senior author elected to perform a 2-stage procedure with correction of the tibial deformity first. Note that on the postoperative AP radiograph, the fibular position has changed. The decreased overlap between the tibia and fibula is due to correction of the rotational deformity. Rotational deformities in the transverse plane are better recognized clinically than on plane radiographs.

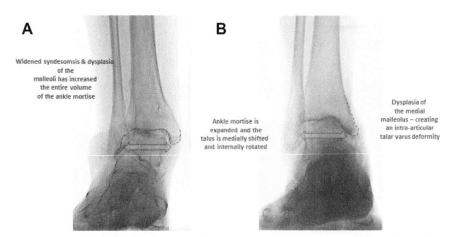

Fig. 5. (A) Long-standing deltoid insufficiency and resultant talar valgus deformity has caused widening (*double arrow*) of the syndesmosis and dysplasia of the fibula. The entire ankle mortise is widened. This needs to be taken into consideration when performing a total ankle arthroplasty. In this case (see **Fig. 1**D), an opening wedge fibular osteotomy and syndesmosis reduction or stabilization was required. (B) Long-standing varus stress has caused dysplasia of the medial malleolus, medial shift of the talus and internal rotation. This has resulted in an increased width (*double arrow*) of the ankle mortise that needs to be taken into consideration with total ankle arthroplasty. It is important to recognize this deformity because intra-articular as an extra-articular correction (supramalleolar osteotomy) can create a Z-type deformity of the distal hindfoot.

After the medial release is performed, the correction of the hindfoot deformity is reassessed. If the hindfoot still does not correct past neutral, consideration is made for performing a SJ arthrodesis (see later discussion).

Intra-Articular Deformity Correction

After a direct-anterior approach is performed, several steps are necessary to correct the intra-articular contributions to the deformity in the varus ankle. First, a thorough debridement of osteophytes is performed (see **Fig. 7**A–C). This includes osteophytes on the anterior aspect of the distal tibia and malleoli. Osteophytes inferior to the tip of the medial malleolus must also be addressed, although these may not be visualized until after further ligament releases are performed. Large osteophytes projecting from the anterior, inferior aspect of the fibula, and lateral aspect of the talus must be addressed to properly reduce the talus into the ankle mortise. This may require a separate lateral incision over the sinus tarsi to adequately decompress the lateral gutter. Osteophytes on the talar neck must also be addressed aggressively. The native talar neck can become obscured by osteophyte formation and the surgeon must recreate the talar neck through boney debridement (see **Fig. 7**B). Most of the new bone formation is on the anterior medial aspects of the talar neck. If this excess bone is not resected it can prevent appropriate placement of the first talar cutting guide for most ankle arthroplasty systems (superior flat cut of the talar body). The lateral gutter needs to be inspected for osteophytes extending off the anterior aspect of the fibular and lateral aspects of the talar body (see **Fig. 7**A–C). In the more severe talar varus deformities, a complete lateral osteophyte resection is obtained through a separate lateral approach.

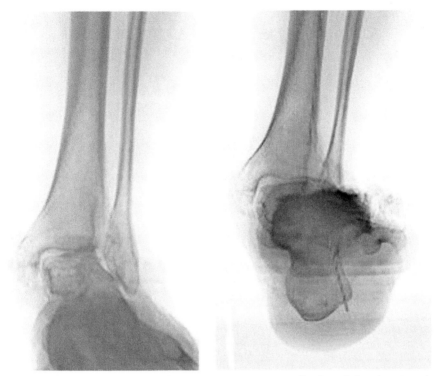

Fig. 6. AP (*left*) and HAV (*right*) of a patient with a stage IV flat foot deformity. The talar valgus is associated with a valgus deformity of the calcaneus. This is best appreciated in the HAV. The orientation of the calcaneus is different than what is observed in **Fig. 3**, in which the patient has compensatory varus of the hindfoot.

After all osteophytes are removed, distraction of the tibiotalar joint is performed. Lamina spreaders are placed into the ankle joint medially and laterally. Sequential distraction of each lamina spreader is performed to release the contracted tissues around the joint. Distraction is left in place for several minutes to allow for creep in the tissues.

Medial and lateral ligament releases are then performed. A periosteal elevator is placed into the medial and lateral gutters. With careful levering on the tibial plafond, complete medial and lateral ligament releases are performed off of the talus and calcaneus. The periosteal elevator must be in contact with the talus or calcaneus at all times to prevent neurovascular structure injury. Palpation posteromedially (just posterior to the medial malleolus) while performing the release helps to ensure a complete release of the posterior deltoid ligament is performed without placing the neurovascular structures at risk. Laterally, the elevator must be slid past the SJ to allow for release of the calcaneofibular ligament (CFL).

Following the ligament releases, deformity correction and ROM are assessed. The goal for ROM before TAR implantation is 45° of motion. If motion was less than this, further osteophyte debridement and ligament releases are performed. The deformity is passively corrected with a valgus and external-rotation force. If the talus is not correctible to neutral alignment, the joint was inspected for the need for further osteophyte resection or ligament releases. If the talus cannot be reduced to neutral

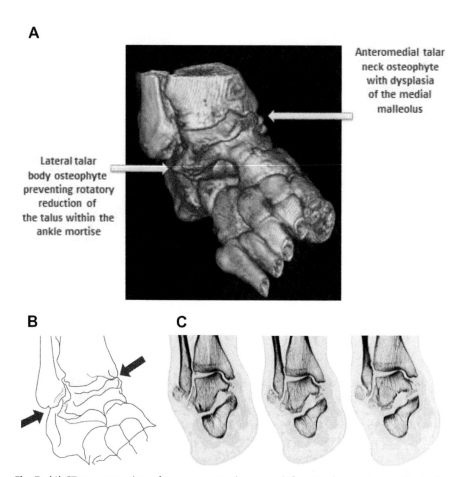

A

Anteromedial talar neck osteophyte with dysplasia of the medial malleolus

Lateral talar body osteophyte preventing rotatory reduction of the talus within the ankle mortise

B

C

Fig. 7. (*A*) CT reconstruction of a congruent talar varus deformity demonstrating the typical location of osteophytes that require debridement. Note the anteromedial talar neck osteophytes and the lateral osteophyte extending of the lateral talar body preventing from rotating into the ankle mortise. (*B*) Artist rendition of typical osteophytes (*arrows*) requiring debridement when reducing a talar varus deformity. (*C*) CT scan demonstrating lateral talar osteophytes typically seen in talar varus deformities.

alignment passively, consideration of conversion to ankle arthrodesis should be considered.

Once a proper anterior intra-articular debridement is performed, a separate lateral incision is made starting proximally at the peroneal tendon sheath and extending distally toward the base of the fifth metatarsal. This extensile lateral approach allows for access to the peroneal tendons, fibula, lateral aspect of the talus, and the lateral ankle ligaments. The peroneal tendons are inspected. In more than 50% of cases with talar varus deformities, 1 or both of the peroneal tendons are diseased or ruptured. The peroneal tendons are prepared for transfer of the peroneus longus (PL) to the peroneus brevis (PB) tendon. In severe talar varus deformities, the PTT has been prepared through the medial incision and transfer laterally for a PTT to PB transfer. The anterior talofibular and CFLs are then lifted off of the fibular and tagged for later imbrication. The lateral fibular and talar body osteophytes are thoroughly debrided. There is often a shelf osteophyte extending off the lateral talar body and, if not debrided, complete correction of the talar varus deformity is not possible. It is important to understand that the talus is internally rotated and extruded anteriorly. Adequate lateral debridement allows the surgeon to externally rotate the talus and reduce it back into the ankle mortise.

Often, at this stage, the senior author reduces the talar deformity. This involves external rotation of the talus and a valgus stress to correct the varus deformity. The talus is then held with 1 or 2 Kirschner (K)-wires extending from the tibia into the talar body. There is often a medial gap that is then filled with cement (see **Fig. 2**B). The K-wires may be removed or left in place. The anterior incision is now closed, followed by performing the lateral tendon transfers (PL to PB plus or minus PTT to PB) and then the lateral ankle ligaments are tightened using a suture anchor (see **Fig. 2**).

The patient is now ready for the second stage, which will be the TAR approximately 8 to 12 weeks later. The sutures are removed at 2 weeks and the patient is allowed to weight-bear in a below knee cast until the second stage is performed.

Tendoachilles Lengthening

A tendoachilles lengthening (TAL) is occasionally necessary to provide adequate dorsiflexion of the TAR. In the senior author's practice, a TAL slide is required in more than 90% of pes planus deformities and less than 10% of cavovarus deformities. This procedure is performed only when necessary during the second stage TAR procedure.

Extra-Articular Deformity Correction

In a 2-stage procedure, some of these procedures are performed in the first stage and others in the second stage. The surgeon needs to be prepared to adjust given the severity of the contractures or deformities and technical difficulty. In most cases, the extra-articular corrections are completed after the TAR has been performed because how much correction is necessary can only be accurately assessed once the TAR has been performed and the ankle joint itself is balanced.

Malleolar Osteotomy

In the varus ankle, over time the talus may erode the medial malleolus and lead to malleolar dysplasia (see **Fig. 5**B). After correction of the talar varus deformity, the medial gutter can be capacious (**Fig. 8**). Rotational instability of the talus can be appreciated as the talus rotates internally into the spacious medial gutter. To restore the static restraint of the medial malleolus, a translational and rotational medial malleolar osteotomy is performed.

A K-wire for the 4.0-mm cannulated screw system is inserted into the medial malleolus, stopping just distal to the level of the tibial tray. A transverse osteotomy is then performed at the distal aspect of the tibial tray, and the medial malleolus is translated laterally and externally rotated to close down the medial gutter (**Fig. 9**). The K-wire is then advanced past the osteotomy site, and a partially threaded 4.0-mm cannulated screw is placed across the osteotomy site for fixation.

First Metatarsal Osteotomy

One of the most common procedures performed at the time of TAR in the varus ankle is a dorsiflexion osteotomy of the first metatarsal. After TAR implantation, the posture of the midfoot and forefoot is assessed clinically and radiographically. A foot-plate can be used intraoperatively to simulate weightbearing. If the first ray is plantarflexed clinically and radiographically (demonstrated by disruption of the lateral talus-first

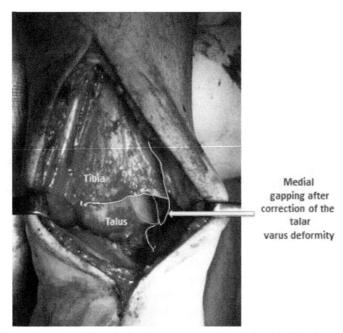

Medial
gapping after
correction of the
talar
varus deformity

Fig. 8. The talar varus deformity has been corrected and the talus has been rotated back into the ankle mortise. Gapping is often seen between the reduced talar body and the dysplastic ankle mortise. In a 2-stage procedure, this gap needs to be filled with cement to prevent the talar deformity from reoccurring when the patient starts to bear weight.

metatarsal line), a dorsiflexion osteotomy is performed. If on preoperative CT-scan, the first tarsometatarsal (TMT) joint demonstrates significant degenerative disease, a dorsiflexion first TMT arthrodesis can also be considered.

A dorsal-medial incision is made beginning at the level of the first TMT joint and extending distally. Approximately 1 cm distal to the first TMT joint, a 5-mm dorsal closing-wedge osteotomy is performed. Ideally, the osteotomy does not breach the plantar cortex of the metatarsal because this enhances stability and reduces the risk of malalignment. Fixation options include staples or plate or screw combinations.

Supramalleolar Osteotomy

A supramalleolar osteotomy (SMO) may be necessary in patients with varus malalignment of the distal tibia of various causes. Extra-articular deformity greater than 10° is an accepted indication for SMO.[5,6,12,21,22] The senior author prefers to perform a lateral closing-wedge osteotomy at the apex of the deformity. This allows for good compression without the need for bone grafting. If the SMO is the only extra-articular deformity correction necessary, it can safely be performed at the time of TAR. If multiple extra-articular procedures are necessary, it is safest to perform the procedures in a staged fashion by correcting deformity before TAR.

Calcaneal Osteotomy

If, after performing a medial release, the hindfoot does not correct past neutral, a calcaneal osteotomy may be considered to achieve a neutral or slightly valgus hindfoot alignment. Options include lateral translational and lateral closing-wedge

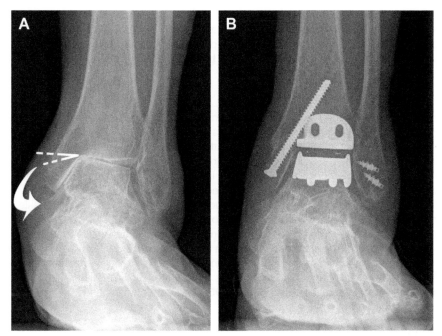

Fig. 9. (*A*) Talar varus with dysplasia of the medial malleolus. Note the medial translation of the talus and the articulation of the medial malleolus on the talar body (*curved arrow*). This causes the deep deltoid fibers to be worn off of their insertion site. (*B*) An anterolateral rotational osteotomy of the medial malleolus to close the anteromedial gap created by correction of the talar deformity. The medial malleolar osteotomy is transverse at the level of the tibial component and then the anterior aspect is rotated in a lateral direction on a posterior hinge.

osteotomies. The senior author's practice is to perform a lateral closing-wedge osteotomy to reduce the risk of a traction injury to the tibial nerve.

To perform the lateral closing-wedge osteotomy, an oblique incision is placed on the posterolateral aspect of the calcaneus, beginning at the level of the insertion of the Achilles tendon and continuing distally at a 45° angle to the sagittal plane. Dissection is carried down to bone and epiperiosteal flaps are raised anteriorly and posteriorly. A 1-cm lateral closing-wedge osteotomy is then performed in line with the skin incision, in between the Achilles insertion and the posterior facet of the SJ. The osteotomy is closed and fixated with 2 6.5 mm cannulated screws inserted from the dorsal aspect of the calcaneus.

Tendon Transfers

Relative weakness of the PB and tibialis anterior muscles compared with the TP and PL muscles may be present in patients presenting with a cavovarus deformity and ankle arthritis. PL to PB transfer may be considered when eversion power is grade 3/5 or less. This transfer will provide a dynamic stabilizer to prevent hindfoot inversion.

A lateral skin incision over the peroneal tendons at the lateral aspect of the calcaneus provides exposure of the peroneal tendons. If a sinus tarsi incision was previously used for ankle joint debridement, this incision can be extended to expose the peroneals. The tendons are isolated. At this level, the PB will be dorsal to the PL as the PL begins to travel into the plantar aspect of the foot. The PL tendon is dissected free of adhesions as distally as possible and then transected. With the foot in dorsiflexion and eversion, the PL is tenodesed to the PB using a Pulvertaft weave.

Lateral Ligament Reconstruction

As previously mentioned, it is important to ensure that the talus sits in a neutral position when the TAR is complete. If the talus has the tendency to invert, a lateral ligament reconstruction is not adequate to reposition the talus, and further bone resection and ligament balancing should be performed as detailed. If the ankle sits in a neutral position at rest but demonstrates significant instability with an inversion stress test (lateral joint opens), then a lateral ligament reconstruction can be performed.

A Broström-type lateral ligament reconstruction is adequate to stabilize the ankle in most situations.[23] A lateral incision directly over the distal fibula and extending over the sinus tarsi is made. Dissection to the extensor retinaculum and joint capsule is performed. These 2 layers are divided in line with the distal fibula, from the anterior aspect of the distal fibula to the inferior tip. Suture anchors placed into the distal fibula at the CFL and anterior talofibular ligament origins are used to repair the lateral ligaments back to the distal fibula (see **Figs. 2**B and **9B**). The repair is tensioned with the foot in dorsiflexion and maximum eversion.

Hindfoot Arthrodesis

In rigid or severe deformity, or in cases of significant degenerative joint disease of the hindfoot, arthrodesis procedures may be necessary. Options for arthrodesis include isolated STJ, double (STJ, TNJ), and triple arthrodesis (STJ, TNJ, CCJ) (**Table 6**). In the setting of TAR, the most common reasons for performing hindfoot arthrodesis are rigid (not correctible) varus deformity or symptomatic arthritis of 1 or more of the hindfoot articulations. Arthrodesis of the hindfoot does not eliminate the need for soft tissue releases to correct deformity and a similar approach is taken whether performing fusions or osteotomies.

If the indication for hindfoot arthrodesis is a not correctible hindfoot varus without significant degenerative changes, an isolated subtalar arthrodesis is performed. The senior author prefers a sinus tarsi approach to prepare the joint surfaces, followed by fixation with 1 or 2 6.5-mm cannulated partially threaded screws. On occasion, a lateral-based closing-wedge osteotomy of the calcaneus is performed in addition to the subtalar fusion to correct the hindfoot varus deformity (**Fig. 10**).

The senior author reserves triple arthrodesis for cases with severe degenerative changes of all 3 joints in the hindfoot complex. This situation is uncommon. The CCJ can usually be preserved and is typically not symptomatic.

Table 6	
Indications of arthrodesis and corresponding procedures	
Indication	**Procedure**
Rigid hindfoot, minimal arthritis	Isolated STJ arthrodesis
STJ arthritis, minimal TNJ or CC arthritis	Isolated STJ arthrodesis
TNJ arthritis	Double (STJ, TNJ) arthrodesis
STJ or TNJ or CCJ arthritis	Triple (STJ, TNJ, CCJ) arthrodesis

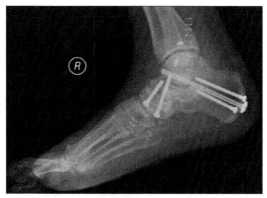

Fig. 10. Patient has undergone a calcaneal osteotomy and subtalar fusion to correct hind-foot deformity.

VALGUS DEFORMITY

Valgus deformity of the talus is less common than varus deformity.[2] Valgus deformities can be broadly placed into 2 categories: valgus arthritis secondary to pes planovalgus (stage IV flat foot) (**see Fig. 6**), and other valgus deformities, such as post-traumatic and chronic medial-sided instability (see **Fig. 3**). As with varus ankle arthritis, all deformities must be considered before proceeding with TAR to obtain a stable, well-positioned implant.

Intra-Articular Deformity

In contrast to varus ankle arthritis in which stiffness and rigidity are common, instability tends to predominate in valgus ankle deformities. Patients with pes planus and ankle arthritis often have widening of the syndesmosis and posterior subluxation of the talus (**Fig. 11**). A similar approach to that previously described is taken to the intra-articular deformity whereby osteophytes are debrided first. Ligaments are assessed for contracture; however, significant releases are less commonly required. Bone defects in the tibial plafond can be corrected with a corrective cut at the proximal aspect of the defect, perpendicular to the shaft of the tibia. Similar principles to the varus ankle are followed to ensure a neutral talus before preparation and component implantation.

Deltoid Ligament Insufficiency

Assessment of the deltoid ligament is paramount in valgus ankle deformities. Deltoid insufficiency is common and must be addressed to stabilize the talus and prevent valgus ankle tilt and rotational instability. In the senior author's experience, deltoid ligament insufficiency is the most challenging issue to address adequately when performing TAR. The deltoid ligament is a large, fan-shaped ligament with multiple attachments distally and no true anatomic reconstruction has yet been described. Many methods of repair and reconstruction of the deltoid ligament have been described; however, no single method has demonstrated superior clinical results thus far.[24–27] The role of deltoid ligament repair or reconstruction remains under investigation in the setting of TAR.

When deltoid insufficiency is suspected, the surgeon must be prepared to address it intraoperatively. This may include the ability to procure autograft or allograft for a ligament reconstruction. If the deltoid ligament is intact and the talar valgus instability is

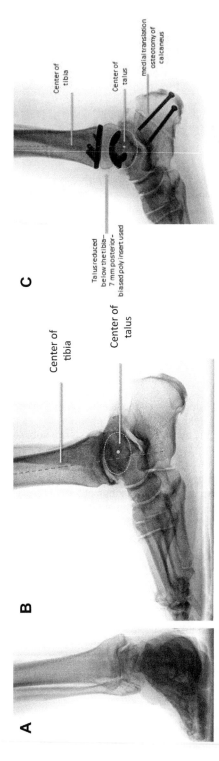

Fig. 11. (A) AP view of a 69-year-old patient with a pes planus deformity and end-stage ankle arthritis. (B) Lateral radiograph of this patient demonstrating the posterior subluxation of the talus due to multidirectional ankle instability. The talus typically subluxes in a posterior and lateral direction with some widening or instability of the syndesmosis. (C) An Integra Cadence (Ascension Orthopedics Inc, Austin, TX) TAR with a posterior-biased polyethylene insert helping to compensate for the posterior instability of the talus and bringing the center of the talus below the center of the tibia. The patient underwent a medial translation osteotomy of the calcaneus and imbrication of the deltoid ligament.

mild, a TAR can be performed with flat foot reconstruction. After appropriate exposure, the medial gutter and medial malleolus are examined. Often the medial gutter and medial malleolus are stripped of their usual soft tissues. Valgus and external-rotation stress tests will demonstrate instability of the talus if the deltoid ligament is incompetent. Repair or reconstruction should be performed after implantation of the TAR. If, however, the talar valgus is greater than 10° and the deltoid ligament is grossly incompetent, a 2-stage procedure or ankle fusion are considered (**Fig. 12**).

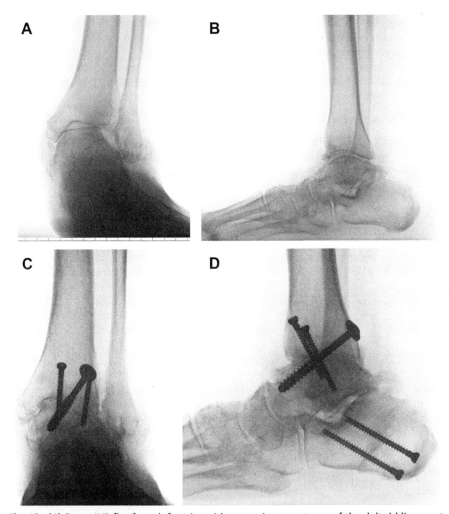

Fig. 12. (*A*) Stage IVB flat foot deformity with severe incompetency of the deltoid ligament. Note the widening of the syndesmosis. (*B*) Lateral radiograph of a Stage IVB flat foot deformity. (*C*) An ankle fusion was performed due to the severe multidirectional ligament instability. If a TAR were considered, a 2-stage approach would have been required with allograft reconstruction of the deltoid ligament and pes planus reconstruction performed in stage 1 and a TAR in stage 2. (*D*) Lateral radiograph of the ankle fusion and medial translation osteotomy of the calcaneus. Often, in stage IV flat foot deformities, fusion of the talonavicular and SJs are not required because correction of the valgus through the ankle joint is sufficient to create a stable pain-free plantigrade foot.

Deltoid ligament repair or reefing is a good option if the tissue quality permits. An incision is placed in the middle of the medial malleolus traveling over the deltoid ligament distally. The soft tissue sleeve of the superficial deltoid ligament is incised and released directly from the medial malleolus. Similar to a Broström reconstruction of the lateral ligaments, the medial malleolus is roughened with a rongeur and 1 to 2 suture anchors are inserted. The superficial deltoid complex is then reefed and repaired to the medial malleolus using the suture anchors. After repair, the stability of the talus can be reassessed. In the author's experience, this repair restores significant stability to the talus to both valgus and external-rotation stresses.

If tissue quality does not permit direct repair or reefing as described previously, deltoid ligament reconstruction with autograft or allograft may be necessary to restore stability. Many methods have been described and usually consist of a 2-tailed graft from a medial malleolar bone tunnel, with 1 tail for the talus and 1 for the calcaneus. The senior author does not perform allograft reconstruction of the deltoid ligament in the same setting as a TAR. If required, this becomes a 2-staged reconstruction.

Lateral Ligament Reconstruction

Patients with valgus ankle arthritis often have lateral ligament insufficiency in addition to deltoid incompetence. The valgus position of the calcaneus leads to calcaneofibular impingement and the lateral ligaments can be ground off of the lateral malleolus. After TAR implantation, the surgeon must assess for lateral ligament insufficiency with an inversion stress test. Any gapping of the lateral joint line of the TAR should be addressed with a lateral ligament reconstruction, as previously described.

Hindfoot Arthrodesis

Most patients with pes planovalgus that has progressed to valgus ankle arthritis have rigid deformity of the hindfoot. In situations in which the hindfoot is rigid or correctible only to neutral, hindfoot arthrodesis is recommended in the form of a double (STJ, TNJ) arthrodesis. This allows for reliable deformity correction and a stable foot beneath the ankle. The authors prefer a dual-incision technique as previously described.

Pes Planovalgus Reconstruction

Occasionally a patient will present with valgus ankle arthritis with a flexible flatfoot beneath (stage II pes planovalgus). If the hindfoot is passively correctible past neutral and into inversion, a flatfoot reconstruction can be considered. Procedures may include calcaneal osteotomies, flexor digitorum longus to TP tendon transfer, and midfoot or forefoot osteotomies or arthrodesis. Again, the goal is to provide a stable, plantigrade foot beneath the TAR.

Malleolar Osteotomy

Valgus ankle deformity may result in lateral malleolar dysplasia (see Fig. 1C and D). Chronic valgus position of the talus can erode the lateral malleolus and after correction of the talus, the lateral gutter may be capacious. The talus may rotate into this space, resulting in rotational instability of the implant. This gutter must be closed down to restore the static restraint of the lateral malleolus.

Lateral malleolus osteotomy is performed through a direct lateral approach over the fibula. Fluoroscopy is used to identify the osteotomy site at the level of the TAR joint line. A transverse, medial opening-wedge osteotomy is then performed, leaving the medial cortex of the fibula intact. Direct visualization of the lateral gutter is necessary to close the gutter to the appropriate width. The osteotomy is fixed with a lateral plate and screw construct, and the bone defect in the fibula is filled with autograft from the tibial bone resection (see **Fig. 1**D).

Syndesmotic Stabilization

Most current TAR systems do not include a syndesmotic fusion. In valgus ankle or hindfoot deformities, chronic stress on the syndesmosis may result in distal tibiofibular instability (see **Fig. 1**C). If not addressed, this can create instability of the TAR, which may lead to early failure (**Fig. 13**). Careful assessment of preoperative imaging can aid in the diagnosis of syndesmotic instability. A bilateral CT scan may be necessary to compare to the contralateral ankle. Intraoperatively, the syndesmosis can be stressed with external-rotation and sagittal stresses. If gapping at the distal tibiofibular articulation is found, debridement of the syndesmosis and stabilization with screw fixation is recommended.

Supramalleolar Osteotomy

Indications for SMO in the setting of valgus ankle arthritis and TAR are similar to those discussed for varus deformity. A medial closing-wedge osteotomy is performed at the CORA of the deformity and fixed under compression with a plate and screw construct (see **Fig. 3**).

THE PING-PONG ANKLE

As previously discussed, some deformities are more complex than may be appreciated on initial assessment. All ankles with valgus deformity are not a result of a pes planovalgus deformity; indeed, some may have an underlying cavovarus foot. Chronic lateral ligament instability is common with cavovarus deformity and may lead to multidirectional instability of the ankle. If the deltoid ligament becomes incompetent, valgus ankle arthritis may develop despite a cavovarus foot deformity. Chronic medial instability results in stress overload to the posterior-lateral aspect of the tibial plafond with gradual erosion and subsequent talar valgus deformity (see **Fig. 3**). The pre-existing hindfoot varus orientation (peek-a-boo heel) associated with compensatory inversion to maintain a plantigrade foot results in a calcaneus or SJ that is in relative varus. This has been referred to as the ping-pong ankle by the senior author and others.

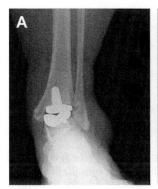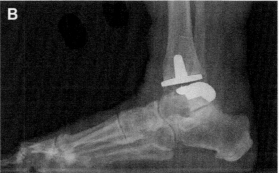

Fig. 13. (*A*) Early failure of a TAR due to unrecognized syndesmosis instability associated with a talar valgus deformity. (*B*) Note the posterior translation of the talus within the ankle mortise. This has occurred because of persistent deltoid insufficiency and instability of the syndesmosis.

It is challenging to appreciate this deformity on clinical examination because the hindfoot may appear to be in a valgus position due to the ankle deformity (**Fig. 14**). The HAV is important in confirming the diagnosis. On the HAV, the position of the calcaneus, talus, and tibia can be assessed. The talus is in a valgus position with respect to the tibia; however, the calcaneus is in a varus or neutral position with respect to the talus (see **Fig. 3**).

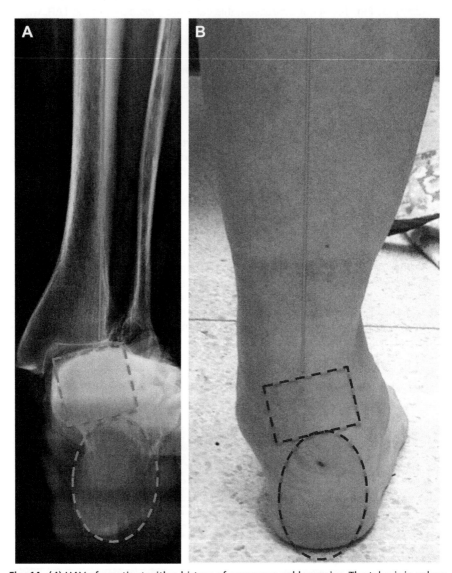

Fig. 14. (A) HAV of a patient with a history of numerous ankle sprains. The talus is in valgus and the calcaneus in relative varus. Note the widening of the syndesmosis. (B) Clinical picture of the same patient. Note that the calcaneus is not in valgus because the SJ complex has compensated for the talar valgus to maintain a plantigrade foot. At a younger age, this patient had a subtle forefoot-driven cavovarus foot with a peek-a-boo sign of the heels when observed from the front. After multiple ankle sprains the deltoid ligament has become insufficient and a talar valgus deformity has evolved.

Appreciating this diagnosis is important preoperatively to avoid intraoperative surprises. In these deformities, after correction of the intra-articular deformity and TAR implantation, the hindfoot will assume a varus position. This may be unexpected if the diagnosis is not made preoperatively. The surgeon may be faced with the opposite deformity than they thought they were dealing with. Correction of the deformity follows the principles previously discussed for the varus hindfoot.

THE ROLE OF STAGING

In severe deformity correction, staged procedures may be necessary to safely perform a TAR. There are no firm rules regarding these decisions. Factors to consider include patient factors (comorbidities, smoking), incision placement (maximize skin bridges), operative time under tourniquet, and the blood supply to the talus. Wound healing complications can be catastrophic in TAR, and the authors advise caution when considering complex deformity and TAR in a single stage. Avascular necrosis of the talus is also a risk and 360° dissection of the soft tissues around the talus in a single stage is hazardous. This is the case when a double or triple arthrodesis is performed with a TAR in a single stage.

In general, if 1 other major boney procedure is being performed for deformity correction (STJ fusion, SMO), it is likely safe to proceed with TAR at the same time. If multiple boney procedures are required, such as double or triple arthrodesis of the hindfoot, correcting the hindfoot deformity first is the safest approach. Each case must be assessed independently; however, if significant deformity correction is necessary one should always consider a staged approach.

SUMMARY

In the past, significant coronal plane deformity of the ankle was considered a contraindication to TAR.[3,4,7,14,15] Improvements in surgical technique and implant design have allowed for successful TAR in coronal plane deformities up to and above 20°.[3,5,16] The importance of obtaining a stable, plantigrade foot beneath the TAR cannot be understated. Understanding the location of deformity and the surgical procedures to adequately correct the deformity is necessary to obtain the desired results.

REFERENCES

1. Colin F, Bolliger L, Horn Lang T, et al. Effect of supramalleolar osteotomy and total ankle replacement on talar position in the varus osteoarthritic ankle: a comparative study. Foot Ankle Int 2014;35(5):445–52.

2. Horisberger M, Valderrabano V, Hintermann B. Posttraumatic ankle osteoarthritis after ankle-related fractures. J Orthop Trauma 2009;23(1):60–7.

3. Queen RM, Adams SB Jr, Viens NA, et al. Differences in outcomes following total ankle replacement in patients with neutral alignment compared with tibiotalar joint malalignment. J Bone Joint Surg Am 2013;95(21):1927–34.

4. Wood PL, Deakin S. Total ankle replacement. The results in 200 ankles. J Bone Joint Surg Br 2003;85(3):334–41.

5. Haskell A, Mann RA. Ankle arthroplasty with preoperative coronal plane deformity: short-term results. Clin Orthop Relat Res 2004;424(424):98–103.

6. Kim BS, Choi WJ, Kim YS, et al. Total ankle replacement in moderate to severe varus deformity of the ankle. J Bone Joint Surg Br 2009;91(9):1183–90.

7. Trajkovski T, Pinsker E, Cadden A, et al. Outcomes of ankle arthroplasty with pre-operative coronal-plane varus deformity of 10 degrees or greater. J Bone Joint Surg Am 2013;95(15):1382–8.

8. Espinosa N, Walti M, Favre P, et al. Misalignment of total ankle components can induce high joint contact pressures. J Bone Joint Surg Am 2010;92(5):1179–87.

9. Daniels TR, Cadden AR, Lim K-K. Correction of Varus Talar Deformities in Ankle Joint Replacement. Oper Tech Orthop 2008;18(4):282–6.

10. Jung HG, Jeon SH, Kim TH, et al. Total ankle arthroplasty with combined calcaneal and metatarsal osteotomies for treatment of ankle osteoarthritis with accompanying cavovarus deformities: early results. Foot Ankle Int 2013;34(1):140–7.

11. Paley D. Principles of deformity correction. Berlin: Springer; 2002.

12. Trincat S, Kouyoumdjian P, Asencio G. Total ankle arthroplasty and coronal plane deformities. Orthop Traumatol Surg Res 2012;98(1):75–84.

13. Saltzman CL, Salamon ML, Blanchard GM, et al. Epidemiology of ankle arthritis: report of a consecutive series of 639 patients from a tertiary orthopaedic center. Iowa Orthop J 2005;25:44–6.

14. Valderrabano V, Pagenstert G, Hintermann B. Total ankle replacement - Three-Component Prosthesis. Tech Foot Ankle Surg 2005;41(1):42–54.

15. Coetzee JC. Management of varus or valgus ankle deformity with ankle replacement. Foot Ankle Clin 2008;13(3):509–20.

16. Hobson SA, Karantana A, Dhar S. Total ankle replacement in patients with significant pre-operative deformity of the hindfoot. J Bone Joint Surg Br 2009;91(4):481–6.

17. Eberhardt RT, Raffetto JD. Chronic venous insufficiency. Circulation 2005;111(18):2398–409.

18. Sieggreen MY, Kline RA. Arterial insufficiency and ulceration: diagnosis and treatment options. Adv Skin Wound Care 2004;17(5 Pt 1):242–51 [quiz: 252–3].

19. Ajis A, Henriquez H, Myerson M. Postoperative range of motion trends following total ankle arthroplasty. Foot Ankle Int 2013;34(5):645–56.

20. Saltzman CL, el-Khoury GY. The hindfoot alignment view. Foot Ankle Int 1995;16(9):572–6.

21. Hennessy MS, Molloy AP, Wood EV. Management of the varus arthritic ankle. Foot Ankle Clin 2008;13(3):417–42, viii.

22. Easley ME. Surgical treatment of the arthritic varus ankle. Foot Ankle Clin 2012;17(4):665–86.

23. Hamilton WG, Thompson FM, Snow SW. The modified Brostrom procedure for lateral ankle instability. Foot Ankle 1993;14(1):1–7.

24. Deland JT, de Asla RJ, Segal A. Reconstruction of the chronically failed deltoid ligament: a new technique. Foot Ankle Int 2004;25(11):795–9.

25. Haddad SL, Dedhia S, Ren Y, et al. Deltoid ligament reconstruction: a novel technique with biomechanical analysis. Foot Ankle Int 2010;31(7):639–51.

26. Hintermann B, Valderrabano V, Boss A, et al. Medial ankle instability: an exploratory, prospective study of fifty-two cases. Am J Sports Med 2004;32(1):183–90.

27. Jeng CL, Bluman EM, Myerson MS. Minimally invasive deltoid ligament reconstruction for stage IV flatfoot deformity. Foot Ankle Int 2011;32(1):21–30.

Current Update in Total Ankle Arthroplasty

Salvage of the Failed Total Ankle Arthroplasty with Anterior Translation of the Talus

Alastair Younger, MB, ChB, ChM, MSc, FRCSC[a],
Andrea Veljkovic, MD, BComm, MPH, FRCSC[b],*

KEYWORDS

- Total ankle arthroplasty • Total ankle replacement • Revision total ankle arthroplasty
- Malposition • Metal component revision • Tibial malunion

KEY POINTS

- Ankle replacement results may be compromised by malposition of the components.
- The anterior displacement can be measured on a lateral standing radiograph.
- The ankle may appear anteriorly translated because the ankle is overstuffed, the heel cord is tight, or the posterior capsule is tight.
- In ankle instability with degenerative arthritis, the talus may be anteriorly translated, internally rotated, and in varus. In an ankle replacement, this deformity may persist and will require correction.
- On occasion, the talus is inserted too anterior; in this case, revision to a flat cut talar component and posterior translation of the talar component will result in correction.

INTRODUCTION

A total ankle arthroplasty has 12 errors of placement for each component: 6 translational and 6 angular. The translational errors are anterior and posterior, proximal and distal, medial and lateral. The angular errors are internal and external rotation, flexion and extension, and varus and valgus. Each component also can be oversized or undersized for a total of 14 errors for each component. There are also 12 potential errors that affect the relationship of each component, resulting in 40 potential errors of placement in each ankle joint replacement.

Disclosure: Dr A. Younger is a consultant with Zimmer, Cartiva, Wright Medical, and Acumed. He has research support from Acumed, Cartiva, Zimmer, Wright Medical, Synthes, and Bioventus. Dr A. Veljkovic has research support from Zimmer and Amniox.
[a] Department of Orthopaedics, University of British Columbia, 560 1144 Burrard Street, Vancouver, British Columbia V6Z 2A5, Canada; [b] University of British Columbia, 1000-1200 Burrard Street, Vancouver, British Columbia V6Z 2C7, Canada
* Corresponding author.
E-mail address: docveljkovic@yahoo.com

Foot Ankle Clin N Am 22 (2017) 301–309
http://dx.doi.org/10.1016/j.fcl.2017.01.014
foot.theclinics.com

In this article, the anterior translation of the talus is addressed. However, like many of these deformities, they are rarely in isolation and are usually combined.

How to measure anterior translation of the talus has recently been published by Veljkovic and colleagues[1] (**Fig. 1**). The anterior position of the talus is referenced off the tibia by measuring the tibial axis on a lateral weight-bearing view and determining the position of the central axis of the talar component. This, therefore, can represent either anterior positioning of the talar component on the talus, anterior translation of the foot on the tibia, or an artifact created by excessive plantar flexion of the foot. Other investigators also have described how to reference this deformity.[2]

Anterior translation of the whole ankle may exist after a tibial nonunion, resulting in an anteriorly translated foot. This should be addressed by a supramalleolar osteotomy.

In a mobile-bearing ankle, anterior slope (extension) of the tibial component can result in an anterior glide of the talar component (**Fig. 2**).[3] If this persists, then an anterior tibial osteotomy correcting the deformity, or a revision of the tibial component can correct the deformity by a combination of a posteriorly directed ankle joint force, as well as a translation of the foot on the tibia.

Within the ankle, a tight posterior capsule or tight posterior structures can result in an equinus deformity with anterior translation of the talus on the tibia. A posterior release will be required to correct the deformity. This tightness may exist after trauma, such as a pilon fracture causing fibrosis of the posterior structures that may not have been recognized at the index arthroplasty. A similar appearance can exist with an overstuffed ankle, resulting in loss of dorsiflexion range and anterior translation of the talar component with respect to the tibial axis.

In some cases, a combined deformity exists after ankle instability. The talus is in varus, internally rotated, in equinus, and anteriorly translated secondary to lateral osteophytes. These can then stretch the lateral collateral ligaments, resulting in subsequent stabilization of the unstable ankle. If this deformity is not corrected at the time of index arthroplasty, then the ankle joint will remain deformed.

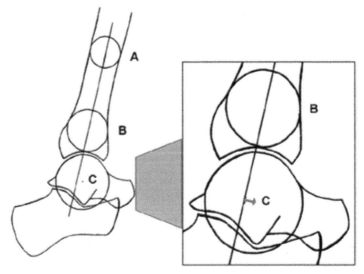

Fig. 1. The measurement of talar station on the lateral view of the ankle. (*A*) Center Tibial graft. (*B*) Center distal tibia. (*C*) Center talus. (*From* Veljkovic A, Norton A, Salat P, et al. Lateral talar station: a clinically reproducible measure of sagittal talar position. Foot Ankle Int 2013;34:1670; with permission.)

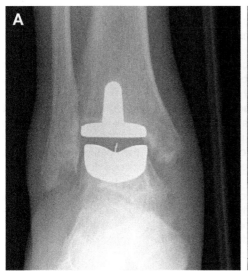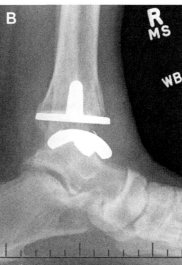

Fig. 2. (A, B) A Mobility ankle with neutral anterior slope and anterior translation of the talar component. At revision, the tibial and talar components were both found to be loose. Both sides of the ankle therefore required revision.

The talar component itself can be anteriorly translated on the talar body. Each ankle system may have different risk factors for failure in this regard. For example, a flat cut talar component, such as a Hintegra (Newdeal SA, Lyon, France) revision talus or an Agility, may be placed too anterior at the time of implantation. However an Inbone (Wright Medical Technology Inc, Memphis, TN) may not be so prone to this because of the jig system. A contoured talar cut from the anterior approach using a prosthesis, such as a Mobility (DePuy, Leeds, UK), Salto (DePuy, Leeds, UK), STAR (Stryker, Mahwah, NJ), or Hintegra standard component, may be anteriorly translated because the surgeon was not able to place the jig posteriorly or did not recognize anterior translation of the cut. A laterally placed ankle such as the Zimmer TM (Zimmer, Warsaw, IN) ankle may not be as prone to anterior translation of the talar component. If an anterior approach is used and the ankle is stiff, the error may be to place the talar component too anterior. The referencing for the talar component anterior to posterior positioning is usually off the posterior side of the initial talar cut. If this is minimal, then the jig will be placed too anterior relative to the central axis of rotation of the talus, resulting in an anteriorly translated talus. This will also cause overstuffing of the ankle, resulting in an anteriorly located talar component with the ankle in equinus. Equally if the posterior talus is not well visualized with the correct gap between the tibia and talus, then the talar guide may be placed too anterior.

Patients with an anteriorly translated talus may present with pain in the ankle, or loss of range of motion. The ankle will lack dorsiflexion rather than plantar flexion range. After clinical examination, a lateral radiograph will typically reveal the deformity. As explained previously, this may be part of a more complex deformity, so a computed tomography (CT) scan will be helpful in assessing the deformity. Then revision surgery can be correctly planned, paying attention to the various potential errors of placement.

CLINICAL EXAMINATION

A history from the patient on the initial complaints and source of ankle arthritis is helpful in determining the cause of malposition. A history of prior tibial fractures, pilon fractures, or ankle instability will help identify the cause.

Physical examination should include watching the patient stand and walk. An equinus gait should alert the surgeon to anterior translation of the talar component as the potential cause.

The tibial alignment should be critically assessed. A recurvatum deformity from a tibial shaft or pilon fracture may be obvious on inspection of the limb from the side, but not so obvious on plain radiographic views.

Recurrent ankle instability can lead to anterior translation, varus, and internal rotation of the talus. Incomplete lateral gutter debridement will result in this position being maintained. Inspection of the position of the foot with respect to the tibia (look for internal rotation of the foot on the long axis of the tibia, varus alignment, and anterior translation) will demonstrate the incomplete correction at the time of index arthroplasty.

An ankle overstuffed and hence in equinus or left with a posterior ankle contracture can give the appearance of an anteriorly displaced talus. In this case, the range of motion and presence of contractures should be recorded.

The old wounds should be inspected for prior or current infection. In a posttraumatic ankle, there may be many old incisions around the ankle, so exposure may be a challenge. A free flap or tissue expansion may be required.

The clinical examination should be completed with an assessment of the surrounding joints, an assessment of the function of the tendons surrounding the ankle, a neurologic examination, and a vascular examination.

PREOPERATIVE INVESTIGATIONS

Standing anteroposterior (AP) and lateral views of the ankle will be required to determine the position of the talus. Several techniques exist to define the talar position from these views.

A CT scan of the failed ankle also is helpful in assessing the position of the components. The foot should be placed in the scanner in a neutral position (foot 90° to the tibial axis) by a jig to allow assessment, as a plantar flexed foot cannot allow correct interpretation of talar position. The CT scan also can be used to determine if lateral talar osteophytes have resulted in the talus being held anterior and internally rotated. A 3-dimensional reconstruction will assist in complex deformities in planning so long as the signal artifact from the components is adequately suppressed.

OPERATIVE MANAGEMENT
Preparation

A clear surgical plan needs to be outlined after the investigations have been performed. A full set of revision components should be available in case the operative plan changes. One or other component might be loose at the time of revision and this needs to be anticipated.

The consent should contain the potential options for revision, including osteotomies (tibial, medial or lateral malleolar, or calcaneal), soft tissue release, lateral ligament reconstruction, and revision of components.

Infection should be ruled out before revision by a history and bloodwork, such as a C-reactive protein or sedimentation rate, and if indicated, an aspiration.

Procedures with Retention of Both Components

In some cases when the talus is anteriorly translated, both components can be preserved. If an equinus deformity exists, or if the ankle is internally rotated and anteriorly translated, a soft tissue procedure alone can be used to posteriorly translate the ankle.

Procedure: equinus deformity
The equinus deformity may require an extensive posterior release. An adequate incision to reach the posterior structures from the medial side is required. Not only will the heel cord require lengthening, but the posterior capsule and the posterior structures also may require release. If the contracture is longer term or posttraumatic, then the deep investing fascia also may be contracted and may require release. Finally, the posterior deltoid ligament may be contracted and also require release.

Procedure: lateral ligament reconstruction
If the lateral ankle is held forward and internally rotated, and otherwise the components are stable, then the ankle may be repositioned from a lateral approach by removing the lateral osteophytes and debriding the lateral gutter. Once the fibula, tibia, and talus have been identified, the lateral collateral ligaments are incised. Once exposed, the osteophytes are removed off the talus and off the fibula. This will then allow the position of the ankle joint to be corrected. For a mobile-bearing and a semiconstrained ankle, this derotation may be possible; however, for a more constrained ankle, the tibial component may require revision too and this will need to be assessed on the table.

If the ankle corrects in position and this is confirmed on the lateral radiograph, then the lateral collateral ligaments are repaired. If severely attenuated, a free graft may be required to perform the repair. The peroneal tendons also may be injured in this deformity, so they should be inspected and treated by repair or tendon transfer at the same procedure.

Procedure: distal tibial osteotomy
On occasion, the anteriorly translated talus can be treated by a tibial osteotomy flexing and extended tibial component and pushing the talar component posteriorly.[3] In this procedure, an anterior approach is used and the stability of the components confirmed. The deformity can be corrected by an opening wedge (which may tighten the posterior structures) or an anterior opening wedge, posterior closing wedge osteotomy that will maintain the same posterior soft tissue tension. This procedure will work for a mobile-bearing prosthesis and may work for a constrained prosthesis depending on the geometry of the components and the anterior translation of the tibial component.

Revision of the Talar Component Alone

This is possible for a mobile-bearing prosthesis if the talus is anteriorly translated on the tibia and can be corrected by a soft tissue procedure.

Procedure: tibial component revision
The prior anterior incision is reopened. The ankle is exposed and the components visualized. Cultures are taken. If the tibial component is solid and correctly placed, then the talus alone can be revised if anterior translated or the ankle is overstuffed, causing anterior translation through equinus.

The old talar component should be removed with careful preservation of bone. To assist, the polyethylene insert should be removed prior.

Care should be taken to avoid fracture of the malleoli during the procedure, and if need be the malleoli prophylactically transfixed with screws before revision.

For a Mobility replacement, a Hintegra revision component can be used with the Mobility tibial component being left in place.

For an STAR, no revision component exists, so the surgeon is faced with recutting a new more posteriorly located component, which may be possible with more bone resection.

After the new component is placed, the position is checked on the lateral view. The talar component should be directly under the long axis of the tibia with the ankle held in zero degrees of plantar flexion.

For a Hintegra ankle, a flat cut revision exists. After removal of the original component, the talar cut is referenced off the tibial jig. The gutters are prepared and the flat cut trial placed and held in an initial position. A lateral view of the ankle will allow determination of the position of the talar component. If malpositioned, it should be repositioned before placement of the drill holes for the fixation pegs of the prosthesis. After placement of the final prosthesis and polyethylene, the wound is closed in layers.

If the ankle is overstuffed and the tibial component well positioned and well fixed to bone, then more bone can be resected from the tibial side so long as that does not lower the joint line.

Revision of Both Components

For most cases, both components will require revision. Most constrained ankles will require revision of both components. For mobile-bearing prostheses, the tibial component will require revision if it is loose or malpositioned. For ankles no longer in production (Agility and Mobility, for example), the surgeon should plan to change both components, as the polyethylene insert will not be revisable and in most cases the tibial and talar components will not match. A device with revision components should be considered, such as an Inbone or Hintegra prosthesis. Most often, a flat cut is required on the talar side. Anterior slope (extension) of the talar component will need to be corrected also.[4]

Procedure: revision both components

The previous anterior ankle wound is opened. The old components are removed with care being taken not to remove too much bone. Revision osteotomes may be required. Care should be taken to avoid damage to the malleoli. They may require prophylactic

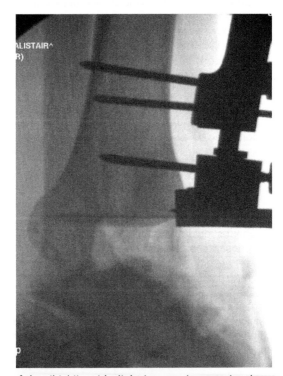

Fig. 3. Placement of the tibial jig with slight increase in posterior slope.

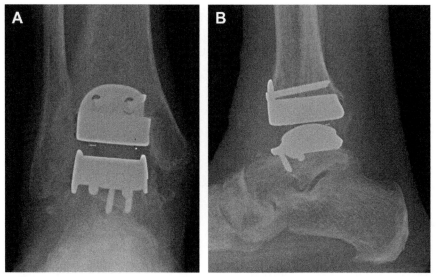

Fig. 4. (*A, B*) The revision components in place with slight increase in posterior slope, and better AP positioning of the talar component.

fixation. In some cases, a fibular shortening osteotomy may be required. If the osteotomy is done early in the procedure, exposure and positioning will be facilitated.

Care should be taken in the revision procedure to ensure that the tibial component is well positioned (**Figs. 3** and **4**), the talar component is well positioned, and the

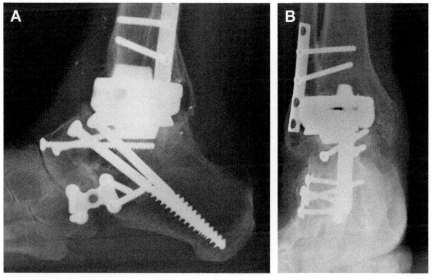

Fig. 5. (*A, B*) An ankle revision with a bimalleolar osteotomy. This Agility is loose, in varus, and the talus anteriorly translated. Often as the talar component subsides, the ankle develops a varus deformity that needs to be corrected.

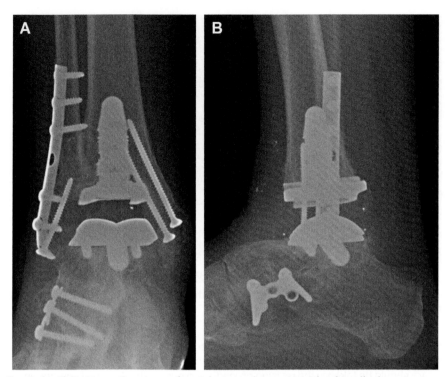

Fig. 6. (*A*, *B*) Postoperative views of an Inbone replacement with a bimalleolar osteotomy allowing correction of the foot position on the long axis of the tibia.

relationship of both components is correct. In our experience, the relationship of both components to each other is complex in the revision ankle and a bimalleolar osteotomy is the only method by which the alignment of both can correctly be addressed (**Figs. 5** and **6**).

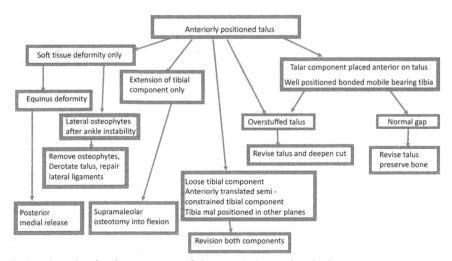

Fig. 7. Algorithm for the treatment of the anteriorly translated talus.

Outcomes

A single article exists on the outcome of revision total ankle arthroplasty.[5] Within this article, the usual reason for revision was loosening rather than malposition and no specific information is outlined on revision for anterior translation of the talar component.

Another article looked at correction in time of talar position and demonstrated that it can improve over the first 6 months after surgery, so an initial anterior translation after surgery may improve in a mobile-bearing ankle.[2]

SUMMARY

This article reviews the techniques required to correct anterior translation of the talus in revision total ankle arthroplasty. An algorithm for the various steps in analysis and treatment is presented (**Fig. 7**).

REFERENCES

1. Veljkovic A, Norton A, Salat P, et al. Lateral talar station: a clinically reproducible measure of sagittal talar position. Foot Ankle Int 2013;34:1669–76.
2. Usuelli FG, Maccario C, Manzi L, et al. Posterior talar shifting in mobile-bearing total ankle replacement. Foot Ankle Int 2016;37:281–7.
3. Veljkovic A, Norton A, Salat P, et al. Sagittal distal tibial articular angle and the relationship to talar subluxation in total ankle arthroplasty. Foot Ankle Int 2016;37(9): 929–37.
4. Cho J, Yi Y, Ahn TK, et al. Failure to restore sagittal tibiotalar alignment in total ankle arthroplasty: its relationship to the axis of the tibia and the positioning of the talar component. Bone Joint J 2015;97-B:1525–32.
5. Hintermann B, Zwicky L, Knupp M, et al. HINTEGRA revision arthroplasty for failed total ankle prostheses. J Bone Joint Surg Am 2013;95:1166–74.

Malalignment Correction of the Lower Limb Before, During, and After Total Ankle Arthroplasty

Taggart T. Gauvain, MD[a], Michael A. Hames, MD[b],
William C. McGarvey, MD[a],*

KEYWORDS

- Deformity • Total ankle arthroplasty • Osteotomy • Alignment procedures
- Soft tissue balancing • Fusion • Tendon transfer

KEY POINTS

- Approximately one-third or more cases of end-stage ankle arthritis present with some degree of deformity.
- These deformities are often multidimensional and present challenges to surgeons to reestablish alignment and provide durable results of arthroplasty procedures.
- Arthroplasty combined with deformity correction is intimidating, but, using basic skills and principles, many of these problems can be met and overcome with good results and longevity of implants.

INTRODUCTION

It is well documented in the literature that the success and survivorship of a total ankle arthroplasty (TAA) is linked to creating a balanced, neutrally aligned, and stable ankle.[1] Clinical and radiographic angular deformity of the ankle from the mechanical axis of the leg that is less than 5° is generally accepted as being within reasonable limits. There is some debate as to the level of deformity that is acceptable, with some investigators advocating that 15° of coronal plane angulation be considered a relative contraindication and some who accept up to 30°.[2] Although coronal plane angulation is a more commonly discussed topic, sagittal plane deformity can exist as well, either independently or as part of a multiplanar misalignment, and must be addressed for

Disclosure: The authors have nothing to disclose.
[a] Department of Orthopaedic Surgery, University of Texas Health Science Center-Houston, 10905 Memorial Hermann Drive, Suite 130 Pearland, Houston, TX 77584, USA; [b] Private Practice Orthopaedics, 1 W Medical Ct Wichita Falls, Wichita Falls, TX 76310, USA
* Corresponding author.
E-mail address: William.c.mcgarvey@uth.tmc.edu

successful TAA. This article discusses various types of deformity and the potential interventions for correction.

Coronal plane deformity can exist in either varus or valgus at the level of the ankle joint and can be either congruent or incongruent. Myerson (personal communication, 2011) has attempted to simplify the thought process by identifying these deformities as either intra-articular or extra-articular.[3] Intra-articular deformities are considered incongruent and the talus and tibial plafond are seen in a nonanatomic alignment. Examples of incongruent ankles are given in **Figs. 6**A and **9**A, showing the alteration in normal ankle alignment. For example, tibial plafond erosion is commonly seen at the medial aspect with varus congruent deformities. This deformity can arise because of lateral joint stabilizers that are deficient or medial structures outside the joint space that have become contracted or altered. The lateral joint line in this case often presents with significant laxity and there can be contracture and derangement of the medial structures. Deformity driven at the extra-articular level is considered congruent. Congruent deformity is usually noted with the talus and tibia remaining in relative anatomic alignment, with surrounding bony deformity, most often within the tibia, along with fairly symmetric existing degenerative changes. A stepwise assessment and correction of all alterations in soft tissues and bony structures must be completed. As with any deformity, the cause driving the deformity must be identified and corrected or there are realistic risks of failure and recurrence. Incongruency has been shown to have a much higher incidence of recurrence.[4] In a study by Reddy and colleagues,[5] preoperatively identified varus incongruent deformity had a 14% recurrence rate. In contrast, no congruent deformity showed recurrence. There are cases of varus and valgus congruent and incongruent deformities that are either intra-articular or extra-articular, respectively. No matter the cause of the deformity, in order to prevent edge loading, instability, subluxation events, and even complete failure of the TAA, the malalignment must be corrected.

A reported 33% to 44% of patients who present for TAA have greater than 10° of coronal plane deformity.[5] Implant survivorship at 8 years decreases from 90% to 48% when deformity is left greater than 10° in the coronal plane.[6] However, if the deformity can be corrected, the success of the TAA approaches the level of TAA performed in anatomically neutral ankles.[7] Implant survivorship has improved vastly based on a collective study of 2240 total ankles arthroplasties and is now reported to range from 70% to 98% at 3 to 6 years and from 80% to 95% at 8 to 12 years.[8]

There exist multiple surgical interventions available to surgeons to assist in the correction of deformity of the ankle. They include soft tissue and bone procedures that can be used preoperatively and intraoperatively. This article discusses some of these current procedures, philosophies, and proposed algorithms in an effort to aid clinicians to develop rational thought processes and approaches in addressing deformity in TAA surgery. The goal is not to present an exhaustive list of procedures or rigid thinking but to provide a thoughtful overview and suggestions for itemizing the problems inherent in deformity management and prioritizing steps to effect correction while minimizing potential complications and pitfalls in this underaddressed area of ankle replacement surgical decision making. Also, consideration is given to whether a deformity correction should be staged or attempted concomitant with the TAA. The hope is that by surveying this article, readers will be able to implement a treatment plan and ultimately perform a successful TAA creating a well-balanced and mechanically aligned ankle joint that provides appropriate functionality and longevity to the patient.

CLINICAL EVALUATION

The perfect patient for TAA has yet to be identified. It has been suggested that patients less than 54 and older than 70 years of age have less favorable outcomes.[9] Health-related factors such as obesity and diabetes have been suggested to negatively influence the outcome of TAA.[9] These factors should be well documented for each patient who is considering a TAA and be a part of the discussion with the patient. Limb alignment and functionality are also important factors in patient assessment. Gaining an understanding of what deformity exists, whether it is static or dynamic, and how to go about reconstruction or repair is paramount to achieving a successful TAA.

All assessment of deformity should begin in the clinical setting. The entire limb should be evaluated as well as the contralateral side for comparison (**Fig. 1**). The patient should be observed walking in the clinic and the gait should be assessed critically. Special consideration to ankle and foot alignment, joint range of motion, rotation of the limb, and leg length should be given (**Fig. 2**). Adjacent joints also need to be evaluated, including the knee and the hip. A clinician must decipher which joints are painful and what structures are not functioning normally. Is the deformity dynamic or static? At what level is the deformity located and how is it affecting the ankle joint? Standing 3-view ankle and foot series and 2 views of the tibia should be obtained as well as full-length limb films for alignment evaluation (**Figs. 3–5**). An axial view of the heel, or Saltzman view, can be of value to determine hindfoot alignment. Computed tomography (CT) scanning has become an integral part of the evaluation as well. CT can help to elucidate the subtleties of the underlying deformity with greater accuracy and detail than routine two-dimensional radiographs. With the current use of three-dimensional printing (available through some implant manufacturers) and weight-bearing CT scans being more prevalent, deformities are able to be evaluated more intricately and effectively to allow better preoperative planning of corrective steps.

Once a thorough evaluation of the patient has been completed, the challenge begins to understand the deformities that may influence the outcomes of the TAA. After identifying the deformity, the clinician must have a treatment plan for addressing the problem and the timing or staging as to when it is appropriate to do so: preoperatively, intraoperatively, or postoperatively.

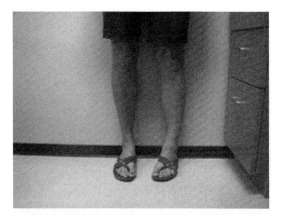

Fig. 1. A patient standing with varus, internal rotation deformity. Note that the relative heights of patellae suggest the left side is short as well.

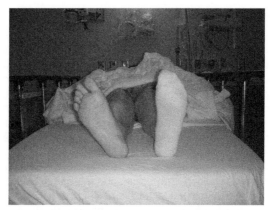

Fig. 2. Rotational assessment is critical in deformity correction. Note the increased external rotation of the right foot relative to the knee.

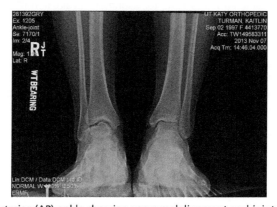

Fig. 3. Anteroposterior (AP) ankle showing varus malalignment and joint irregularities.

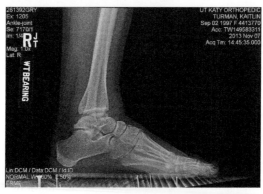

Fig. 4. Lateral ankle revealing incongruency and morphology changes.

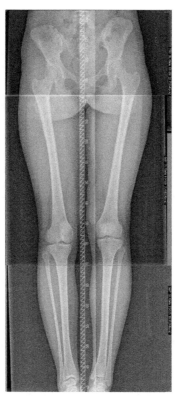

Fig. 5. Long-standing radiographs are helpful in assessing not only leg length inequality but also its effect on the mechanical axis and overall influence on skeletal balance.

TREATMENT AND CONSIDERATION OF DEFORMITY

The first step in treating deformity about the ankle is to recognize that a malalignment exists. This step is best done on weight-bearing views of the ankle and foot. The malalignment may be in the coronal or sagittal plane or both. Once a deformity is noted in the coronal plane, representing either varus or valgus, the next step is to assess the joint and identify congruent versus incongruent tibiotalar alignment.

Full-length standing limb films provide insight into more proximal sources of deformity, which may include hip or knee abnormalities (arthritis or deformity), rotational anomalies of the femur or tibia, as well as angular deformities (in both the coronal or sagittal plane) of the femur or tibia. Any or all of these may drive malalignment of the foot and ankle complex. Standing foot films and clinical assessment of the foot with regard to laxity and stiffness of joints and ligaments may provide evidence of a distal source of deformity driving the ankle malalignment. More common abnormalities, including pes planus, pes cavus, and deltoid or lateral ligament insufficiency, are encountered in the clinic. Sagittal plane deformity is less readily discussed as a major source of deformity and usually results from either anterior plafond erosion or posterior malleolar insufficiency. However, this condition must be identified and treated for proper mechanical function of the planned implant. Armed with this knowledge, surgeons may then follow an algorithm appropriate for the deformity noted.

DEFORMITY PROXIMAL TO THE ANKLE JOINT

If deformity of any kind or degenerative changes at the hip, femur, and/or knee are noted that may be influencing the alignment of the ankle and foot, it is recommended that these be addressed first. The reasoning pertains to the propensity for the proximal joint alignment and length to have a higher degree of impact on more distal manipulations. Distal alignment is based generally on proximal references. Degenerative hip or knee disease should be addressed first, particularly if these contribute to identifiable deformity leading to proximal malalignment. Ankle arthroplasty performed in the presence of existing proximal deformity is done with aberrant proximal references and landmarks that can alter good surgical decision making. In addition, should the deformity require later correction, the implanted ankle may no longer assume the desired alignment because of the alteration of the mechanical axis inherent in hip, and especially knee, arthroplasty. There have been case reports of concomitant knee and ankle arthroplasty that had good outcomes; however, these are limited and provided a significant challenge to the surgeons involved.[10] The authors recommend these be approached by experienced surgeons only. In general, these should be considered staged procedures with the more proximal of those done primarily (**Figs. 6** and **7**).

Other proximal sources of deformity, such as tibial angulation, should be addressed preoperatively as well. Tibial deformity may be developmental, congenital, or posttraumatic. Sagittal plane deformity may be either apex anterior (procurvatum) or apex posterior (recurvatum). The deformity may occur anywhere along the tibia, but has a more pronounced effect on the ankle when it occurs in the distal one-third.[11] Sagittal plane deformity of 15° (either anterior or posterior) in the distal one-third of the tibia can yield changes in ankle joint contact pressures of 40%.[12] Recurvatum deformity typically produces erosion of the anterior tibial plafond and some degree of subluxation of the talus anteriorly. It is often accompanied by functional equinus contracture that is driven by the proximal deformity as the foot finds the ground. It is generally accepted that coronal deformity greater than 5° should be corrected to avoid edge loading.[13] In either plane of tibial deformity, the authors recommend correction of deformities greater than 5° and recommend doing so before proceeding with TAA.

The correction of tibial malalignment is accomplished via osteotomy, which may be closing wedge, opening wedge, dome osteotomy, or an osteoplasty using distraction osteogenesis principles. Wedge osteotomies either shorten (closing wedge) or lengthen (opening wedge) the limb and require intraoperative translation to maintain alignment. Opening wedge osteotomies may require bone grafting to heal as well. Dome osteotomies provide correction without translation or lengthening and provide the greatest contact surface. This type of osteotomy is much more technically challenging than the closing or opening wedge. Osteoplasty using distraction osteogenesis principles can realign the tibia in any plane needed without unwanted translation or lengthening. This procedure is challenging and requires extended time in a frame and should be done only by surgeons with experience and understanding of this process. Regardless of the type of correction, the surgeon's goal is to create a mechanically well-aligned tibia that is neutral both in angulation as well as in translation with regard to the mechanical axis.

Fixation may be accomplished by internal means or by external fixator frame application. Multiplanar spatial frame application has the advantage of allowing slow and controlled correction of the deformity with smaller wounds and less soft tissue insult at the osteotomy site. This advantage comes at the cost of increased time for

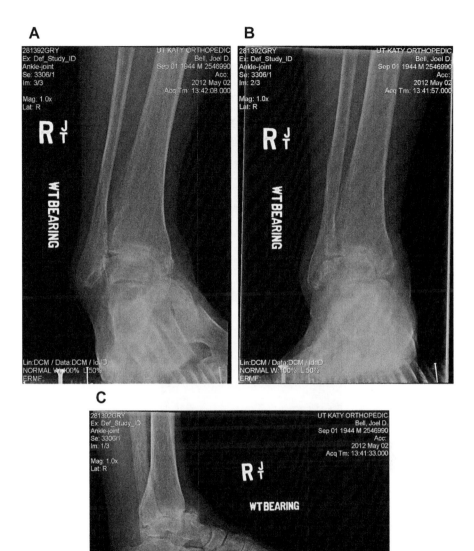

Fig. 6. A 59-year-old man with long-standing history of ankle pain and instability. He presented requesting ankle replacement. Seen are (*A*) AP, (*B*) mortise, and (*C*) lateral views of his arthritic ankle.

correction as well as the potential for pin site issues, need for secondary surgery for removal, and the cumbersome nature of a frame. During correction of sagittal plane recurvatum deformity in which there is pronounced equinus, consideration for soft tissue management must be made. Concomitant tendo Achilles lengthening with frame application spanning both procedures allows gradual correction and may help to prevent posterior soft tissue compromise caused by tension.

A

B

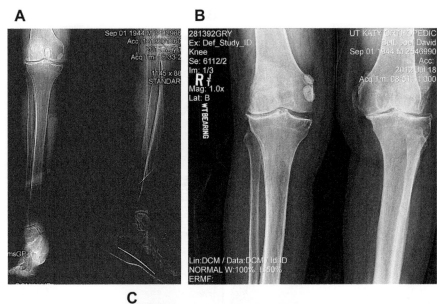

C

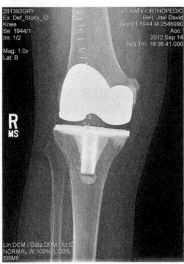

Fig. 7. The same individual as in the previous figures also had some degree of knee pain. (*A*) Arthritic changes and valgus alignment. (*B*) The comparative alignment. The patient first underwent proximal realignment with total knee arthroplasty (*C*) with good relief of knee pain and improvement in gait.

DEFORMITY OF THE FOOT DISTAL TO THE ANKLE

After addressing considerations to proximal contributions to the deformity of the ankle joint, consideration of distal deformities or those about the foot should be undertaken. The foot generally (but not always) finds the ground and therefore deformity at the foot distal to the ankle may be compensatory to any proximal deformity, be it at (intra-articular) or above the ankle. It may also be the driving force of deformity about the ankle.

Regardless of whether or not the foot deformity is the cause of, or response to, the deformity at the ankle, a clinical and radiographic assessment thereof and a plan to correct it must be made.

Consider the following questions:

- Is the foot plantigrade?
- Is there cavus or planus present? If so, is the deformity supple and flexible or rigid and fixed?
- Are there degenerative changes in the transverse tarsal and/or subtalar joints?
- Is there ligamentous laxity at either the medial or lateral side of the ankle?
- Is there laxity of the first ray (tarsometatarsal joint) or is it fixed in either dorsiflexion or plantarflexion?
- What is the alignment of the heel?

Flexible deformities about the foot may be approached in much the same way that they would without ankle arthritis and deformity. The hindfoot tends to be in the position of the talus. Valgus ankle (talar) alignment tends to yield pes planus (**Fig. 8**), whereas varus talus tends to yield cavus hindfoot. Flexible pes planus, presenting with hindfoot valgus and possibly dorsiflexion through the first ray, may be addressed with corrective calcaneal and cuneiform osteotomies, recreation of the medial arch sling, and posterior tibial tendon reconstruction as indicated. Correctable cavus feet, with varus hindfoot and possible fixed plantarflexed first ray, may be addressed with calcaneal osteotomy, plantar fascial release, and dorsiflexion first ray osteotomy as appropriate.

These procedures may be addressed concomitantly with the TAA or in a separate procedure before undertaking the TAA (**Figs. 9** and **10**). Approaching these procedures along with TAA should be done with caution, because they may add considerable time under tourniquet as well as increasing the risk of vascular embarrassment caused by the multiple incision placement, dissection, and manipulation of all vasculature. The counterpoint to this caveat is that achieving neutral alignment of the foot may be easier with the ankle appropriately reduced after the arthroplasty has been completed. In an

A   **B**

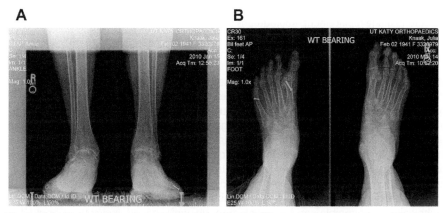

Fig. 8. This 69-year-old woman presented with inability to walk further than 1.5 to 3 m (5–10 feet) at a time because of ankle pain. She shows valgus alignment (A) of the ankle. However, there also exists a moderate abduction of the midfoot, as shown by the uncovering of the talus on weight-bearing AP views of the feet (B). This finding may need to be factored into the decision making for the surgery.

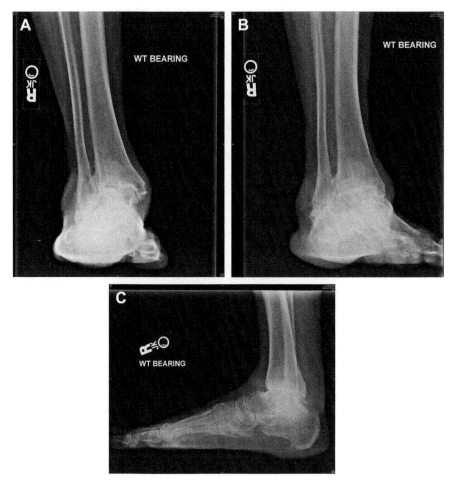

Fig. 9. This 73-year-old man presented with moderate valgus ankle arthritis and severe pain, requesting ankle replacement. Radiographs of his ankle only were obtained with (A) AP, (B) mortise, and (C) lateral views.

effort to merge perspectives, Haddad (personal communication, 2012) suggested using cement injected into the collapsed side of the incongruous joint to achieve level balance and hold the ankle in relative neutral alignment while allowing the performance and healing of corrective foot surgeries as well as allowing weight bearing on the now plantigrade foot once appropriate. Once the foot procedures are healed and stable, the surgeon may return to perform the arthroplasty, which is now a fairly uniform implantation in a nondeformed extremity, thus reducing the time in surgery and the risk of multiple procedures outlined earlier.

In general, most surgeons are comfortable performing procedures that are brief, technically reproducible, and low risk through well-spaced incisions. Should the foot realignment be estimated to require protracted surgical time, the surgeon should consider staging the procedures to avoid potential complications, including wound healing issues, infection caused by prolonged exposure, and/or neurovascular damage from multiple and simultaneous insults. Typically, a calcaneal osteotomy and/or

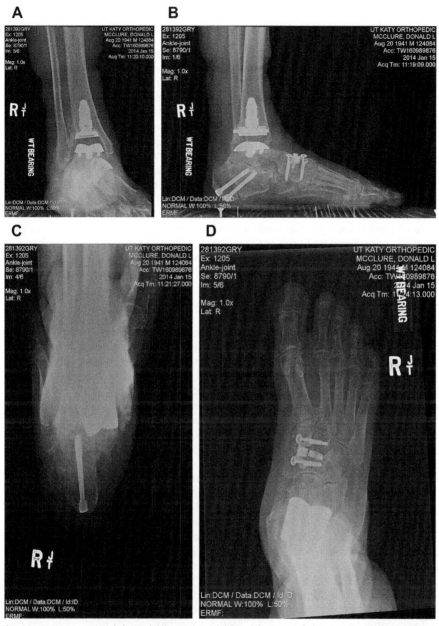

Fig. 10. Intraoperative (*A*) AP, (*B*) lateral, and (*C*) axial views of the previously featured patient, who was identified to have a compensatory adductus of the foot that was exaggerated after the correction of the ankle valgus. (*D*) An abduction-producing osteotomy and medial column fusion to reposition the foot in better alignment with this ankle correction. Better preoperative assessment would have allowed better planning and less stress to the surgical team at the time of surgery.

forefoot osteotomy, single-joint arthrodesis, or isolated soft tissue procedure constitutes low risk. Stacking procedures, even simple versions, can produce hyperbolic increases in risk.

Rigid deformities of the foot are addressed with a similar algorithm. The procedures appropriate to achieve a plantigrade foot should be considered after the disorder present at each joint causing a fixed deformity is identified. If the hindfoot lacks flexibility, the ankylosed joint should be taken down, prepared, aligned in appropriate position, and fused. This process may require fusion of the subtalar, talonavicular, and/or calcaneocuboid joints. However, selective hindfoot fusions can have a significant effect on the remaining motion about the triple complex. A cadaver study simulating arthrodesis of the various hindfoot joints found that fusion of the subtalar joint alone can limit talonavicular joint motion to approximately one-quarter of its motion, and talonavicular fusion essentially eliminated hindfoot motion.[14] When deciding which joints to fuse, attention should be paid to radiographic findings as well as clinical examination of motion and location of pain. In general, in patients with deformity about the hindfoot, joints displaying radiographic evidence of arthritis as well as clinical signs of pain should be considered for fusion of the affected joints. Rigid deformity or multiple joint arthrodesis, in the authors' opinion, are indications for staging the arthroplasty after correction.

CONSIDERATIONS WHEN PERFORMING ADJUNCTIVE PROCEDURES

It is accepted among many foot and ankle surgeons that extra-articular bony deformity in the coronal or sagittal plane involving the tibia should be corrected preoperatively. However, Colin,[15] DeOrio,[16] and others have refuted that assertion and have suggested that reasonable results can be achieved through simultaneous, well-performed supramalleolar osteotomies,[15,16] which becomes an issue of soft tissue envelope viability and surgeon experience. Greater degrees of prior injury and surgery leading to soft tissue scarring, adhesion, and vascular compromise preclude extensive combined procedures. Similarly, surgical expertise should dictate the opportunity to attempt these procedures simultaneously. Only clinicians who are facile enough to proceed efficiently and with enough experience and confidence to navigate the potential pitfalls of this magnitude of procedure should entertain this type of endeavor.

Correction of mechanical axis deformity in the tibia in the sagittal and/or coronal plane and correction of severe equinus contractures can be accomplished by use of osteotomy with internal fixation, spatial frame application, or a combination of techniques as previously stated. These problems can be addressed at the same time or in isolation depending on the presentation of the patient. **Fig. 21A–C** shows a tibia with both coronal and sagittal plane deformity. This disorder was a chronic deformity that was addressed preoperatively with an osteotomy of the tibia and frame application. Correction in a frame provides the ability to correct other deformities as well. In this patient there was a concomitant severe equinus contracture that was corrected at the same time. After the mechanical axis of the tibia was corrected and the osteotomy site healed, the total ankle operation was performed without complication and the patient is now more than 3 years from operation and has shown no signs of failure.

Numerous subtleties exist in implantation of TAA after deformity correction of the tibia. The surgeon must align the prosthesis correctly with the mechanical axis of the limb in both the coronal and sagittal planes. The surgeon cannot become distracted by callous formation or abnormal bone morphology that would cause implantation in an inappropriate position. A disastrous outcome, including early catastrophic failure, can occur if special attention is not given to placing the TAA implants in mechanically accurate positions with respect to the mechanical axis of the limb. Should the surgeon think that this cannot be done reliably, staging should be considered to alleviate the stress of the surgeon and the risk to the patient.

Similarly, subtalar joint fusions, difficult fusions including midfoot joints and triple arthrodesis,[3] as well as multiple simultaneous soft tissue procedures, are fraught with inherent and increased risks. Accordingly, it has been suggested that the presence of painful arthritic changes in joints other than the ankle should be addressed by appropriate fusion procedures preoperatively.[7] These procedures are discussed separately later.

The triple arthrodesis has shown long-term satisfaction ratings for patients of around 95%.[17] The nonunion rate is noted to be between 5% and 15% and along with malunion are considered two of the most common complications of this procedure.[17] The talonavicular joint is commonly thought to be the most frequent site of nonunion.[17] Because of the difficulty of obtaining 3 well-healed fusion sites, especially when requiring deformity correction maneuvers, this procedure is recommended to be done preemptively, which allows powerful correction of malalignment and resolution of degenerative joint arthritis in the foot before undertaking a TAA.

Some clinicians have suggested that all hindfoot fusion procedures be completed before TAA.[6,7] However, that suggestion has been contested by Lewis and colleagues,[18] who state that, despite lower scores in overall outcome measures, pain relief, and implant survivorship compared with TAA alone, performing subtalar fusion at the same time as TAA leads to reliable improvement in pain profile, functionality, and quality of life despite failure rates of 10%. Usuelli and colleagues[19] substantiated this and reported a 92% fusion rate of the subtalar joint based on CT studies of 25 patients who underwent simultaneous subtalar fusion and TAA.

Controversy persists over whether to fuse a subtalar joint in conjunction with TAA. Advocates for preoperative fusions have pointed to the tenuous talar blood supply, which may sustain a massive insult when performing both procedures in the same operative setting.[7,15] With the anterior approach to the ankle and the implantation of the TAA, the extraosseous blood supply to the talus is often disrupted independent of which type of implant the surgeon may use.[20] Adding further vascular insult to the talus with a complete subtalar fusion that will possibly interfere with the blood supply to the talus because of damage to the artery of the tarsal canal can induce avascular necrosis. Surgeons must be careful not to promote avascular necrosis of the talus because this may result in subsidence of the talar implant and ultimate failure.[21] To avoid this potential catastrophe, it has been anecdotally suggested to fuse only the posterior facet of the subtalar joint to avoid intrusion on the blood supply to the talar neck.

Kim and colleagues[21] showed that staged subtalar fusion and TAA had higher resultant soft tissue scarring and bony impingement but also that there was a higher rate of instability or dislocation if the two procedures were performed at the same time. Lewis and colleagues[18] supported performing the procedures simultaneously, showing no difference in radiographic talar component subsidence versus control groups at 2 years after surgery. However, the experimental group had a significantly lower survivorship rate of 90% compared with the control group with 97.6% at 3.2 years after surgery.[18] With evidence for both sides of the argument, there is no clear consensus.

The authors propose that any joint fusion that would require a lengthy surgical time or predictably increased morbidity be accomplished before attempting a TAA. The limitations of weight bearing and motion that are needed to promote fusion of joints about the foot are potentially in contrast with the general goals of arthroplasty postoperative protocols and should be taken into account before proceeding to ensure optimal outcomes. Appropriately rigid and unobtrusive fixation must be used such that, after sufficient soft tissue healing occurs, range of motion to tolerance and early weight bearing may be implemented.

From a soft tissue standpoint, severe equinus contractures that cannot be anticipated to be adequately corrected with a tendo Achilles lengthening or gastrocnemius recession should be addressed preoperatively. Some ankles, particularly those having experienced remote trauma and posttraumatic gait disturbances leading to contracture, require not only superficial releases but the addressing of the deep capsular layers as well. Severe equinus that is acutely corrected can pose risks to soft tissue and neurovascular structures that would be left under tension when the foot is returned to neutral. Drastic Achilles equinus correction can be accomplished with the use of a spatial frame, which allows for measured correction over a time period that will allow soft tissues and neurovascular structures to slowly accommodate the new foot position without generally causing any compromise. Other soft tissue procedures, particularly those that are required for ligament balancing and can be performed through the same anterior approach, should be performed at the time of ankle implantation to ensure adequate stability of the implant. These procedures include deltoid release and lateral ligament advancement and repair (Brostrom) for the varus ankle and superficial deltoid reefing with lateral release as necessary for patients with valgus.

In addition, the authors propose that, if a surgeon is to undertake any procedures to correct deformity at the same time as TAA, the procedures should be limited to those that can be completed successfully within the confines of the tourniquet time and those that do not require large incisions leaving thin skin bridges that have the potential to complicate healing and soft tissue survival. Surgeons should respect their own limitations with regard to speed and experience when making these decisions.

INTRAOPERATIVE CONSIDERATIONS
Varus Ankle

It is generally accepted that varus incongruent alignment, especially when greater than 10° to 15°, is most likely to lead to failure of the TAA.[21] Approach to the varus ankle should be systematic and inclusive. The considerations have been described earlier and include tibial deformity, intra-articular disorder, and cavus or cavovarus foot anomalies. Proximal tibial deformity should be addressed by knee arthroplasty when appropriate or high tibial osteotomy. Once the mechanical axis is normalized, the ensuing procedure can be entertained (see **Figs. 6** and **7**; **Fig. 11**). Of note, a percentage of patients are relieved of more distal symptoms and elect to forego further procedures at the ankle.

More distal tibial deformities, as already identified, are more controversial in the timing and necessity of correction. Up to 10° of distal tibial varus can still be compensated for through corrective intra-articular adjustment at the time of arthroplasty. Beyond that, a separate tibial osteotomy should be performed. Closing wedge is most reliable (**Figs. 12** and **13**) and reportedly faster to heal but opening wedge and dome-shaped osteotomies work as well, depending on the surgeon's familiarity and the timing of the osteotomy with respect to the implantation of the TAA. Should more than a tibial osteotomy be necessary or anticipated for correction, it is our recommendation to perform these at separate sittings.

Once proximal realignment is completed or deemed unnecessary, the ankle can be implanted. This implantation may require release of superficial and even deep deltoid

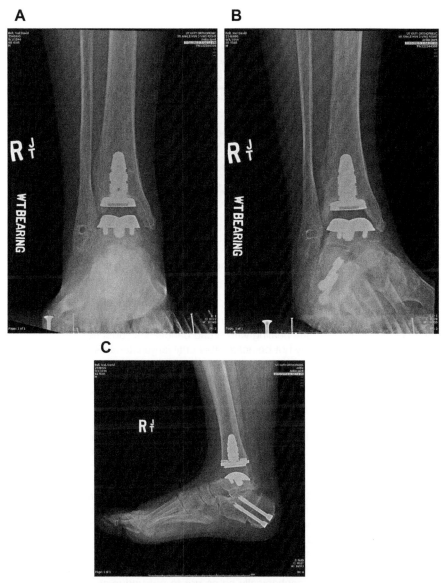

Fig. 11. This patient first underwent proximal realignment surgery (see **Figs. 6** and **7**). Persistent ankle pain necessitated valgus-producing calcaneal osteotomy and lateral ligament reconstruction with the peroneus brevis (Evans procedure) along with his ankle replacement, as seen on postoperative (*A*) AP, (*B*) mortise, and (*C*) lateral views.

restraints. The former can be performed by passing an elevator subperiosteally along the inferior and medial edges of the medial malleolus to elevate as much deltoid as needed to effect correction back to neutral with manipulation of the hindfoot into valgus. An alternative is a vertical sliding medial malleolar osteotomy, as described by Doets and colleagues,[6] to allow distal migration of the medial side, thus providing functional lengthening to that side without stripping the soft tissues from bone. This

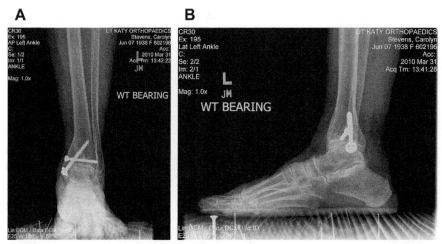

Fig. 12. A 73-year-old woman with posttraumatic arthritis after distal tibial fracture that healed with a metaphyseal malunion reaching 25° of varus seen here on (*A*) AP and (*B*) lateral views.

technique has the advantages of maintaining direct vascular attachments of the deltoid and direct bone-to-bone healing with broad cancellous surfaces.

Corrected positioning may not be achievable until large lateral osteophytes, which are seemingly reproducibly present in severe varus ankles, are removed from the talar shoulder and distal tibia and fibula. This removal is essential. Consideration must then be given to lateral ligament stabilization if varus stress under fluoroscopy shows more than 10° of lateral opening greater than the normal side. Anatomic repairs are often ineffectual because there is no remaining lateral ligament. Several procedures are available, including lateral tendon weaves, allograft reconstructions, or even synthetic graft supports. This author prefers a modification of the Evans procedure in which the peroneus brevis is transferred, either wholly or split, to the fibula. Coetzee[22] proposed a variation in which this tendon is transferred to the anterior tibia for fixation. Either method allows good sagittal plane motion while restricting the potentially hazardous varus instability. While there, consideration should be given to a peroneus longus to brevis transfer to reduce the dynamic plantarflexion of the first ray and promote further eversion moment, and this can either be sutured to the Evans repair or directly to the base of the fifth metatarsal. It should be emphasized that, although the preparation and necessary graft harvesting can be performed at this point, the foot must be addressed and corrected mechanically so as not to put undue stress on either the ankle implant or the ligament reconstruction, as identified later.

In addition, the foot should be addressed to minimize or eliminate any remaining varus. Valgus-producing osteotomy of the calcaneus, and/or dorsiflexion of the first metatarsal, depending on the degree of forefoot-driven hindfoot varus, are staples in this correction and can be performed immediately or at some point more remotely if tourniquet time, incisions, and swelling are of growing concern (**Figs. 14** and **15**). It is far more desirable to return later when conditions are more favorable rather than chancing a major complication like nonunion, inability to close wounds, or vascular spasm.

Postoperatively, patients are held non–weight bearing depending on the most tenuous procedure performed. Soft tissues alone allow for weight bearing in a brace

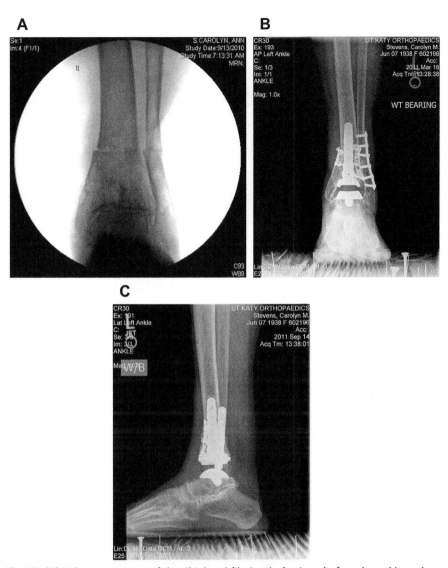

Fig. 13. (*A*) Valgus osteotomy of the tibial and fibular shafts done before the ankle replacement, shown in (*B*) AP and (*C*) lateral radiographs.

at 2 weeks, assuming incisional stability. Closing wedge osteotomies require 4 weeks. Tibial osteotomies mandate a minimum of 6 weeks non–weight bearing. Range of motion can begin with any of these as soon as wounds look healthy.

Valgus Ankle

In the past, the varus ankle was thought to be the most challenging of all of the deformities, but, in recent years, surgeons with arthroplasty experience have begun to prefer identifying the larger valgus deformities as those with greater difficulty in correction and less predictable outcomes. However, the same general principles apply to these

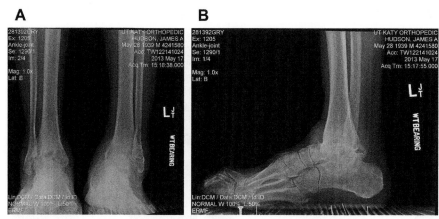

Fig. 14. A 74-year-old man with moderate to severe varus as a result of ankle osteoarthritis, seen on (A) AP and (B) lateral preoperative radiographs.

deformities as to their varus counterparts. Surgeons typically begin with deformity analysis and work proximal to distal.

Proximal deformity is again addressed first. Arthroplasty or proximal osteotomy is performed as needed and as previously discussed. Tibial deformity is considered next. This time, a medial closing wedge is favorable, provides good and predictable healing, and can be done through the same incision if planned adequately.

Any concern about overstripping the intercalary distal tibial fragment should obviate the simultaneous procedure and this should be reserved for another time. However, if vascularity is maintained, then total ankle implantation can be performed simultaneously.

In this case, after the implant is placed, the need for ligament balancing must be assessed. Most often, the deltoid ligament has some attachment and does not require reconstruction. Lateral ligaments are most often not tight, may be damaged by fibular impingement on the lateral calcaneus with chronic deformity, and rarely require release. Most often the joint will accept a larger polyethylene insert to absorb the laxity resultant from the deltoid attenuation. Should there still be valgus at the ankle, consideration has to be given to deltoid reconstruction (**Figs. 16** and **17**).

As with the varus ankle, soft tissue reconstruction may be performed, this time medially, using native soft tissue advancement of the superficial deltoid, which tends to be more robust than its lateral counterpart. If not present or substantial, the deltoid can be substituted with autograft or allograft. This author's preference is to use the posterior tibialis tendon, if present and healthy, to insert through a drill tunnel into the medial malleolus. If not present or healthy, then allograft works nicely, but requires more dissection. There is the advantage of providing tissue for reconstruction of both superficial and deep components of the deltoid by attaching the distal end to the talus (or navicular for short talar necks). Then the graft is woven proximally through the anterior medial malleolus, out through the posterior portion, and then down into the medial talar body or calcaneus (again, depending on bone stock and quality).

Again, similar to its varus counterpart, the foot is then reassessed. This author has a low threshold for realignment in the foot, particularly in a deltoid ligament reconstruction. The natural tendency of the foot to create a valgus moment is potentially deleterious to the ankle implant stability and the philosophy is to err toward slight overcorrection to maintain a more vertical weight-bearing axis. In an effort to do so,

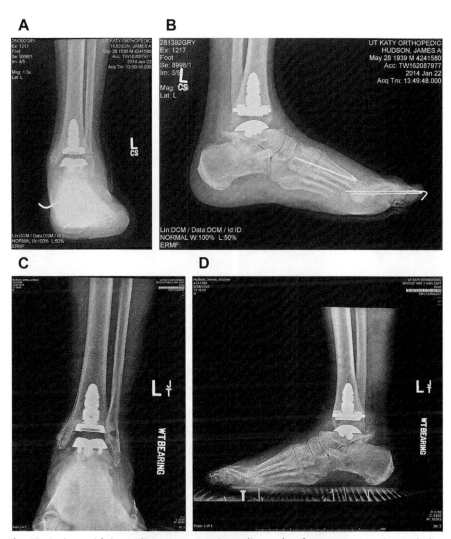

Fig. 15. Patient with immediate postoperative radiographs after varus correction including ankle realignment through the joint, lateral ligament reconstruction with peroneal tendon rerouting, and first metatarsal elevation osteotomy. (*A*, *B*) AP and lateral radiographs with metatarsal fixation in place. (*C*, *D*) The same views after hardware has been removed.

a medial displacement calcaneal osteotomy is often added with a generous medial shift to seat the tuber under the tibia. In addition, a medial column procedure can be extremely helpful. A stiff first tarsometatarsal joint allow an opening wedge medial cuneiform osteotomy with intention to depress the first ray. However, unless the first tarsometatarsal joint is fairly stiff, a medial column fusion may be necessary (**Fig. 18**). Medial column stability may be unclear at the time of correction. One tip is to sequentially pin the medial joints and determine which are necessary to fix in order to maintain a plantarflexed first ray. Consideration to a peroneus brevis transfer to the longus for dynamic improvement of first ray plantarflexion may be useful. The Achilles is often recessed in addition to the aforementioned procedures. Once again, the soft tissue

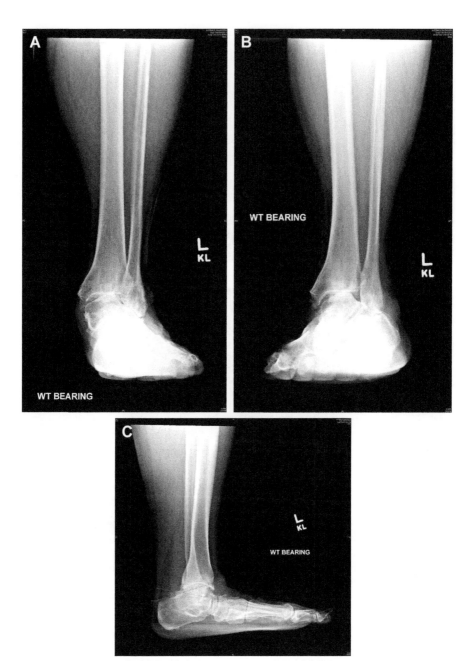

Fig. 16. Ankle series of 61-year-old with long-standing progressive valgus ankle perceived as flattening of his foot on (A) AP, (B) mortise, and (C) lateral views.

balancing may be prepared, but securing the procedures is withheld until bony balance is established.

Like the varus ankle, any signs of unfavorable or untoward events should signal the surgeon to reevaluate whether staging should be considered.

A   **B**

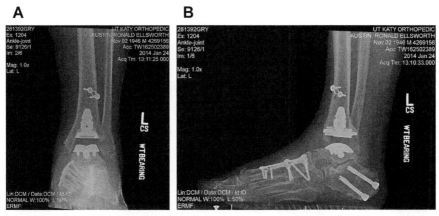

Fig. 17. Reconstruction of patient featured in **Fig. 16** with ankle arthroplasty, medial displacement calcaneal osteotomy, medial column fusion with plantarflexion of first ray, and deltoid ligament reconstruction using the posterior tibial tendon through a drill hole in the medial malleolus, as seen on (A) AP and (B) lateral views.

Postoperatively, the patients are mobilized early, unless a deltoid reconstruction is performed. Under these circumstances, the patient undergoes prolonged immobilization of no less than 6 weeks in a non–weight-bearing cast. Gradual weight bearing ensues with a medially posted orthotic device within the postoperative boot or brace for an additional 6 weeks and the patient is advised to have a medially posted orthosis for at least 6 months in the regular shoe.

Recurvatum

This deformity typically occurs in the setting of the stiff arthritic ankle leading to anterior plafond wear as a result of the talus being repetitively driven into the anterior tibia. It also occurs as avascular bone at the anterior tibia from prior trauma disintegrates from repetitive intrusion of the talar body into the tibial plafond. Both of these scenarios combine with a tight posterior capsule and tendo Achilles to allow anterior talar escape. The resultant deformity is not only anterior subluxation, but frequently involves some degree of shortening from a few millimeters to more than a centimeter (**Fig. 19**).

Proximally based recurvatum typically involves not only angulatory deformity but most often some degree of translation as well. As such, these are in the category of multiplanar and are discussed in detail later in this article. Intra-articular recurvatum is more simply addressed through the joint by performing appropriate resection for the arthroplasty at the level of the anterior ledge of cortical tibial bone. This procedure may leave a large resection of posterior bone that can be challenging to remove. The resultant anteriorization caused by deformity necessitates relief of the posterior capsule, which can be done from the anterior approach with great care to avoid traveling medial to the identifiable flexor hallucis longus tendon. After trial component placement, Achilles lengthening may be necessary because of the degree of preoperative shortening. Often, these patients develop significant medial and lateral adhesions, osteophytes, or both. This condition requires aggressive debridement of the so-called gutters to relieve the obstacle to posterior translation such that the lateral process of the talus sits beneath the dome of the implant and this centers on the intramedullary canal on lateral fluoroscopy.

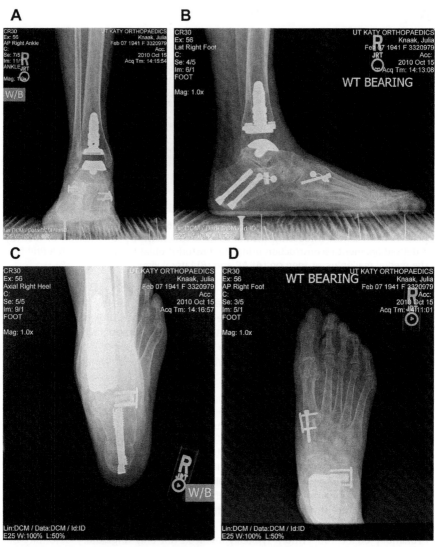

Fig. 18. Corrected ankle and foot of patient shown in **Fig. 8**. She had ankle valgus and compensatory heel valgus and midfoot abduction. Correction was achieved with lateral column lengthening and first tarsometatarsal plantar flexion arthrodesis, as seen on (A) AP, (B) lateral, (C) axial, and (D) AP foot radiographs.

Postoperatively, these patients are typically mobilized after wound stability is checked at 5 to 7 days to prevent recurrent posterior capsular adhesion and stiffness or restriction to dorsiflexion. Weight bearing begins at 10 to 14 days.

Procurvatum

This deformity is probably the least common of the unifocal deformities. It usually results from posterior bony wear allowing posterior escape and some proximal migration. The Achilles is often contracted as a result.

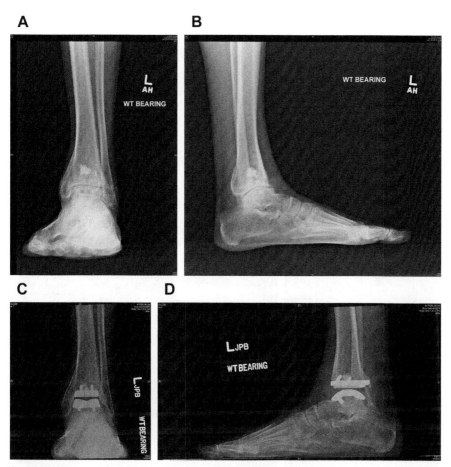

Fig. 19. A 41-year-old with posttraumatic arthritis shown with anterior subluxation in (A) AP and (B) lateral views. He failed multiple prior attempts at treatment, including ankle arthroscopy and distraction arthroplasty. (C, D) Postoperative radiographs of the previously anteriorly subluxated ankle joint. Note the lateral process of the talus repositioned and centered on the midline of the tibial shaft on the lateral view.

Initial deformity assessment and principles are performed as discussed earlier. Angular distal tibial deformity implies multifocal correction options, which are discussed later.

This deformity, similar to recurvatum, is often corrected through the joint. Tibial resection is based on the posterior ledge of tibial cortical bone at its lowest level. Posterior capsular release and tendo Achilles lengthening are mandatory to allow for distal and anterior migration. Gutter debridement should also be performed to provide freedom of mobility and to enhance sagittal plane motion once the components are implanted. Lateral alignment should follow a line centered in the medullary canal through the center of the dome of the implant, the lateral process of the talus, and the angle of Gissane (**Fig. 20**).

Postoperatively, early motion and weight bearing facilitate rehabilitation and restoration of motion and function as described earlier.

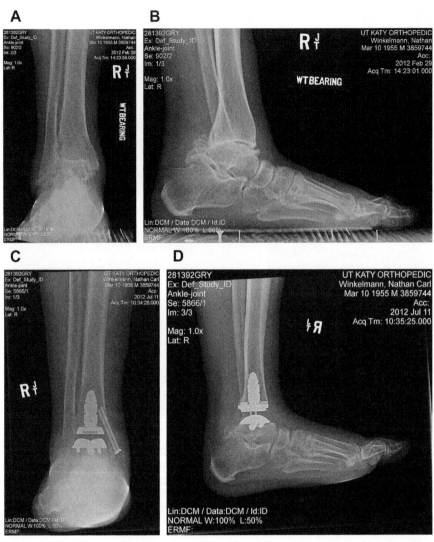

Fig. 20. (A, B) A 57-year-old with progressive ankle arthritis and posterior subluxation. Note the procurvatum that results from the posterior positioning of the ankle. (C, D) Corrected position of ankle after arthroplasty with anteriorization to more mechanically appropriate position. Note that the lateral process of the talus now sits in more anatomic position near the center of a vertical line centered in the tibial canal.

Multiplanar

Any deformity requiring consideration of correction in more than 1 radiographic view, by definition, is multiplanar. These deformities usually occur as a result of prior trauma but may also be present as a result of congenital deformity, previous infection, or metabolic bone disorder. These deformities should be addressed before undertaking any bony or articular correction to avoid postoperative deformity.

The variety of deformities is too diverse to address each of them because these, like fractures, tend to have individualized characteristics. These deformities must be reviewed carefully with the tools and guidelines described throughout this article. All facets of deformity must be considered and factored into the planning, and include alterations in length, angulation, rotation, and translation, as well as joint posture or position. Soft tissues, especially neurovascular structures, are also included in the deformity and must be considered when contemplating a method of correction, because these may be the deciding factor based on risk per individual procedure.

Options include traditional osteotomy at the apex of the deformity, which may be difficult to accurately assess if the deformity plane is not in line with the two-dimensional orthogonal radiographs. Other treatments include multilevel osteotomies and osteoplasty with external fixation. All of these require a fairly comfortable knowledge of the method of calculation and identification to the center of rotation and angulation, which is the apex or apices of deformity in multiple planes (**Fig. 21**).

With more than 1 plan of deformity, this author's preference is to perform gradual correction with external multiplanar circular external fixation. The advantages are fewer and smaller incisions, lower risk to the neurovascular structures, and ability to

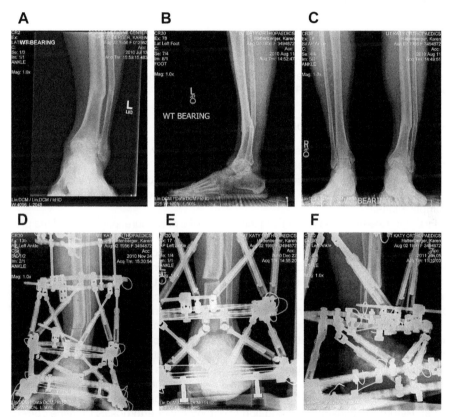

Fig. 21. A 54-year-old woman with deformity since nonoperative treatment of a tibia fracture at age 17 years. Deformity is multiplanar, as noted by the varus and recurvatum on (*A*) AP and (*B*) lateral radiographs respectively. (*C*) Bilateral AP views are also shown for side by side comparison. What is not easily seen is the length inequality (shortening) and internal rotation, which was better assessed by CT scanning. The radiographs also suggest evidence of ankle arthritis with asymmetric joint space narrowing, osteophytes, and sclerosis. (*D*) The initial application of a multiplanar small wire external fixator and corrective osteotomy. (*E, F*) The corrected position of the tibia in the frame.

adjust the deformity correction based on progression to make it as accurate as possible and not lose length or bone stock.

Disadvantages are the length of time in the frame, the inevitable pin tract problems that affect these patients in long-term devices, and the risk of delayed union or nonunion with overly rapid correction or premature frame removal.

Nevertheless, this provides powerful correction capability and is, in this surgeon's experience, the most accurate and effective tool for this purpose.

Once corrected, weight bearing begins in the frame until CT evidence reflects circumferential healing. If this is delayed, some level of stimulation may be required. Bone grafting the defect seems to be effective, reliable, and fairly reproducible to stimulate the necessary biological reactivity. This procedure is often performed by packing harvested autograft into the osteotomy site if no radiographic progress is seen between 6 and 8 weeks from the completion of the correction program.

Once healing is initiated as identified by radiographic progression, the frame is gradually dismantled by removing 1 or more pieces every few weeks as tolerated by the patient. Parameters for further reduction of frame support include no change in pain perception, no increase in swelling, no increase in remaining pin drainage, and improvement (or at least no negative changes) in radiographs. After complete removal of the frame, the patient undergoes rehabilitation. In some instances, the alignment provides satisfactory relief and the patient no longer wishes to proceed with arthroplasty. If not, the limb alignment is restored and a less complicated, better mechanical outcome can be expected (**Fig. 22**).

AVOIDING POSTOPERATIVE DISASTER

General and more global considerations common to many, if not all, major reconstructive lower extremity surgeries apply to this category of anticipated problems. The following highlight the most common concerns and provide an overview of considerations and concepts for use in managing and, it is hoped, preventing the inherent complications.

First and foremost, if at any time in the course of a procedure, particularly if the procedure was planned as a single-stage operation with TAA and deformity correction, the conditions become unfavorable for that degree of procedure, the recommendation is to amend the treatment plan and abbreviate the surgery. Avoiding complications is imperative and although risk is not able to be eliminated, it is reducible. Surgeons must not be so rigid in thought that their patients are at risk because of failure of recognition of a potential threat or hazardous course. Deformity correction following successful implant arthroplasty can be completed or refined at some later date with lower risk and successful outcome. Alternatively, surgeons may perform a plan to perfection but, because of unforeseen or unrecognizable features, still notice malalignment postoperatively on initiation of weight bearing. This situation is the scenario for postimplant deformity correction as well, and typically involves some level of fine tuning of foot posture after the patient has begun weight bearing and persistent deformity is recognized. Return for adjustment or addition of osteotomy or arthrodesis to refine correction is useful to provide longevity to a well-fixed and otherwise satisfactory arthroplasty. The potential for this type of procedure should be discussed and the patient made aware as part of the preoperative discussion, so that it comes as little surprise and the patient appreciates the surgeon's attention to detail and wish to provide a maximal result.

These patients with greater degrees of deformity have more incisions, leading to more swelling, higher risk of infection, greater degrees of nerve irritation, and

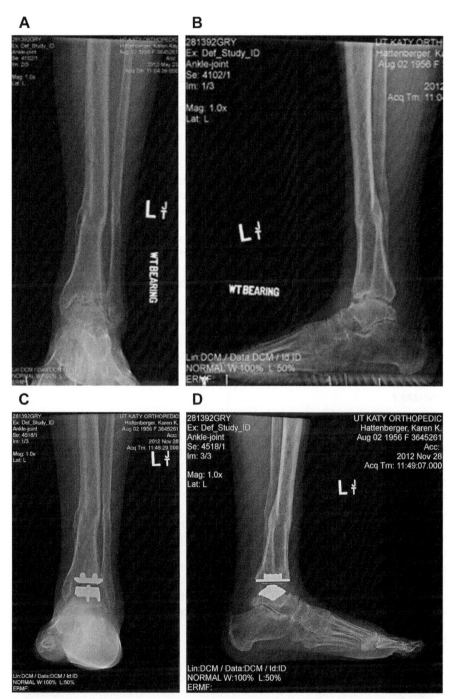

Fig. 22. (*A*, *B*) The final outcome of the tibial and fibular correction of the patient shown in **Fig. 21**. Although mechanical alignment was improved and clinical symptoms relieved, the patient still complained of pain and stiffness specific to the ankle joint. (*C*, *D*) Ultimate treatment with ankle arthroplasty, simplified by previously realigning the proximal bone.

enhanced venous stasis. Incisional management is very individualized. Compressive, flexible bandages are helpful in maintaining a reduced level of swelling in the limb. Reduced swelling means less drainage and typically translates into lower infection risk.

Thromboembolic prophylaxis is controversial and individualized. There is no proof that these patients show any higher risk than any other patients undergoing foot and ankle surgery. The overall risk of deep vein thrombosis is low. As a result, unless the patient has an identifiable systemically mediated disorder that routinely increases the risk, these patients are managed expectantly with mechanical prophylaxis and aspirin as thought to be needed.

Rehabilitation and weight-bearing progression is probably the most difficult item to address as a protocol because these patients vary so greatly in their degrees of deformity, bone quality, number of procedures, and soft tissue integrity. Concordantly, each case must be managed with all of these factors individually and collectively considered to mobilize the patient effectively, but safely. Because of the amount of surgery, rehabilitation is typically slower and more tedious. Range of motion is usually tolerable for most and probably the most important parameter to restore as early as feasible, depending on the soft tissues. If motion is restored, the remaining function, balance, and power are fairly easily regained at variable times after the procedure. This is therefore the primary goal of early therapy, regardless of extent of surgery and within reasonable limits of healing. Regaining range of motion most often requires assistance and supervision to be effective, so formal therapy is recommended as early as possible for this purpose, with the addition of functional proprioception, gait training, and strengthening later as indicated and tolerated based on the healing of structural procedures.

SUMMARY

Addressing the arthritic ankle with deformity is extremely complex. Treating these deformities with arthroplasty requires a broad skill set and even more expansive experience with complicated reconstructions and arthroplasty. The implications of these deformities are sometimes limb threatening from the outset and so not only a working knowledge of deformity correction and arthroplasty implantation but also a level of anticipation and flexibility along with some creativity are necessary features of the surgeons who care for these patients.

However, newer implant designs; improved, more efficient surgical techniques; and more skilled and experienced surgeons participating in the management of these difficult situations have evolved into a domain in which deformities and problems previously considered untreatable with ankle arthroplasty are now being more frequently evaluated and successfully cared for. Only time will tell how much deformity will be able to be corrected in future, but a strong foundation currently exists with which to increase the capabilities that were not present as recently as the last decade.

REFERENCES

1. Choi WJ, Kim BS, Lee JW. Preoperative planning and surgical technique: how do I balance my ankle? Foot Ankle Int 2012;33(3):244–9.
2. Sung K-S, Ahn J, Lee K-H, et al. Short-term results of total ankle arthroplasty for end-stage ankle arthritis with severe varus deformity. Foot Ankle Int 2014;35(3): 225–31.
3. Ryssman DB, Myerson MS. Total ankle arthroplasty: management of varus deformity at the ankle. Foot Ankle Int 2012;33:347–54.

4. Haskell A, Mann RA. Ankle arthroplasty with preoperative coronal plane deformity: short-term results. Clin Orthop Relat Res 2004;424:98–103.
5. Reddy SC, Mann JA, Mann RA, et al. Correction of moderate to severe coronal plane deformity with the STAR ankle prosthesis. Foot Ankle Int 2011;32(7): 7659–64.
6. Doets HC, van der Plaat LW, Klein J. Medial malleolar osteotomy for the correction of varus deformity during total ankle arthroplasty: results in 15 patients. Foot Ankle Int 2008;29(2):171–9.
7. Kim BS, Choi WJ, Kim YS, et al. Total ankle replacement in moderate to severe varus deformity of the ankle. J Bone Joint Surg Br 2009;91B:1183–90.
8. Easley ME, Adams SB Jr, Hembree WC, et al. Current concepts review: results of total ankle arthroplasty. J Bone Joint Surg Am 2011;93:1455–68.
9. Schipper ON, Denduluri SK, Zhou Y, et al. Effect of obesity on total ankle arthroplasty outcomes. Foot Ankle Int 2016;37(1):1–7.
10. Pagenstert GI, Hintermann B. Simultaneous bilateral total knee and ankle arthroplasty as a single surgical procedure. Case Report. BMC Musculoskelet Disord 2011;12:233.
11. Tarr RR, Resnick CT, Wagner KS, et al. Changes in tibiotalar joint contact areas following experimentally induced tibial angular deformities. Clin Orthop Relat Res 1985;199:72–80.
12. Ting AJ, Tarr RR, Sarmiento A, et al. The role of subtalar motion and ankle contact pressure changes from angular deformities of the tibia. Foot Ankle 1987;7(5): 290–9.
13. Espinosa N, Walti M, Favre P, et al. Misalignment of total ankle components can induce high joint contact pressures. J Bone Joint Surg Am 2010;92(5):1179–87.
14. Astion DJ, Deland JT, Otis JC, et al. Motion of the hindfoot after simulated arthrodesis. J Bone Joint Surg Am 1997;79(2):241–6.
15. Colin F, Bolliger L, Horn Lang T, et al. Effect of supramalleolar osteotomy and total ankle replacement on talar position in the varus osteoarthritic ankle: a comparative study. Foot Ankle Int 2014;35(5):445–52.
16. DeOrio JK. Total ankle replacement with malaligned ankles: osteotomies performed simultaneous with TAA. Foot Ankle Int 2012;4:344–6.
17. Thordardson D. Foot and ankle. 2nd edition. Philadelphia: Lippincott Williams & Wilkins; 2012. Print.
18. Lewis JS Jr, Adams SB Jr, Queen RM, et al. Outcomes after total ankle replacement in association with ipsilateral hindfoot arthrodesis. Foot Ankle Int 2014;35(6): 535–42.
19. Usuelli FG, Maccario C, Manzi L, et al. Clinical outcome and fusion rate following simultaneous subtalar fusion and total ankle arthroplasty. Foot Ankle Int 2016; 37(7):696–702.
20. Tennant JN, Rungprai C, Pizzimenti MA, et al. Risks to the blood supply of the talus with four methods of total ankle arthroplasty: a cadaveric injection study. J Bone Joint Surg Am 2014;96:395–402.
21. Kim BS, Knupp M, Zwicky L, et al. Total ankle replacement in association with hindfoot fusion: outcome and complications. J Bone Joint Surg Br 2010;92: 1540–7.
22. Coetzee JC. Surgical Strategies: lateral ligament reconstruction as part of the management of varus ankle deformity with ankle replacement. Foot Ankle Int 2010;31(3):267–74.

Revision of Stemmed Agility Implants

Michael M. Brage, MD[a], MAJ Uma E. Ramadorai, DO[b],*

KEYWORDS

- DePuy Agility • Stemmed • Revision • Arthroplasty • Ankle • INBONE

KEY POINTS

- The talus is a challenge in the case of revision total ankle arthroplasty.
- Revision of the stemmed agility implant requires careful patient selection and surgical planning.
- Bone loss is common and should be considered in the surgical planning.
- Removal of the component can be difficult because of bony ingrowth.
- The INBONE (Wright Medical, Memphis, TN) system offers options to address loss of talar bone stock.

INTRODUCTION

Total ankle arthroplasty (TAA) has evolved over the last 20 years. The DePuy Agility (Warsaw, Indiana) TAA is a second-generation implant that uses a 3-surface reconstruction to include the medial and lateral articular surfaces in addition to fusion of the syndesmosis. Several of these were implanted with subsequent failure via a variety of mechanisms, one of the most common being failure of the talar component. Revision using a custom stemmed talar component served as a treatment option for adjacent subtalar arthrosis and component subsidence. Although these implants allowed retention of the tibial component, eventual need for revision arthroplasty or conversion to arthrodesis necessitates removal of this stem. This removal can prove to be difficult, especially when the stem will generally enjoy excellent ingrowth into the cancellous bone of the calcaneus.

Disclosure: Dr M.M. Brage is a paid consultant for Wright Medical. Dr U.E. Ramadorai has no financial disclosures.
[a] Department of Orthopaedics and Sports Medicine, Harborview Medical Center, University of Washington, 325, 9th Avenue, Seattle, WA 98104, USA; [b] Department of Orthopaedic Surgery, San Antonio Military Medical Center, 3551 Roger Brooke Drive, San Antonio, TX 78219, USA
* Corresponding author.
E-mail addresses: uramador@gmail.com; uma.e.ramadorai.mil@mail.mil

Foot Ankle Clin N Am 22 (2017) 341–360
http://dx.doi.org/10.1016/j.fcl.2017.01.005
1083-7515/17/Published by Elsevier Inc.

BACKGROUND

The incidence of osteolysis following TAA using the Agility implant has been well described and is cited as occurring from 37% to 85% and occurs at follow-up of less than 5 years[1-3] (**Figs. 1–3**). The reoperation rate following primary Agility TAA has been investigated and ranges from 9% to 39% and is generally defined as revision arthroplasty, conversion to arthrodesis, or below-knee amputation.[2,4,5] A US Department of Agriculture clinical trial performed in 2012 found a revision rate of 6% at the 24-month follow-up with subsidence of the talar component occurring in 10 of 48 patients.[6] Despite radiographic evidence of osteolysis and component complications, an investigation of 33 worldwide joint registries using a Kaplan-Meier estimator produced a prosthesis survivorship of 81% at 10 years.[7] When considering the use of a stemmed implant, failure of the talar component is the most common indication; this mode of failure is relatively common in the Agility implant. Ellington and colleagues[8] performed a retrospective review on 53 patients who underwent revision arthroplasty and found talar subsidence to be the most common indication for revision (63%). The investigators also proposed a classification system for talar subsidence following TAA to which Roukis[9] has proposed modifications to address coronal plane deformity in the grade 3 group[8,9] (**Tables 1 and 2**).

When there is significant loss of talar bone stock, whether that is in a primary or revision setting, the custom stemmed Agility implant offers an option to address the talus by spanning the subtalar joint with a large stemmed component aimed at stability and the prevention of subsidence (**Figs. 4 and 5**). The indications for this range from stage IV flatfoot to failed primary arthroplasty. The classification system described earlier offers guidance in the treatment of talar subsidence and can guide implant choice. For example, McCollum and Myerson[10] advocated the use of stemmed implants in the case of grade 3 talar subsidence. In the revision setting, the implant was commonly used to address talar subsidence after a previous TAA, with several investigators describing the technique and publishing outcomes following the use of a stemmed implant in primary and revision settings[11-14] (**Table 3**).

Although arthrodesis following a failed TAA is an option, the results are reported as inferior to that of primary arthrodesis with respect to life quality and function despite

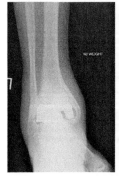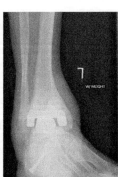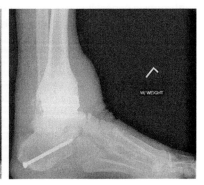

Fig. 1. A 65-year-old man who underwent TAA and lateralizing calcaneal osteotomy in 1995 followed by curettage and bone filler placement 4 years later. He presented to clinic 10 years after index procedure for evaluation of his now painful ankle.

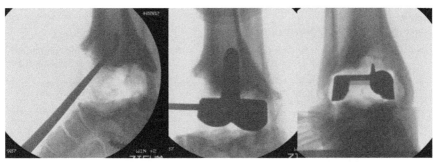

Fig. 2. Same patient undergoing revision to a stemmed implant in 2006.

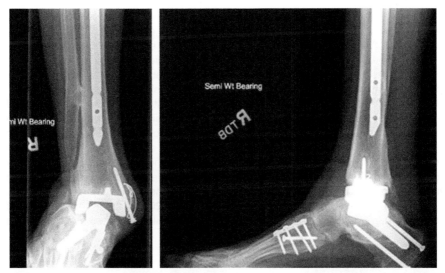

Fig. 3. A 57-year-old patient 9 years status post (s/p) index Agility implantation. Infection workup positive.

Table 1	
Ellington classification of talar subsidence	
Grade 1	No subsidence
Grade 2	Subsidence but not to the level of the subtalar joint
Grade 3	Subsidence to or below the level of the subtalar joint

From Roukis TS. Revision of primary agility and agility LP total ankle replacements. Gewerbestrasse (Switzerland): Springer International Publishing; 2016; and Ellington JK, Gupta S, Myerson MS. Management of failures of total ankle replacement with the agility total ankle arthroplasty. J Bone Joint Surg Am 2013;95(23):2112–8.

Table 2
Roukis modifications of Ellington grading system

Grade 3	A: component has migrated onto or through the subtalar joint	B: talus has fractured and component has migrated onto or through the subtalar joint
	VARUS A: primary implant was inserted in varus	VALGUS A: primary implant was inserted in valgus
	VARUS B: lateral ligamentous structures and peroneal tendons are incompetent	VALGUS B: syndesmosis nonunion and tibial component has subsided into valgus
	VARUS C: talus has subsided into varus	

From Roukis TS. Revision of primary agility and agility LP total ankle replacements. Gewerbestrasse (Switzerland): Springer International Publishing; 2016; and Ellington JK, Gupta S, Myerson MS. Management of failures of total ankle replacement with the agility total ankle arthroplasty. J Bone Joint Surg Am 2013;95(23):2112–8.

fusion rates approaching 89%.[15–18] Berkowitz and colleagues[19] retrospectively reviewed all failed total ankles converted to fusion of either the ankle joint only or a tibiotalocalcaneal (TTC) fusion. There were 5 nonunions, 4 of which occurred in the subtalar joint. The authors present a case later wherein arthrodesis was attempted that eventually went on to nonunion requiring revision arthrodesis (**Figs. 6–19**). The decision for arthrodesis versus revision arthroplasty can be a difficult one and requires careful discussion with patients concerning their expectations. The decision to proceed with arthrodesis is made when there is an ongoing infection that cannot be cleared, in which case an external fixator to achieve arthrodesis is useful. In addition, poor quality or quantity of bone can preclude the placement of arthroplasty components, as there are limits in the sizes of polyethylene spacers and metal augmentation. More recently, cage and trabecular metal implant reconstructions have been introduced to act as a void filler[20,21] (**Fig. 20**). Carlsson[22] reported on 3 patients whereby, at revision surgery, the cage was filled with necrotic debris and

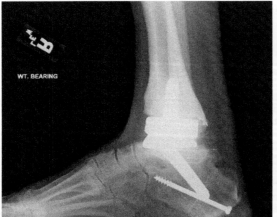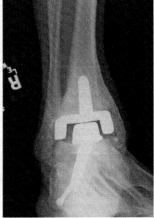

Fig. 4. A 2-year follow-up after stemmed implant.

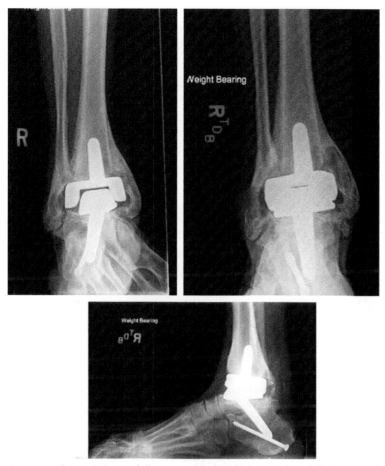

Fig. 5. Four years later, at 6-year follow-up with significant tibial and fibular osteolysis.

Table 3
Outcomes following stemmed implant

Study	Number of Patients	Follow-up	Outcome Measures	Outcomes
Alvine & Alvine,[11] 2016 retrospective review	30 Primary and revision stemmed implants	Mean 54.0 mo	Retention of implant AOFAS scores	88% retention AOFAS improved 55–71
Ketz et al,[12] 2012 retrospective review	33 Primary and revision stemmed implants	Mean 58.6 mo	ROM radiographic results SF-36 AOFAS MFS	ROM: 21.3° ± 14° to 32.2° ± 11°; AOFAS: 41 ± 16 to 68 ± 12

Abbreviations: AOFAS, American Orthopedic Foot and Ankle Society; MFS, Maryland Foot Scale; ROM, range of motion; SF-36, 36-Item Short Form Health Survey.
  Data from Refs.[11–14]

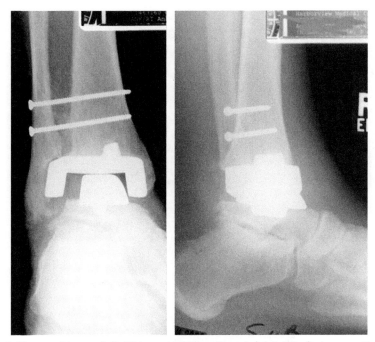

Fig. 6. A 50-year-old man, 6 ft, 10 in and 350 lb with painful Agility first-generation prosthesis in 2001.

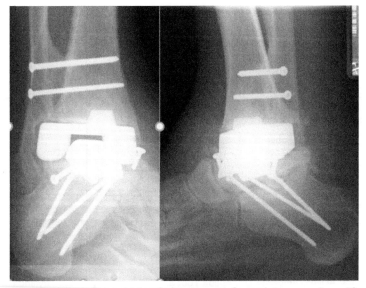

Fig. 7. 2002: Follow-up after subtalar fusion was performed 1 year prior with subtalar nonunion and talar subsidence.

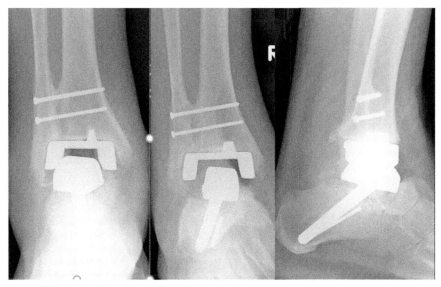

Fig. 8. 2003: Revised to stemmed Agility implant.

no osseous union was noted. Infection of a TAA can be addressed with antibiotic spacer placement; but at the time of revision, the amount of bone loss is a challenge (**Figs. 21–23**).

SURGICAL TECHNIQUE

Patients are placed supine with a bump under the operative hip. A thigh tourniquet is placed. An anterior approach to the ankle joint is performed, and the polyethylene portion is removed. Curved osteotomes can be introduced between the tibial tray and polyethylene, and the polyethylene can be removed using a shoehorn technique. If this is not possible, the polyethylene can be broken into pieces with an

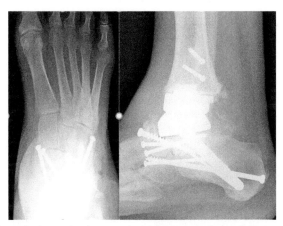

Fig. 9. 2004: Talonavicular and calcaneocuboid fusions performed for continued pain and deformity.

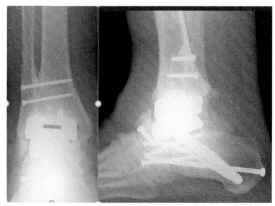

Fig. 10. 2005: Midfoot fusion nonunion and Agility stem fracture; patient opted against any more surgery at this point.

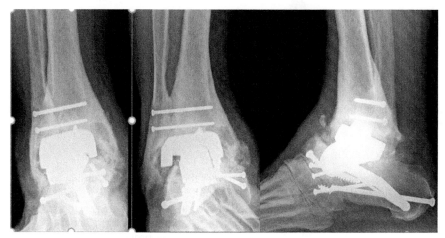

Fig. 11. Six years later in 2011, multiple areas of hardware failure, stem fracture again evident, and osteolysis present surrounding prosthesis.

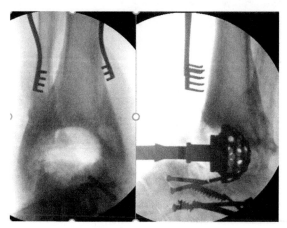

Fig. 12. Fusion with femoral head allograft and hindfoot nail.

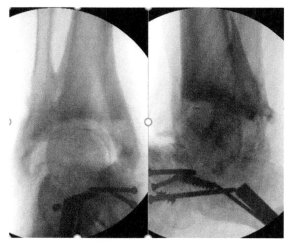

Fig. 13. Fusion with femoral head allograft.

osteotome or saw and then removed piecemeal. The tibial component is then removed using thin-bladed osteotomes. The size of the tibial component is noted, and the osteotome is marked using the same sized trial component to avoid over-penetration and neurovascular or tendon damage (**Figs. 24** and **25**). Removal of a stemmed Agility tibial component necessitates the use of an anterior corticotomy, which should be done in a fashion facilitating fixation following implantation of

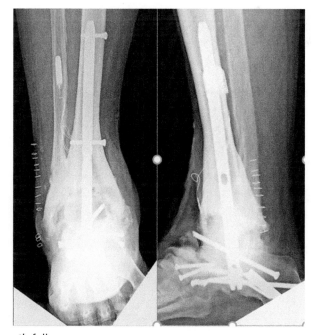

Fig. 14. Six-month follow-up.

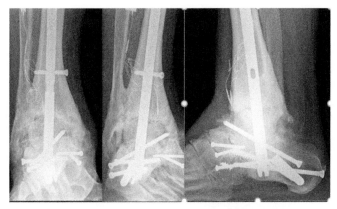

Fig. 15. One-year follow-up.

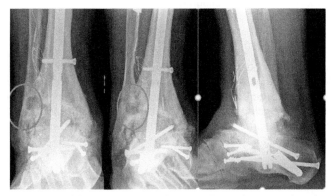

Fig. 16. Eighteen-month follow-up, increased pain and osteolysis noted. Red circle denotes osteolysis.

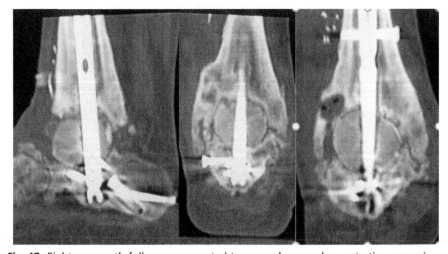

Fig. 17. Eighteen-month follow-up computed tomography scan demonstrating nonunion.

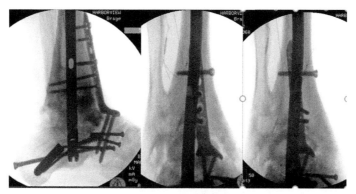

Fig. 18. Revision fusion with anterior fusion plate and iliac crest bone graft/tricalcium phosphate.

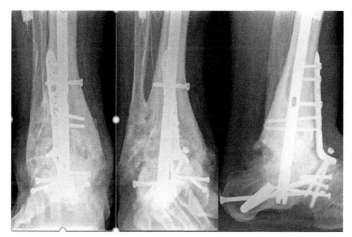

Fig. 19. Eighteen-month follow-up, doing well.

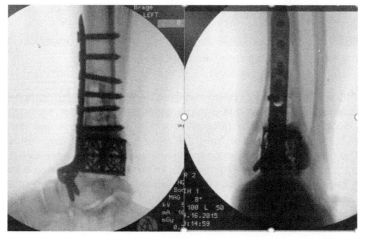

Fig. 20. Porous tantalum cage with autograft and anterior plate for ankle arthroplasty salvage.

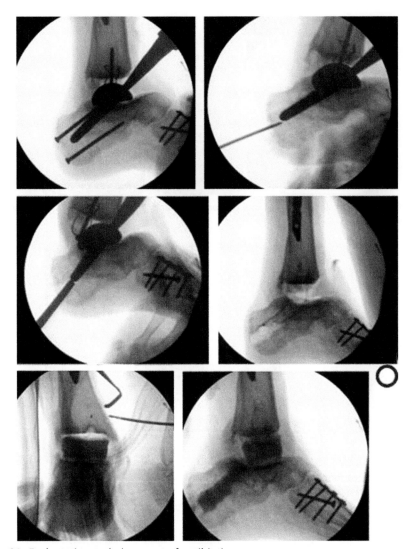

Fig. 21. Explantation and placement of antibiotic spacer.

the INBONE II (**Fig. 26**). In order to remove the stemmed talar component, the removal tool is threaded into the component from the anterior incision and the vice grip is placed around the removal tool (**Fig. 27**). Fluoroscopic guidance is then used to place a guidewire from the posterior heel, abutting the stemmed implant. The guidewire is checked on the lateral view and axial heel view to ensure appropriate placement. A tunnel to the tip of the prosthesis is created with the use of a large cannulated drill bit over the guidewire. This is followed by the use of curved osteotomes, which is used to disengage bony ingrowth around the talar stem. A blunt bone tamp is applied to the tip of the stem, and the talar component is delivered it out of the ankle joint by mallet (see **Fig. 21; Fig. 28**). Once the Agility components have been removed, the ankle is irrigated and the gutters debrided. If there is a significant amount of osteolysis of the malleoli, this is addressed via

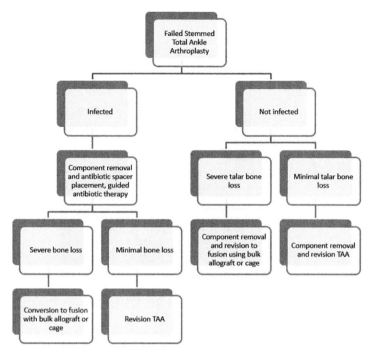

Fig. 22. Algorithm guiding surgical decision making in the case of an infected versus non-infected arthroplasty.

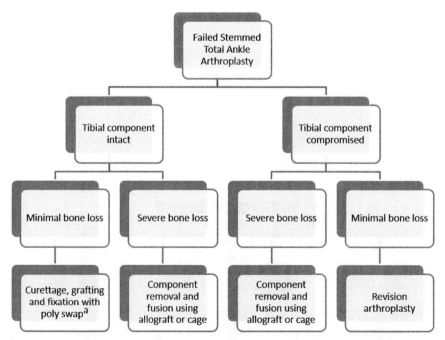

Fig. 23. Algorithm guiding surgical decision making in the case of failed stemmed arthroplasty without infection present. [a] Johnson and Johnson will soon no longer support the Agility™ implants making a polyethylene exchange impossible and thus necessitating revision arthroplasty despite well fixed components.

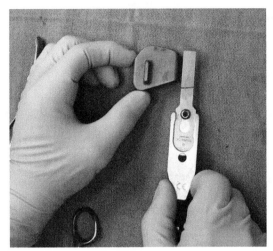

Fig. 24. Measuring the tibial component based on size and marking the osteotome to avoid overpenetration.

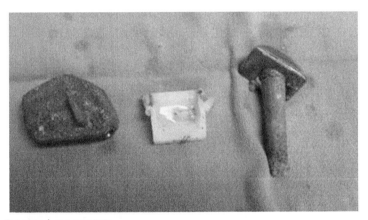

Fig. 25. Extracted components.

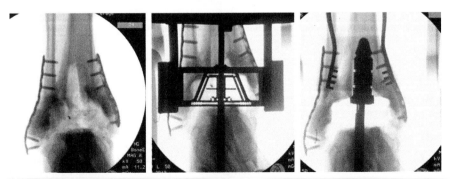

Fig. 26. Curettage and fixation of tibial and fibular cysts, INBONE II guide, anterior corticotomy, and placement of stemmed implant.

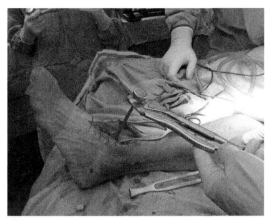

Fig. 27. Talar removal tool and vice grip placement to facilitate removal of the stemmed component.

prophylactic plate fixation followed by curettage and placement of PRODENSE (Wright Medical, Memphis, TN) or a similar calcium phosphate bone filler. The foot is now placed in the foot holder for the INBONE II cuts, and the revision ankle arthroplasty is completed (**Figs. 29–31**). Range-of-motion films in dorsiflexion and plantar flexion are taken to allow for an objective baseline to look at patients' range of motion in the postoperative period (**Fig. 32**). Patients are placed in a splint and kept non–weight bearing with follow-up in 2 weeks for transition to a cast for an additional 4 to 5 weeks of non–weight bearing. Radiographs are obtained at the 6-week mark, and patients are either allowed to begin a gradual weight-bearing protocol and range of motion with physical therapy or weight bearing is delayed and range of motion is started. This decision depends on radiographic findings and extent of bone loss discovered during surgery (**Fig. 33**).

OUTCOMES

There is a paucity of literature with regard to the long-term outcomes of revision TAA. It is a technically demanding procedure with a high rate of intraoperative and perioperative complications to include mechanical loosening, osteolysis, periprosthetic fracture, and dislocation.[23] Hintermann and colleagues[24] reviewed 117 revision total

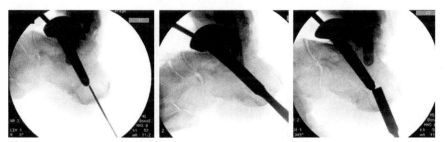

Fig. 28. Intraoperative removal of stemmed component. A guidewire is placed followed by a cannulated drill and then osteotome disimpaction of the component.

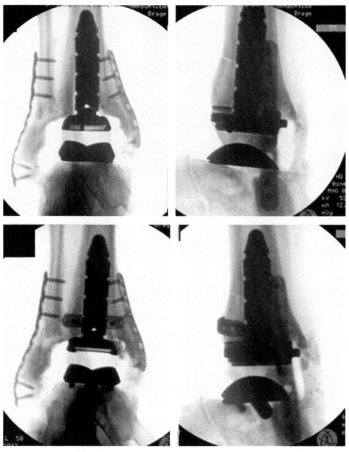

Fig. 29. Final stem and tibial component placement, talar component placement, and fixation of anterior corticotomy.

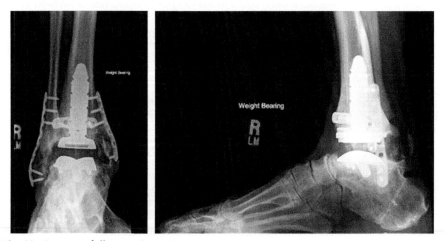

Fig. 30. Two-year follow-up in 2015.

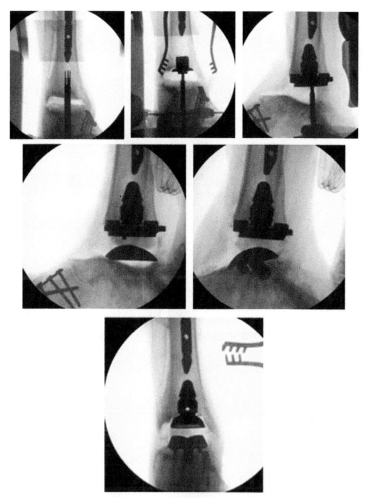

Fig. 31. Revision to INBONE II after antibiotic therapy completed.

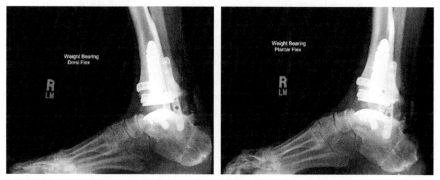

Fig. 32. Two-year follow-up flexion and extension films demonstrating limited range of motion.

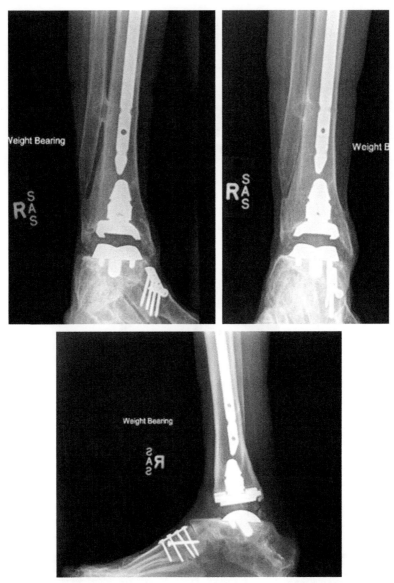

Fig. 33. Two-year follow-up.

ankles at a mean follow-up of 6.2 years and found results similar to primary arthroplasty. With respect to conversion from the Agility implant to the INBONE, DeVries and colleagues[25] described their experience with this procedure using both the anterior approach and the posterior approach for patients with an inadequate anterior soft tissue envelope. Their series of 14 patients at an average follow-up of 2.4 ± 1.4 years revealed a 64.3% complication rate, with roughly half of those requiring a secondary operative intervention. There were 2 cases considered failures, with one patient ultimately undergoing TTC arthrodesis and one undergoing below-knee amputation.[25]

SUMMARY

Revision of a custom stemmed Agility TAA to the INBONE prosthesis is a challenging undertaking and requires extensive preoperative planning, surgical experience, and possibly adjunct procedures. Conversion to fusion can be a difficult undertaking as well and is further complicated by concomitant subtalar fusion. Extensive bone loss often requires bulk allograft to fill the defect. Further studies are needed to investigate the long-term outcomes in these patients.

REFERENCES

1. Kopp FJ, Patel MM, Deland JT, et al. Total ankle arthroplasty with the agility prosthesis: clinical and radiographic evaluation. Foot Ankle Int 2006;27(2):97–103.
2. Knecht SI, Estin M, Callaghan JJ, et al. The agility total ankle arthroplasty. Seven to sixteen-year follow-up. J Bone Joint Surg Am 2004;86-A(6):1161–71.
3. Yoon HS, Lee J, Choi WJ, et al. Periprosthetic osteolysis after total ankle arthroplasty. Foot Ankle Int 2014;35(1):14–21.
4. Criswell BJ, Douglas K, Naik R, et al. High revision and reoperation rates using the agility total ankle system. Clin Orthop Relat Res 2012;470(7):1980–6.
5. Roukis TS. Incidence of revision after primary implantation of the agility total ankle replacement system: a systematic review. J Foot Ankle Surg 2012;51(2):198–204.
6. JG. A. Agility LP ankle arthroplasty outcomes. ClinicalTrialsgov 2014; Registration #NCT01366872.
7. Bartel AF, Roukis TS. Total ankle replacement survival rates based on Kaplan-Meier survival analysis of national joint registry data. Clin Podiatr Med Surg 2015;32(4):483–94.
8. Ellington JK, Gupta S, Myerson MS. Management of failures of total ankle replacement with the agility total ankle arthroplasty. J Bone Joint Surg Am 2013;95(23):2112–8.
9. Roukis TS. Revision of primary agility and agility LP total ankle replacements. Gewerbestrasse (Switzerland): Springer International Publishing; 2016.
10. McCollum G, Myerson MS. Failure of the agility total ankle replacement system and the salvage options. Clin Podiatr Med Surg 2013;30(2):207–23.
11. Alvine GF, Alvine FG. Total ankle arthroplasty using the agility stemmed talar revisional component: three to eight year follow-up. S D Med 2016;69(4):151–4.
12. Ketz J, Myerson M, Sanders R. The salvage of complex hindfoot problems with use of a custom talar total ankle prosthesis. J Bone Joint Surg Am 2012;94(13):1194–200.
13. Roukis TS. Salvage of a failed DePuy Alvine total ankle prosthesis with agility LP custom stemmed tibia and talar components. Clin Podiatr Med Surg 2013;30(1):101–9.
14. Myerson MS, Won HY. Primary and revision total ankle replacement using custom-designed prostheses. Foot Ankle Clin 2008;13(3):521–38, x.
15. Rahm S, Klammer G, Benninger E, et al. Inferior results of salvage arthrodesis after failed ankle replacement compared to primary arthrodesis. Foot Ankle Int 2015;36(4):349–59.
16. Gross C, Erickson BJ, Adams SB, et al. Ankle arthrodesis after failed total ankle replacement: a systematic review of the literature. Foot Ankle Spec 2015;8(2):143–51.
17. Doets HC, Zurcher AW. Salvage arthrodesis for failed total ankle arthroplasty. Acta Orthop 2010;81(1):142–7.

18. Kitaoka HB, Romness DW. Arthrodesis for failed ankle arthroplasty. J Arthroplasty 1992;7(3):277–84.
19. Berkowitz MJ, Clare MP, Walling AK, et al. Salvage of failed total ankle arthroplasty with fusion using structural allograft and internal fixation. Foot Ankle Int 2011;32(5):S493–502.
20. Henricson A, Rydholm U. Use of a trabecular metal implant in ankle arthrodesis after failed total ankle replacement. Acta Orthop 2010;81(6):745–7.
21. Palmanovich E, Brin YS, Ben David D, et al. Use of a spinal cage for creating stable constructs in ankle and subtalar fusion. J Foot Ankle Surg 2015;54(2):254–7.
22. Carlsson A. Unsuccessful use of a titanium mesh cage in ankle arthrodesis: a report on three cases operated on due to a failed ankle replacement. J Foot Ankle Surg 2008;47(4):337–42.
23. Williams JR, Wegner NJ, Sangeorzan BJ, et al. Intraoperative and perioperative complications during revision arthroplasty for salvage of a failed total ankle arthroplasty. Foot Ankle Int 2015;36(2):135–42.
24. Hintermann B, Zwicky L, Knupp M, et al. HINTEGRA revision arthroplasty for failed total ankle prostheses. J Bone Joint Surg Am 2013;95(13):1166–74.
25. DeVries JG, Scott RT, Berlet GC, et al. Agility to INBONE: anterior and posterior approaches to the difficult revision total ankle replacement. Clin Podiatr Med Surg 2013;30(1):81–96.

Management of Talar Component Subsidence

Shu-Yuan Li, MD, PhD*, Mark S. Myerson, MD

KEYWORDS

- Total ankle arthroplasty (TAA) • Talar subsidence • Bone loss • Revision

KEY POINTS

- Total ankle arthroplasty has, over the past decade, increased in popularity, but as a consequence there are an increasing number of failures that require revision.
- Component subsidence has been found to be the most frequent complication; the cause of subsidence is unclear, and seems to be multifactorial, including component loosening, osteolysis, malalignment of the components, disruption of the extraosseous and/or intraosseous blood supply of the talus, avascular necrosis of the talus, and component design.
- Talar subsidence is more frequently encountered than tibial subsidence; in many cases there is massive bone loss, which is more difficult to manage because the anatomy of the talus makes it difficult to augment.
- A newly introduced revision system, the Salto XT, has the ability to solve the dilemma of bone loss through flat cuts on the talus and impaction bone grafting.

INTRODUCTION

For end-stage ankle arthritis, total ankle arthroplasty (TAA) is now considered a very useful treatment option, with the advantages of preserving ankle joint movement, and possibly better function than arthrodesis. With the development of prosthesis design and improvements in surgical technique, the survival rate of TAA has been improved in recent years. However, prosthesis failure and the subsequent need for revision remain critical problems that foot and ankle surgeons face. Among the several known failure patterns, prosthesis subsidence is a common complication of TAA, with the incidence varying from 1% to 15%.[1,2] According to a systematic review of 20 studies, a short-term and intermediate-term failure rate of 12.4% (1.3%–32.3%) at 64 months (24–144 months) was reported in 2386 ankles. Subsidence and aseptic loosening were the most common complications encountered, occurring at a rate of 10.7% and 8.7% respectively.[3]

Disclosure: The authors have nothing to disclose.
The Foot and Ankle Association, Inc., 1209 Harbor Island Walk, Baltimore, MD 21230, USA
* Corresponding author.
E-mail address: drshuyuanli@gmail.com

In cases of component subsidence, there is always uneven distribution of the load, and loosening and increased movement of the involved component, which might cause further erosion of the bone, shift of the load-bearing axis, impingement of the talomalleolar facets, and prosthesis failure.[4,5] Based on the literature review, Glazebrook and colleagues[3] classified the subsidence as a medium-grade complication, which was proposed to lead to failure less than 50% of the time. In contrast, in a retrospective review of 15 years of a single-center database, subsidence was found to be the highest risk and resulted in 100% of TAA failure.[6] Another literature review, with 10 TAA primary studies in 852 patients, showed that the intermediate-term and long-term revision rate following TAA was 7% (3.5%–10.9%) with loosening and/or subsidence being the primary reason for TAA revisions (28%).[7] Spirt and colleagues[8] noted that component migration and failure occurred almost exclusively with the talar component.

To a large extent, this literature must be viewed according to the prostheses involved in these studies, because some of the earlier generation of implants had a much higher rate of talar component subsidence than others. Although failure of these earlier implants had a lot to do with flaws in the design of the prostheses, the principles that are discussed later in this article apply to all types of implant system.

It is widely proved and accepted that successful TAA has a very good functional outcome. The patients are able to walk faster, with their gait parameters significantly better than the preoperative status,[9] and similar to a healthy ankle.[10,11] A literature review also showed that the intermediate outcome of TAA was similar to that of ankle arthrodesis, in clinical evaluation and revision rate.[7]

CAUSE OR RISK FACTORS FOR SUBSIDENCE
Component Migration

Fong and colleagues[12] defined implant migration as "the longitudinal movement of an implant with respect to the bone in which it is imbedded over time." During the first couple of months after the TAA placement, slight migration of the components is normal and an acceptable phenomenon as the components get to their final positions and achieve a solid combination with the bone; this movement is small and can be considered physiologic prosthetic component migration.[12,13] In contrast, continuous subsequent migration is considered to be pathologic with much larger magnitudes of migration, and was proved to be able to predict premature failure within 10 years in total knee arthroplasty.[14] It was proposed that continuous migration for TAA may still predict premature failure within 10 years, as seen in total knee arthroplasty.[15,16] The threshold of acceptable early migration between the 1-year and 2-year follow-ups in total knee arthroplasty was proposed to be 0.2 mm, but there have been no quantified data for pathologic component migration in TAA.[16,17] A study using a modular stem fixed-bearing TAA prosthesis showed that the mean implant migration was 0.7 mm at 1 year and 1.0 mm at 2 years. Time and gender were significant predictors of implant migration.[18]

Osteolysis

Periprosthetic osteolysis can be asymptomatic, but progressively increasing in size and eventually leading to component loosening, subsidence, and implant failure.[19] The exact cause of osteolysis is still unknown, because it can be mechanically related to stress shielding, biochemically because of the wear particles of the prosthesis, or biologically caused by bone remodeling. In the earlier literature, there was a high incidence of osteolysis reported with different TAA models, including 76% of ankles with the Agility implant (DePuy, Warsaw, IN),[20] and a 12.5% incidence of aseptic loosening after Scandinavian Total Ankle Replacement (STAR).[21] More frequent osteolysis occurrence was found with the (Ankle Evolutive System [AES] Transystem, France) prosthesis in the short and medium term, such as a 21% severe lesion rate at 31 months,[22] a 24% rate of significant lesions at 58 months,[23] a 77% rate of cysts on radiographs and 100% on computed tomography (CT) scans at 39 months,[19] and a 79% rate of osteolysis and 40% rate of severe cysts at 28 months.[24] According to another case series study, at a mean 40 months' follow-up the functional and clinical results of the AES ankle prosthesis were good, with 96% implant survivorship, but bone-implant interface abnormality rates were high, with rapid adverse evolution. There were tibia/implant interface cysts (>5 mm) in 62% of cases, and talar/implant interface cysts in 43%. Talar osteolysis mostly began and predominated at the anterior implant anchorage. Although functional outcomes were comparable with the other mobile total ankle arthroplasty (TAA) in the literature, bone lysis with the AES prosthesis was more frequent with risk of subsidence, and this implant was removed from the market for these reasons.[25]

Component Design Factors

The design of TAA is highly relevant to its biomechanical behavior, and therefore influences overall results,[26,27] and is even associated with some complications.[28] Early prosthesis models had a high revision rate of 28% to 39% at 3 to 4 years of follow-up, caused by the nonanatomic design, excessive osseous resection, increased constraint, and poor joint congruency.[8,29] In recent years, with the improvement of implant design, a higher survivorship and good clinical outcome have been reported.[30–32] Moreover, it was shown in a study on revision TAA that design plays an important role in determining whether larger bone grafts should be used to bridge the gap for bone loss. The more resurfacing the TAA has, the less bone loss and the easier the reconstruction of the revision TAA.[33] The drawbacks of some implant designs in their early versions, and relevant modification in recent new generations, are listed here.

Increasing of Talar Surface Coverage: Agility/Agility LP

Before 2006, the Agility was the only 2-component, fixed polyethylene bearing TAA implant with US Food and Drug Administration (FDA) approval in the United States, and therefore has the longest follow-up data of any fixed-bearing device to date.[34] Before the introduction of the Agility LP TAA system,[35] the original Agility TAA system's talar component covered only 38% of the cut talar surface. Earlier versions of the prosthesis had a narrower posterior dimension of the talar component, giving it a trapezoidal shape when viewed from below. Focal load through the small undersurface led to a high incidence of subsidence into the body of the talus. This phenomenon was even worse in smaller implants and a failure rate of 43% in patients who received a size 1 prosthesis was reported.[36] The Agility LP TAA design was introduced in 2006, with an increase of the talar surface coverage to 85% by adding medial and lateral flares to the base of the implant. This modification helped to counteract subsidence by both distributing the load more evenly and increasing the potential for bone ingrowth.[35,37,38]

Improvement of Talar Component Articulating Design: INBONE I/INBONE II

In a case cohort study with 59 primary TAA using INBONE I or II implants, 5 cases (4 with INBONE I implants and 1 with INBONE II implants; 8% of the entire cohort) required revision surgery at a mean of 32.4 months (15–48 months) because of symptomatic talar subsidence. Talar subsidence was the main postoperative complication that led to revision, and predominantly affected the first-generation INBONE I implants.[39]

The INBONE II TAA system has a sulcus articulating geometry of the talar component with a central stem with 2 4-mm anterior talar dome pegs to its distal surface. The sulcus articulating geometry provides increased coronal plane stability, and the talar component's central stem and anterior pegs provide 3 points of fixation resulting in increased rotational stability.[40]

Blood Supply of the Talus

Theoretically, any compromise of the vascularity of the talus could lead to early component subsidence and malposition.[41] The following relevant issues are discussed: ipsilateral hindfoot arthrodesis, disruption of the intraosseous talar blood supply during the surgery, disruption of the extraosseous talar blood supply during the surgery, and performing TAA on cases with avascular necrosis (AVN).

There is concern that placement of an arthroplasty component on a talus previously instrumented by hindfoot arthrodesis may further compromise the vascularity of the talus and lead to early component subsidence and malposition.[41] Recently, a study compared the outcome of isolated TAA with outcomes of TAA with ipsilateral hindfoot arthrodesis, with 70 patients (17.3%) having had a hindfoot fusion before, after, or at the time of TAA, and 334 isolated TAAs as the control group. At a mean of 3.2 years' follow-up, no significant difference was found in terms of talar component subsidence between the fusion and control groups. However, the failure rate in the hindfoot fusion group (10.0%) was significantly higher than that in the control group (2.4%; $P<.05$). Furthermore, the investigators looked into the rate of different kinds of prosthesis usage in this study, and noted that all 7 (100%) failures in the hindfoot fusion group had an INBONE prosthesis. The INBONE system uses an intramedullary referencing system for the tibial component positioning, which involves drilling through the calcaneus, talus, and tibia with a 6-mm drill. The investigators suspected that increased instrumentation of the talus with this system might predispose patients to aseptic loosening and early failure in patients with an ipsilateral hindfoot fusion.[42] Another study from the same institution looked into the early to midterm outcomes of the INBONE system in 194 primary TAA cases, and reported that, in addition to a 6% revision rate for metallic components, 5% of the ankles had stable subsidence of the talar component, and 5% had unstable subsidence and impending failure of the prosthesis. The investigators were concerned that osteolytic processes or avascular changes within the talar body, and the introduction of instruments through the subtalar joint, may risk injury to the extraosseous and intraosseous talar vascular network through the plantarposterior aspect of the talar neck.[43,44]

Disruption of the extraosseous talar blood supply during the surgery is considered to be another factor contributing to talar component subsidence. A study on freshfrozen cadaveric specimens evaluated the risk of injury to specific extraosseous arteries supplying the talus associated with 4 contemporary TAA systems: STAR, INBONE II, Salto Talaris, and Trabecular Metal Total Ankle (TMTA). All 4 implant types subjected the extraosseous talar blood supply to the risk of injury. The INBONE subtalar drill hole directly transected the artery of the tarsal canal in 3 of 4 specimens. The lateral approach for the TMTA transected the first perforator of the peroneal artery in 2 of 4 specimens. The STAR caused medial injury to the deltoid branches in all 4 specimens, whereas the other 3 systems did not directly affect this supply ($P<.005$). The Salto Talaris and STAR implants caused injury to the artery of the tarsal canal in 1 of 4 specimens. This finding presents theoretic risks of aseptic loosening and implant failure caused by talar osteonecrosis.[45]

Avascular Necrosis of the Talus

There is a paucity of literature on performing TAA in patients with AVN of the talus. Historically, it was thought that a cementless TAA to treat AVN of the talar body was contraindicated because the potential for ingrowth and component fixation was poor. In the 1970s, there was a case report of TAA with bilateral AVN secondary to steroid medication with improvement of function.[46] Devalia and colleagues[47] used a 2-stage approach in 7 patients having subtalar arthrodesis followed by TAA for ankle arthritis and AVN of the talus. At a 3 years' mean follow-up, there was a significant improvement in pain, stiffness, and function, with radiological signs of talar subsidence noted in 2 patients at year 1, and no progress at 3 years' follow-up. Lee and colleagues[48] described successful cementless TAA in 2 cases of AVN following revascularization of the talus through conservative treatments, which included nonsteroidal antiinflammatory drugs, protective weight bearing in an ankle-foot orthosis, and a decrease in activity. TAA was only performed after revascularization of the talus was confirmed on MRI and radionuclide bone scanning results.[48] The authors have had varied experiences and outcomes with primary and revision TAA in the setting of talar AVN. From a practical standpoint, it does not make sense to attempt to implant a component on top of avascular bone, because there will not be bone ingrowth into the prosthesis and therefore inevitable loosening and subsidence will develop. In most of the revision cases in which talar subsidence has occurred, some degree of AVN of the talus is present as a result of the sclerosis and loosening that has taken place. It is always preferable to have the revision talar component seated on vascularized bone. However, in practice is not always possible because a flat cut of the talus made correctly leaves areas of the talus that are well vascularized and in which punctate bleeding is visible, and other areas where there is clearly no bleeding and the bone remains sclerotic and avascular. The authors do not think that this is a contraindication to the revision procedure, provided there is some potential for bone ingrowth into the talar component.

Malalignment

Malalignment has been considered a major risk factor for early failure of TAA.[49–52] It increases the focal stress and leads to edge loading, which increases the risk of prosthetic component aseptic loosening and eventual TAA failure. According to a study of 196 second-generation TAAs, of the ankles with preoperative varus or valgus deformities, approximately 50% (29 out of 55 varus and 23 out of 46 valgus) retained some malalignment after the procedure. Those retaining 15° of frontal plane deformity after the index TAA surgery had a significant increase in failure rates.[53] Any deformity should be corrected at the time of the index TAA surgery with an osseous and/or soft tissue balance procedure.[50,51,54–56] A preoperative deformity in the coronal plane of more than 10° is not easily correctible, and has been considered a relative contraindication for total ankle arthroplasty, because of a very low component survival rate. The authors do not agree with this statement, nor does the literature support this finding, because correction of either varus or valgus of up to 30° is feasible and technically possible with a good predictable outcome provided that the deformity of the foot, as well as the ankle, is corrected.[52,57] Malposition of the component placement always leads to failure. An ideal position of the talar component has the same goal that implanting the prosthesis with a good alignment of the ankle has, otherwise there would be increased focal stress and edge loading, and subsequent increased risk of subsidence.[58]

Gender has been found to be a concern. Implant migration was proved to be greater in men than in women. The investigators proposed that this discrepancy arises from the greater compressive forces at the ankle and larger anatomy in men, resulting in greater implant migration.[18,59] However, there are too many additional factors that may contribute to this gender difference, including lifestyle, daily activities, average weight, and occupation, and the authors caution the reader to assume a gender difference unless all these factors are accounted for.

TREATMENT OF TALAR COMPONENT SUBSIDENCE

Management of talar component subsidence is a challenge, because there is always bone loss, and sometimes massive loss, which can be caused as noted earlier by direct mechanical erosion, periprosthetic osteolysis, or necrotic changes of the underlying trabecular bone.[4] The subsidence can be severe, with complete erosion of the talar body and migration of the talar component into the subtalar joint, which may be difficult if not frustrating to correct. For a failed TAA with subsidence, possible treatment options are revision with another TAA, conversion to an ankle arthrodesis or tibiotalocalcaneal arthrodesis with bone graft, or a below-knee amputation.[58,60]

Revision Total Ankle Arthroplasty or Arthrodesis

Regardless of the decision to perform a revision TAA or an arthrodesis, the goal of the treatment is always to relieve pain, restore a plantigrade foot and ankle with normal mechanical alignment, and ideally to restore anatomic height. Unlike primary surgery for end-stage ankle arthritis, the salvage surgery of a failed TAA with either a revision TAA or an arthrodesis is much more difficult because of the problems of bone loss.

Although an ankle or tibiotalocalcaneal arthrodesis seems to have more predictable outcomes than ankle replacement, especially in primary surgeries, it also has many limitations, including substantial stiffness, limitation of activities, and adding high levels of stress on adjacent joints, which lead to pain, eventual arthritis, and dysfunction of the joints.[58,61–63] Any revision surgery when converting a failed TAA to an arthrodesis is much more difficult than doing a primary arthrodesis, primarily because of bone loss and deformity. Furthermore, the nonunion rate of a salvage arthrodesis in failed TAA is greatly increased because of the need for large structural bone grafts for restoring limb length, and this risk is even higher in patients who have had previous hindfoot fusions.[64] In a case series of failed TAA patients who were treated with ankle arthrodesis using compression screw fusion with use of tricortical iliac crest grafts, all patients but 1 achieved solid union and no complications were reported.[65] Berkowitz and colleagues[66] compared 12 patients who had an ankle fusion with 12 patients who had tibiotalocalcaneal arthrodesis for the treatment of failed TAA. In the group with tibiotalocalcaneal arthrodesis, nonunions occurred in a high rate and were identified as a risk factor for worse outcome. Jeng and colleagues[67] and Myerson and Won[68] showed that the results of tibiotalocalcaneal arthrodesis using femoral heal allografts were poor, with a fusion rate of 50%. The problem with all these studies is the type of prosthesis used and the size of the defect present that requires arthrodesis. For example, in the study by Culpan and colleagues,[65] it is not known what the size of the bone defect was, what type of bone graft was necessary to fill the void, what type of fixation was used, and whether any biologic adjuvants were used during the arthrodesis.

A high nonunion rate was found after salvage ankle arthrodesis in patients with inflammatory joint disease. Eleven of the 18 ankles healed after a first attempt, and the remaining 7 nonunions occurred in patients with inflammatory joint disease (mainly rheumatoid arthritis). Four nonunions underwent a second attempt at salvage arthrodesis, resulting in union in 2 patients, with 1 ankle that failed to unite after a third attempt.[69] Meanwhile results from the same institute and several other institutes showed that, in patients with rheumatoid disease, primary TAA can achieve a satisfactory survival rate.[36,57] In Hurowitz and colleagues'[36] retrospective study, patients with rheumatoid arthritis had a statistically significant lower rate of failure. However, there has been no study on survival rate of revision TAA in rheumatoid arthritis cases.

At present, information regarding revision TAA is limited.[68,70–72] The largest series of literature was published in German by Hintermann and colleagues[73] with 83 revision surgeries in 79 patients and a 5-year follow-up. Eighty-three percent of patients were satisfied with the result, 14% judged the result as fair, and 2% as poor. Fifty-nine percent were pain free at the time of follow-up with an acceptable range of motion at the ankle joint.[73] Ellington and colleagues[74] reported the results of managing failed TAA with the Agility TAA prosthesis and a minimum of 2 years' follow-up. Among the 41 patients who were available for follow-up, there were 5 patients who had been converted to an arthrodesis. Twenty-two patients (54%) had a subtalar arthrodesis performed at the time of the revision arthroplasty, with 19 of those having a custom-designed long-stem talar component. There were satisfactory outcomes for pain and function improvement, with no significant change on radiographic measurements of component position. The investigators concluded that revision arthroplasty may be considered as an alternative to arthrodesis when treating patients with a failed Agility total ankle implant. Our study on short-term results of revision TAA with Salto XT showed that, among the 40 revised TAA cases, with an average of 24.2 months (range, 12–36 months), an 85% survivorship of the revision was achieved, with 6 cases of revision, which included 4 cases of suspected postoperative infection and 2 cases of implant loosening (Li SY, Myerson MS, Coetzee JC, et al. Management of a failed total ankle replacement with a revision prosthesis. A multicenter study of the indications, surgical techniques and short term outcomes. Unpublished data, 2016).

Treating Talar Component Subsidence with Revision Total Ankle Arthroplasty: Surgical Tips and Techniques

A failed TAA with symptomatic talar component subsidence can be revised either by just changing the talar component or changing all the implants, depending on the status of the tibial component and the polyethylene insert. The ideal revision components need to have sufficient surface area, cortical contact, and stability, and various options with the tibia, talus, and polyethylene inserts.[60] However, TAA prostheses for revision purposes are limited, with few implant systems able to meet requirements mentioned earlier. As discussed repeatedly earlier, to manage the bone loss in failed TAA is very demanding, and the situation worsens following removal of the implants, debridement of necrotic bone, and resection of the talus to a stable, flat configuration for the placement of the talar component. According to a previously published radiographic grading system of talar component subsidence that guides treatment and correlates with outcome following revision TAA, subsidence of grades 2 and 3 could not be treated with a standard technique because there is not adequate bone stock left to maintain the stability of the revision talar component.[74] In the past, facing a situation with absent bone, either a hindfoot arthrodesis[58,75] or a custom long-stemmed talar component was used.[58,73,75] Hintermann and colleagues[73] described a different method of grading subsidence: if the osseous defect is less than 18 mm with the talar dome intact, a standard replacement component can be used; in the case of an osseous defect between 18 and 25 mm with the talar dome intact, revision replacement components need to be used; if the osseous defect size is larger than 25 mm, a custom replacement component is necessary.[73]

The custom long-stemmed talar component was always used in conjunction with subtalar joint arthrodesis but this long-stemmed component is no longer available even as a custom device in the United States. Kim and colleagues[41] showed a tendency toward higher soft tissue scarring and bony impingement with staged TAA and hindfoot fusion, and a higher rate of instability or dislocation of the polyethylene component with simultaneous procedures. In cases combined with subtalar joint degeneration, arthritis, or a hindfoot deformity, a combined subtalar joint arthrodesis is necessary and acceptable.[75] However, in cases with a normal subtalar joint, the remaining hindfoot motion may need to be sacrificed in order to get a stable fixation of the talar component. Moreover, the long-stem components are no longer approved by the FDA and have not been used for more than 7 years.

A new revision replacement system, the Salto XT prosthesis, was introduced into use in recent years. It has the ability to solve the dilemma of bone loss through flat cuts on the talus and impaction bone grafting; that is, a resurfacing technique. Moreover, the Salto XT offers a range of polyethylene insert sizes up to 21 mm thick, and allows for mismatching the tibial and talar components based on patient anatomy by selecting the tibial component of the same or 1 size larger than the talar component. The authors have found that this system is feasible for revision of each of the TAA systems available for use in the United States.

The preoperative evaluation and preparation work is as outlined earlier. Preoperative weight-bearing radiographs, including anteroposterior (AP), lateral, mortise views, hindfoot alignment view, flexion, and extension views, as well as CT scans of the ankle, must be obtained to define the status and alignment of the failed prosthesis, condition of residual bone stock of the tibia and talus (quality, bone loss, necrosis, cyst formation), deformity of the ankle and hindfoot, mobility of the ankle, and the condition of the adjacent talonavicular joint and subtalar joint. It has been shown that, on average, CT scans show osteolytic lesions 3 times larger than those seen on radiographs. Moreover, CT can provide more reliable information on implant loosening than radiographs, especially in cases with persistent pain and no evidence of loosening on standard radiographs.[60,76] Standard blood work-up is necessary to exclude infection preoperatively. Careful assessment of the vascularity, skin viability, and prior surgical incisions is essential to decision making, and noninvasive arterial vascular studies need to be performed if there are any concerns about the status of 1 or both of the vessels.

During the revision surgery, a standard anterior approach using the prior incision is used with careful protection of the neurovascular bundle. A dilemma arises if a poor incision was used previously, which limits full exposure of the joint. Clinicians should never make a separate adjacent incision, but the incision distally can be made much longer and, with retraction, can give more exposure with less tissue risk. Deep specimens need to be taken before giving prophylactic antibiotics and proceeding to full revision. Some of the following issues are extremely important with respect to implant removal and joint surface preparation. Prophylactic guide pins placed in both the medial and lateral malleolus before implant removal are very helpful to protect against intraoperative fracture. First remove the polyethylene liner, then remove the talar component, which is always loose in cases of subsidence, followed by the tibial component removal. Placing the ankle in plantarflexion can help with talar implant removal, by prying it out with an osteotome. Because this component is always loose, further bone loss with implant removal does not occur. The tibial component is then removed, and here the surgeon has to be more careful because this component may be firmly secured with good bone ingrowth. If the tibial component is in excellent position, and stable, the surgeon may consider leaving it in place and letting the tibial component guide the position of the talar trial. If the tibial component has to be removed, then preserve as much bone as possible using thin, fine osteotomes. The next step is to do an extensive medial and lateral gutter release and debridement, starting with a rongeur and then, if necessary, with a reciprocating saw to remove all pathologic bone and soft tissue overgrowth in the gutters before proceeding with the revision. This step often frees the movement in the ankle. A 4-mm gap in each gutter is necessary to help increase the range of motion of the ankle. The next step is to remove the posterior scar because there is frequently a hard posterior shell of fibrous scar and bone that limits the range of ankle motion. It needs to be peeled off the posterior tibia and then the talus. Attention needs to be paid when operating medially to avoid neurovascular injury, and this step commences with debridement posterior-laterally. Further debridement of the bone is performed, focusing on cyst formation using angled curettes. All cystic and necrotic bone is excised, until bleeding bone is exposed.

Depending on the magnitude of the bone loss, the authors generally perform free-hand bone cuts and do not make the cuts through the cutting block jig. The tibial bone cut is performed first, and, once the tibia is in a neutral position, the talus is evaluated. Talar component subsidence is rarely flat with respect to the floor. Usually there is more bone loss presenting posteriorly, with further collapse presenting medially or laterally, which tilts the talus into varus or valgus, and causes deformity and ultimately more edge loading. The coronal plane deformity needs to be evaluated and addressed first, which is strongly related to the outcome of the revision. Any soft tissue imbalance needs to be treated before proceeding further with preparation of the talar surface. After that, a flat bone cut is performed to treat the irregularity of the talar surface caused by component erosion. When doing this, the foot is held reduced with a laminar spreader in place centrally, with the forefoot in a plantigrade position. The bone is cut into a plantigrade coronal plane position. If there is posterior subsidence of the talar surface, then a cut is initiated from the talonavicular joint articular surface so as to remove more bone anteriorly and create a talar surface that is parallel with the ground. The cut on the talus can be performed either freehand or by using the cutting jigs.

In cases of severe bone loss with very little bone of the talar body and a small portion of the talus head left, the talus head is removed completely to facilitate making a flat cut on the calcaneus, and the talar component can be placed directly on to the calcaneus. The authors have not found that removing the head of the talus has any influence on the stability of either the prosthesis or the midfoot. Next, check the correct position of the bony cuts with AP and lateral fluoroscopic examination. However, the angle of Gissane indicates that the talar component cannot be inserted directly on to the calcaneus, because there would be a sagittal plane deformity. Therefore, it is useful to slightly notch the posterior edge of the calcaneus so that the talar component can sit directly on the posterior calcaneus, and then the anterior talar component can be supported by bone graft.

Bone loss can be corrected with impaction grafting using a mixture of allograft and/or autograft to achieve a flat surface for prosthesis implantation.[60] The bone graft is inserted loosely between a large osteotome and the defect on the talus, and then the osteotome is hit with a mallet to apply a forcible impact to the bone graft.

Cement has been used as a method for bone augmentation. The authors have had a lot of experience with the use of cement, but have not found that it is predictable enough around the tibia or the talus because it adheres very well to the component, but not always as well to the bone. The use of cement under the talar component is acceptable, especially in a very-low-demand patient with poor-quality bone who needs to be able to weight bear early. In a study of metal-reinforced cement augmentation for treating complex talar subsidence, the investigators introduced a new technique by placing the talar component on 3 or 4 metallic supports placed into the remaining talus, across the subtalar joint, and into the calcaneus, with cement leveled up to the top of the metal supports for augmentation. Then the final talar component with the attached stem was coated with cement inferiorly, and inserted onto the metal support–cement combination. The preliminary results from a series of 17 patients with a mean follow-up of 1.3 years (range, 6–48 months) were satisfactory. In 2 cases there was some separation of the cement from the talocalcaneal bone mass at 6 months postoperatively; however, these interfaces have remained stable at 1 year and 18 months, respectively. No lysis around the metal-bone interface has been observed in any of the other 15 patients. Two of the fixation devices (1 acetabular screw, 1 fusion rod) underwent fatigue failure. However, the cement interface in these patients had remained stable for 2 years and 9 months, respectively, without subsequent migration of any of the components. In the other 15 patients there was no loosening of the cement-metal-bone interfaces and the components have remained congruent at the polyethylene interface as well.[77]

After checking the trial implants under fluoroscopy, the definitive implants are placed. The tibial component can be the same or 1 size larger than the talar component, allowing for mismatching the tibial and talar components based on patient anatomy; this is often necessary given the change in the dimensions of the working surface for the components. In addition, the ankle is assessed for stability, range of motion, as well as coronal plane balance. An Achilles lengthening is performed at this stage if further dorsiflexion is required. A lateral ligament reconstruction is performed as required for instability with either a modified Brostrom procedure or a peroneal augmentation. Any hindfoot deformity must be addressed in order to prevent failure of the revision surgery. In the case series reported by Hintermann and colleagues,[73] in addition to exchange of the metallic components, 36 concomitant procedures (ie, arthrodesis, osteotomies, ligament repairs, and peroneus longus to peroneus brevis transfers) were performed to balance the hindfoot.

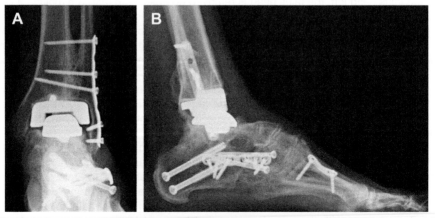

Fig. 1. Preoperative AP (A) and lateral (B) views of the ankle joint. Note the subsidence of the talar component with bone buildup circumferentially around the joint.

TYPICAL CASES
Case 1: Conversion Agility to Salto XT

This patient was a 55-year-old woman who presented with a failed Agility LP replacement. There was severe subsidence of the talar component. There was no range of motion of the ankle at all as a result of the excess bone growth (**Fig. 1**).

During the surgery, after making the incision, retracting the soft tissue, and dissecting to the joint, the entire anterior joint was not visible, because it was obliterated by

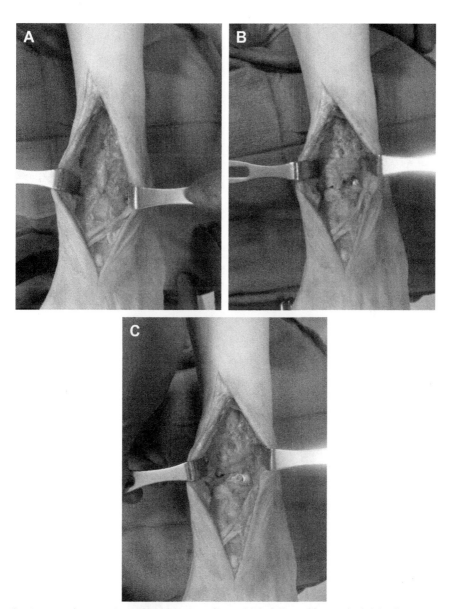

Fig. 2. A regular anterior approach was performed (*A*), followed by gradual debridement to expose the ankle joint and the failed prosthesis (*B, C*).

bone and scar. In order to visualize the joint, debridement was performed with a large rongeur. Care was taken to visualize and protect the neurovascular bundle, which is typically encased in scar. With gradual debridement the prosthesis eventually became visible (**Fig. 2**).

An osteotome was inserted to lever the polyethylene component out from the tibial component. The polyethylene from this Agility LP prosthesis was easy to retrieve because it was wedged out anteriorly. With the polyethylene removed, the talar component was then removed. Because the talar component was likely to be loose,

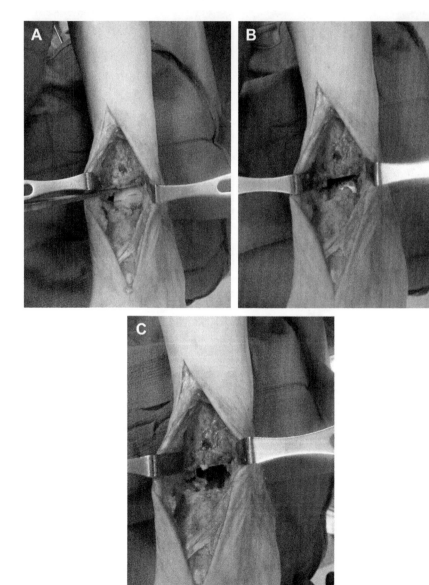

Fig. 3. Removing the polyethylene insert (*A*, *B*) and the talar component (*C*).

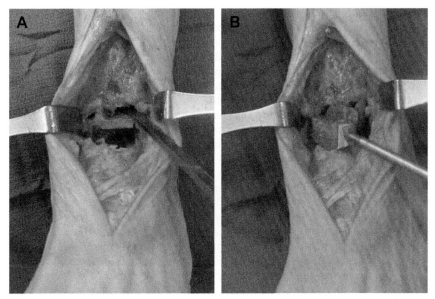

Fig. 4. Removing the tibial component with an osteotome (*A*) and the threaded inserter tool from the Agility set (*B*). Care must be taken to preserve the anterior cortical rim of the distal tibia.

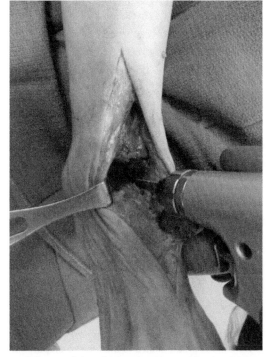

Fig. 5. Debridement of the medial and lateral gutters with a sagittal saw.

a fine 6-mm osteotome was inserted under the talar component to loosen it further and pry it out. It was useful to insert the threaded guide from the Agility replacement into the talar component to help facilitate its removal (**Fig. 3**).

It was imperative for as much anterior tibial cortex to be preserved as possible to support the revision component, but this was not always possible if there was solid bone ingrowth, in which case a fine osteotome was inserted under the tibial component to loosen it further and pry it loose without creating a defect in the anterior tibial cortical rim. The Agility tibial component has a fin that is on the medial side of the prosthesis and is generally buried beneath 8 mm of anterior bone, hiding its position. It was ideal to preserve this anterior rim of bone, which increased the anterior cortical rim for support of the revision prosthesis. It was generally possible to do so by using an osteotome under the visible portion of the tibial component and gradually loosening it. Once the tibial component was loose then a tamp was used to push the component out inferiorly. In this way most of the anterior cortical rim was preserved. It was helpful to be able to remove the tibial component with the threaded inserter tool from the Agility set (**Fig. 4**).

Debridement of the medial and lateral gutters was then performed with a sagittal saw. All heterotopic bone and hypertrophic thickened soft tissue scar was removed so that there was smooth, unimpeded range of motion of the ankle. There should be about 4 mm of space in each gutter following this debridement with the saw (**Fig. 5**). Care must be taken on the medial gutter not to cut into the apex of the medial joint, which would weaken the medial malleolus.

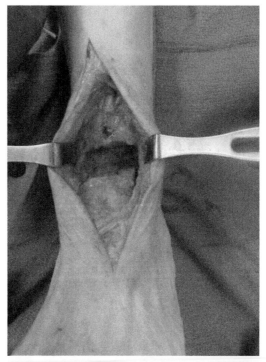

Fig. 6. Freehand cuts were made on the tibia and the talus to prepare for the implants. Note the flat surfaces of bleeding bone.

The distal tibial bone could be cut in 2 ways, one being through the tibial cutting guide, and the other a freehand cut. In this case, freehand cuts were made on the tibia to prepare for the tibial component. The talar bone was cut into a plantigrade coronal plane position (**Fig. 6**).

The talar and tibial trial components were inserted together with the appropriate-sized polyethylene and the ankle range of motion evaluated. It was important to ensure that the talar component was centered correctly over the body of the talus. The tibia would follow the talus and must be centered on the tibia. When inserting the tibial trial component, the position laterally was important to assess fluoroscopically to ensure that it was centered and not lifting off either anterior or posteriorly (**Fig. 7**).

The anterior talar positioning pins were inserted after predrilling. Before inserting these pins, the position of both components was checked fluoroscopically. There was a tendency for the trial components to shift with range of motion of the ankle, and the foot should be kept in maximum dorsiflexion to lock the components in place, check the position under fluoroscopy, and then maintain this position before drilling and insertion of the anterior talar pins. Once the talar positioning pins were inserted, the ankle was again checked under fluoroscopy before making the tibial drill holes. The tibial drill holes were made and the small rongeur used to remove bone between the 2 drill holes. The rasp should be used to prepare the tibia for the component (**Fig. 8**).

It was far easier to drill the talus for the talar stem (**Fig. 9**A) and the posterior slotted holes (see **Fig. 9**B) once the tibial trial component was removed. This stage was done

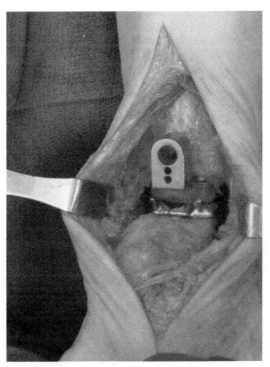

Fig. 7. The trial implant was inserted. Note that the talar component was centered correctly over the body of the talus.

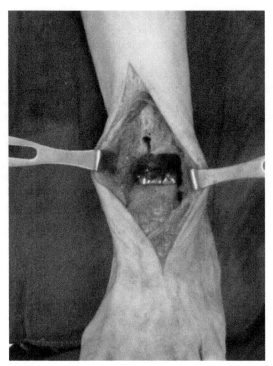

Fig. 8. Preparation of the distal tibia for the tibial component.

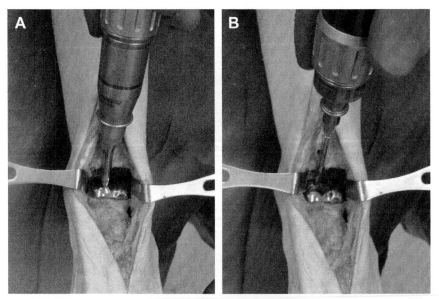

Fig. 9. Preparation of the talar bone for the talar component with drilling for the talar stem (*A*) and the posterior slotted holes (*B*).

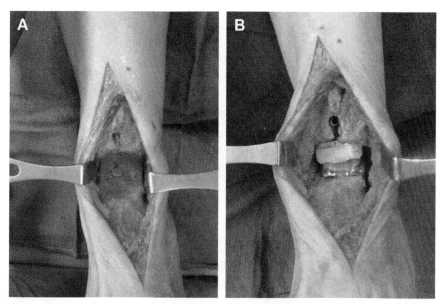

Fig. 10. Checking the final bone surface. It is important to remove any remaining bony or scar tissue in the gutters and the posterior capsule that might block the range of motion (*A*). Insertion of the components (*B*).

with the foot in maximum plantarflexion otherwise the anterior tibial cortex would have been in the way and would have blocked the reamer.

At the completion of the bone preparation, the gutters were checked to make sure they contained no debris, that the gutters were completely decompressed, and that there was no scar tissue remaining in the posterior capsule that would block range of motion. Following insertion of the components, the range of motion was checked and a percutaneous lengthening of the Achilles was performed if 10° of dorsiflexion had not been achieved (**Fig. 10**).

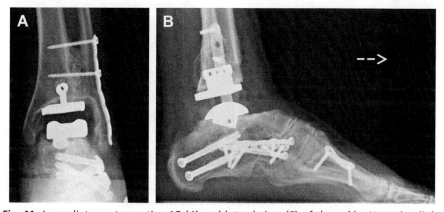

Fig. 11. Immediate postoperative AP (*A*) and lateral view (*B*) of the ankle. Note the slight extension position (opening) of the tibia component on the lateral view (*B*) for a larger bone surface and to prevent sizing problems.

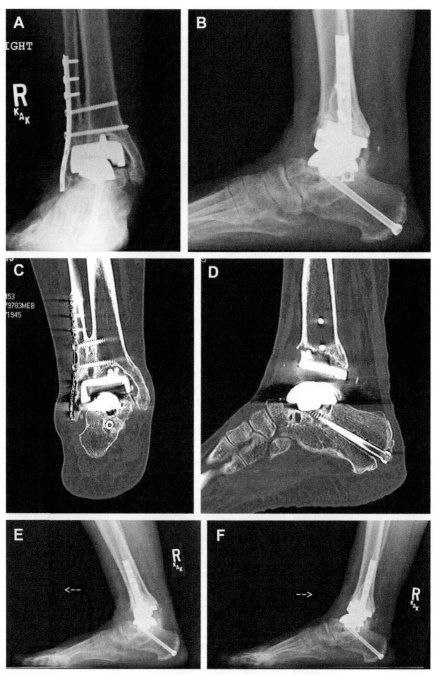

Fig. 12. Preoperative radiological examination results. Note the component subsidence on both tibial and talar sides on radiographs (*A*, *B*) and CT scan (*C*, *D*), and a good movement of the ankle with about 20° dorsiflexion and 15° plantarflexion (*E*, *F*).

The immediate postoperative radiographs showed the clearance of bone in the gutter. The tibial component was slightly extended relative to the axis of the tibia. However, this was not the ideal position for the component. The tibia was very narrow further proximally, and with a plantigrade cut on the tibia this would have caused

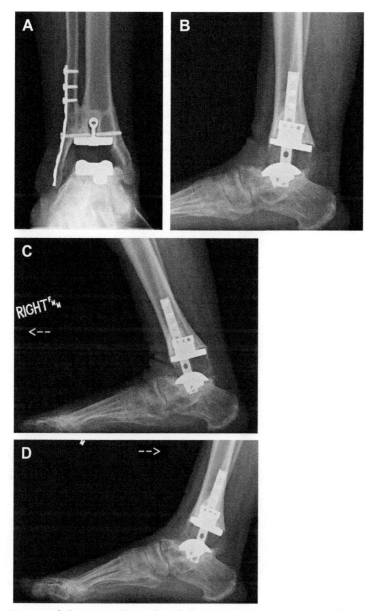

Fig. 13. Two-year follow-up radiographs of the revision TAA. Note the stable position of both tibial and talar side components (*A, B*), the slight extension position (opening) of the tibial component for a larger bone surface to avoid sizing problems (*top right*), and a very good range of motion of the joint (*C, D*).

problems with sizing. This extended (open) position of the tibia in most cases increases dorsiflexion of the ankle (**Fig. 11**).

Case 2: Both Tibial Side and Talar Side Subsidence

This was a 68-year-old woman presenting with a failed Agility TAA and severe ankle pain. The subtalar joint had been fused previously. There was a good movement of the ankle with about 20° dorsiflexion and 15° plantarflexion (**Fig. 12**E, F). Radiographs (see **Fig. 12**A, B) and CT scan (see **Fig. 12**C, D) showed that there were both tibial component subsidence and talar component subsidence with moderate erosion of the talus (see **Fig. 12**B, C), severe erosion of the anterior cortical rim of the distal tibia (see **Fig. 12**D), and large cysts underneath both the tibial and the talar components (see **Fig. 12**C, D).

A revision TAA was performed by removing the Agility prosthesis, removing the hardware from the subtalar joint, and inserting a Salto XT prosthesis into the joint. Both the distal tibia and the top of the talus were cut into flat surfaces for placing the revision components. After debriding the necrotic bone of the distal tibia, in order to maintain a plantigrade neutral position of the tibial component, the cut was made

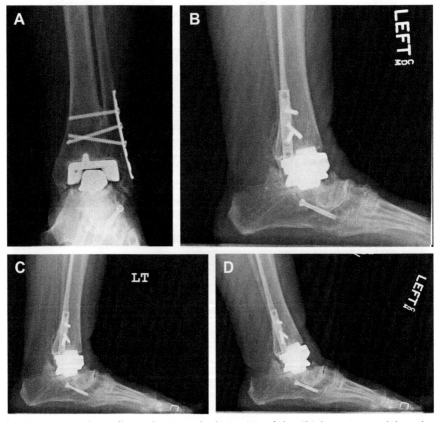

Fig. 14. Preoperative radiographs. Note the loosening of the tibial component (A), and severe talar component subsidence on the lateral view with surrounding bone overgrowth (B), which blocked the movement of the ankle joint. (C) Dorsiflexion of the joint; (D) plantar flexion of the joint.

proximally where the diameter of the tibia was narrow. In order not to cause a problem with sizing and mismatch of the components, the anterior tibia was cut in a slight extension position (opening), for a larger bone surface (**Fig. 13**B). At 2 years of follow-up the patient had a very good outcome, with a stable position of the prosthesis (see **Fig. 13**A, B) and a very good range of motion of the joint (see **Fig. 13**C, D).

Case 3: Severe Talar Component Subsidence

This was a 59-year-old woman, presenting with a failed left TAA. An Agility prosthesis was placed 10 years previously, which had been progressively causing swelling and pain in her ankle. Her ambulation was severely limited and she could only walk in an Arizona brace. On examination, there was 10° of dorsiflexion and 10° of plantar flexion

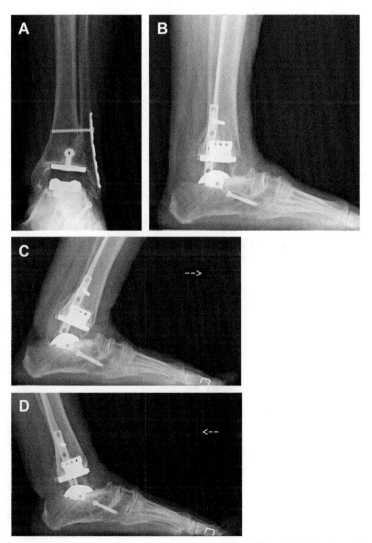

Fig. 15. Two-year follow-up radiographs. Note the stable position of the implants (*A, B*), and good ankle movement (*C, D*).

in the ankle. Radiographs showed loosening of the tibial component and a considerable amount of talar component subsidence with collapse of the talus (**Fig. 14**).

A revision TAA with Salto XT prosthesis was performed. Because there was very little talar bone stock left, after the flat cut, the talar component was sitting directly on the calcaneus with cancellous bone graft impacted underneath (**Fig. 15B**). The implants were mismatched, with a size 2 tibia component, a size 1 talar component, and a

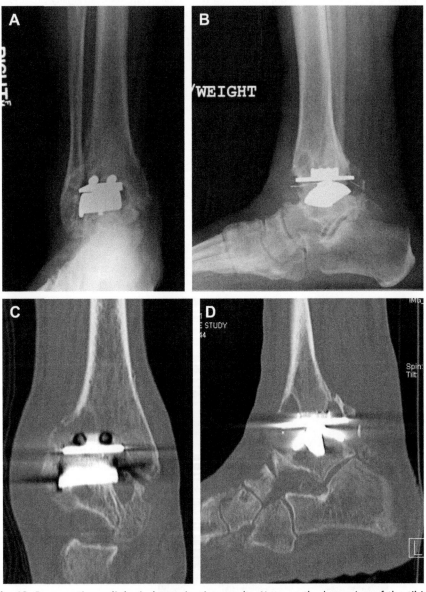

Fig. 16. Preoperative radiological examination results. Note on the loosening of the tibial component, the subsidence of the talar component (*A, B*), with large cysts underneath both components (*C, D*).

size 13 polyethylene insert. Two years' follow-up showed a very satisfactory outcome, with a painless ankle, good ankle movement, and a stable position of the implants (see **Fig. 15**).

Case 4: Talar Component Subsidence and Polyethylene Fracture

A 70-year-old man presented with right ankle problems 3 years following a TAA with the STAR system. On the radiological and CT scan results there was fractured polyethylene with loosening of both the tibial and the talar components (**Fig. 16**).

After the joint surfaces were prepared, the implants were inserted with cement used to fill the smaller bone defects. There was good alignment of the ankle and a stable position of the prosthesis (**Fig. 17**A, B), and satisfactory movement of the ankle (see **Fig. 17**C, D).

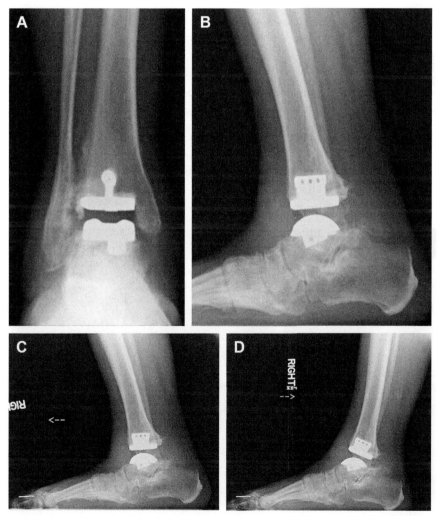

Fig. 17. Postoperative radiographs. Note the stable position of the prosthesis (*A, B*), and the satisfactory movement of the ankle (*C, D*).

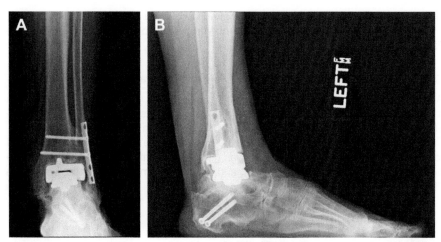

Fig. 18. Preoperative radiographs. Note the significant talar component subsidence on both AP (*A*) and lateral (*B*) views.

Case 5: Revision with Long-stemmed Custom Prosthesis

This patient underwent a replacement with the Agility system several years previously. She presented with pain in the ankle and slowly changing range of motion to the extent that anterior ankle pain was present as a result of subsidence of the talar component. It is important to recognize that the bone in the anterior ankle is not new bone, osteophytes, or heterotopic bone, but followed subsidence from a previous normal level at which the bone cut was made (**Fig. 18**).

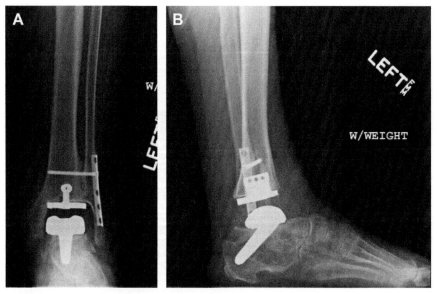

Fig. 19. Four-year follow-up radiographs. Note the good position of the components on both AP (*A*) and lateral (*B*) views.

Because of the marked collapse of the talar component and the questionable quality of the remaining bone, a long-stem custom Tornier prosthesis, designed consistent with the Salto Talaris, was chosen. The advantage of the long talar stem has been proved in previous publications.

We had to anticipate the diameter of the tibial component relative to the talar component preoperatively, because this was a custom prosthesis, and there would be no room for error, particularly with respect to the width of the talus, which must be measured on CT scan. The tibial component can be the same size or 1 size bigger than the talar component, and again the diameter of the tibia at the level of the new bone cut must be anticipated preoperatively for seating the tibial component.

The postoperative AP and lateral positions of the components are noted here, and the patient continued to have a good outcome at her final follow-up 4 years following the revision surgery (**Fig. 19**).

SUMMARY

A successful midterm to long-term TAA revision is based on strict indication selection, thorough preoperative evaluation and preparation, choosing a reliable anatomically and biologically designed revision prosthesis system, careful surgical process with correction of the bony deformity, balancing the soft tissue instability, impacting any bony defect, and an appropriate postoperative rehabilitation plan. However, with time, gradual implant migration and osteolysis changes are still inevitable. It is widely accepted that serial radiographs are useful to document progression.

In summary, talar subsidence is a common and severe complication of TAA, and is highly relevant to TAA failure. The cause of subsidence formation is unclear, and is multifactorial. Management of the talar subsidence with severe bone loss is highly demanding on the salvage surgeries, like revision TAA or salvage arthrodesis, with a high risk of complication and failure. Compared with salvage arthrodesis procedures, revision TAA has the advantage of preserving joint function with at least no worse survival rate. As a newly introduced specific revision prosthesis system, the Salto XT has the ability to treat most of the TAA systems available for use in the United States.

REFERENCES

1. Bonnin M, Judet T, Colombier JA, et al. Midterm results of the Salto total ankle prosthesis. Clin Orthop Relat Res 2004;(424):6–18.
2. Buechel FF Sr, Buechel FF Jr, Pappas MJ. Twenty-year evaluation of cementless mobile-bearing total ankle replacements. Clin Orthop Relat Res 2004;(424): 19–26.
3. Glazebrook M, Arsenault K, Dunbar M. Evidence-based classification of complications in total ankle arthroplasty. Foot Ankle Int 2009;30:945–9.
4. Castro MD. Insufficiency fractures after total ankle replacement. Techniques Foot Ankle Surg 2007;6:15–21.
5. Espinosa N, Wirth SH. Revision of the aseptic and septic total ankle replacement. Clin Podiatr Med Surg 2013;30:171–85.
6. Gadd RJ, Barwick TW, Paling E, et al. Assessment of a three-grade classification of complications in total ankle replacement. Foot Ankle Int 2014;35:434–7.
7. Haddad SL, Coetzee JC, Estok R, et al. Intermediate and long-term outcomes of total ankle arthroplasty and ankle arthrodesis. A systematic review of the literature. J Bone Joint Surg Am 2007;89:1899–905.
8. Spirt AA, Assal M, Hansen ST Jr. Complications and failure after total ankle arthroplasty. J Bone Joint Surg Am 2004;86-A:1172–8.

9. Queen RM, Butler RJ, Adams SB Jr, et al. Bilateral differences in gait mechanics following total ankle replacement: a two year longitudinal study. Clin Biomech (Bristol, Avon) 2014;29:418–22.

10. Roselló Añón A, Martinez Garrido I, Cervera Deval J, et al. Total ankle replacement in patients with end-stage ankle osteoarthritis: clinical results and kinetic gait analysis. Foot Ankle Surg 2014;20:195–200.

11. Detrembleur C, Leemrijse T. The effects of total ankle replacement on gait disability: analysis of energetic and mechanical variables. Gait Posture 2009; 29:270–4.

12. Fong JW, Veljkovic A, Dunbar MJ, et al. Validation and precision of model-based radiostereometric analysis (MBRSA) for total ankle arthroplasty. Foot Ankle Int 2011;32:1155–63.

13. Carlsson A, Markusson P, Sundberg M. Radiostereometric analysis of the double-coated STAR total ankle prosthesis: a 3-5 year follow-up of 5 cases with rheumatoid arthritis and 5 cases with osteoarthrosis. Acta Orthop 2005;76:573–9.

14. Ryd L, Toksvig-Larsen S. Early postoperative fixation of tibial components: an in vivo roentgen stereophotogrammetric analysis. J Orthop Res 1993;11:142–8.

15. Dunbar MJ, Fong JW, Wilson DA, et al. Longitudinal migration and inducible displacement of the mobility total ankle system. Acta Orthop 2012;83:394–400.

16. Ryd L, Albrektsson BE, Carlsson L, et al. Roentgen stereophotogrammetric analysis as a predictor of mechanical loosening of knee prostheses. J Bone Joint Surg Br 1995;77:377–83.

17. Kärrholm J, Borssén B, Löwenhielm G, et al. Does early micromotion of femoral stem prostheses matter? 4-7-year stereoradiographic follow-up of 84 cemented prostheses. J Bone Joint Surg Br 1994;76:912–7.

18. Brigido SA, Wobst GM, Galli MM, et al. Evaluating component migration after modular stem fixed-bearing total ankle replacement. J Foot Ankle Surg 2015; 54:326–31.

19. Rodriguez D, Bevernage BD, Maldague P, et al. Medium term follow-up of the AES ankle prosthesis: high rate of asymptomatic osteolysis. Foot Ankle Surg 2010;16:54–60.

20. Knecht SI, Estin M, Callaghan JJ, et al. The Agility total ankle arthroplasty. Seven to sixteen-year follow-up. J Bone Joint Surg Am 2004;86-A:1161–71.

21. Wood PL, Prem H, Sutton C. Total ankle replacement: medium-term results in 200 Scandinavian total ankle replacements. J Bone Joint Surg Br 2008;90:605–9.

22. Koivu H, Kohonen I, Sipola E, et al. Severe periprosthetic osteolytic lesions after the Ankle Evolutive System total ankle replacement. J Bone Joint Surg Br 2009; 91:907–14.

23. Morgan SS, Brooke B, Harris NJ. Total ankle replacement by the Ankle Evolution System: medium-term outcome. J Bone Joint Surg Br 2010;92:61–5.

24. Kokkonen A, Ikävalko M, Tiihonen R, et al. High rate of osteolytic lesions in medium-term followup after the AES total ankle replacement. Foot Ankle Int 2011;32:168–75.

25. Besse JL, Brito N, Lienhart C. Clinical evaluation and radiographic assessment of bone lysis of the AES total ankle replacement. Foot Ankle Int 2009;30:964–75.

26. Cracchiolo A 3rd, Deorio JK. Design features of current total ankle replacements: implants and instrumentation. J Am Acad Orthop Surg 2008;16:530–40.

27. Saltzman CL, Mann RA, Ahrens JE, et al. Prospective controlled trial of STAR total ankle replacement versus ankle fusion: initial results. Foot Ankle Int 2009;30: 579–96.

28. Deorio JK, Easley ME. Total ankle arthroplasty. Instr Course Lect 2008;57: 383–413.
29. Criswell BJ, Douglas K, Naik R, et al. High revision and reoperation rates using the Agility™ total ankle system. Clin Orthop Relat Res 2012;470:1980–6.
30. Easley ME, Adams SB Jr, Hembree WC, et al. Results of total ankle arthroplasty. J Bone Joint Surg Am 2011;93:1455–68.
31. Nunley JA, Caputo AM, Easley ME, et al. Intermediate to long-term outcomes of the STAR total ankle replacement: the patient perspective. J Bone Joint Surg Am 2012;94:43–8.
32. Schweitzer KM, Adams SB, Viens NA, et al. Early prospective clinical results of a modern fixed-bearing total ankle arthroplasty. J Bone Joint Surg Am 2013;95: 1002–11.
33. Hopgood P, Kumar R, Wood PL. Ankle arthrodesis for failed total ankle replacement. J Bone Joint Surg Br 2006;88:1032–8.
34. Guyer AJ, Richardson G. Current concepts review: total ankle arthroplasty. Foot Ankle Int 2008;29:256–64.
35. Cerrato R, Myerson MS. Total ankle replacement: the Agility LP prosthesis. Foot Ankle Clin 2008;13:485–94.
36. Hurowitz EJ, Gould JS, Fleisig GS, et al. Outcome analysis of agility total ankle replacement with prior adjunctive procedures: two to six year followup. Foot Ankle Int 2007;28:308–12.
37. Roukis TS. Incidence of revision after primary implantation of the Agility™ total ankle replacement system: a systematic review. J Foot Ankle Surg 2012;51: 198–204.
38. McCollum G, Myerson MS. Failure of the Agility total ankle replacement system and the salvage options. Clin Podiatr Med Surg 2013;30:207–23.
39. Hsu AR, Haddad SL. Early clinical and radiographic outcomes of intramedullary-fixation total ankle arthroplasty. J Bone Joint Surg Am 2015;97:194–200.
40. Abicht BP, Roukis TS. The INBONE II total ankle system. Clin Podiatr Med Surg 2013;30:47–68.
41. Kim BS, Knupp M, Zwicky L, et al. Total ankle replacement in association with hindfoot fusion: outcome and complications. J Bone Joint Surg Br 2010;92: 1540–7.
42. Lewis JS Jr, Adams SB Jr, Queen RM, et al. Outcomes after total ankle replacement in association with ipsilateral hindfoot arthrodesis. Foot Ankle Int 2014;35: 535–42.
43. Adams SB Jr, Demetracopoulos CA, Queen RM, et al. Early to mid-term results of fixed-bearing total ankle arthroplasty with a modular intramedullary tibial component. J Bone Joint Surg Am 2014;96:1983–9.
44. Miller AN, Prasarn ML, Dyke JP, et al. Quantitative assessment of the vascularity of the talus with gadolinium-enhanced magnetic resonance imaging. J Bone Joint Surg Am 2011;93:1116–21.
45. Tennant JN, Rungprai C, Pizzimenti MA, et al. Risks to the blood supply of the talus with four methods of total ankle arthroplasty: a cadaveric injection study. J Bone Joint Surg Am 2014;96:395–402.
46. Manes HR, Alvarez E, Llevine LS. Preliminary report of total ankle arthroplasty for osteonecrosis of the talus. Clin Orthop Relat Res 1977;(127):200–2.
47. Devalia KL, Ramaskandhan J, Muthumayandi K, et al. Early results of a novel technique: Hindfoot fusion in talus osteonecrosis prior to ankle arthroplasty: A case series. Foot (Edinb) 2015;25:200–5.

48. Lee KB, Cho SG, Jung ST, et al. Total ankle arthroplasty following revascularization of avascular necrosis of the talar body: two case reports and literature review. Foot Ankle Int 2008;29:852–8.

49. Haskell A, Mann RA. Ankle arthroplasty with preoperative coronal plane deformity: short-term results. Clin Orthop Relat Res 2004;(424):98–103.

50. Hobson SA, Karantana A, Dhar S. Total ankle replacement in patients with significant pre-operative deformity of the hindfoot. J Bone Joint Surg Br 2009;91:481–6.

51. Kim BS, Choi WJ, Kim YS, et al. Total ankle replacement in moderate to severe varus deformity of the ankle. J Bone Joint Surg Br 2009;91:1183–90.

52. Wood PL, Deakin S. Total ankle replacement. The results in 200 ankles. J Bone Joint Surg Br 2003;85:334–41.

53. Henricson A, Ågren PH. Secondary surgery after total ankle replacement. The influence of preoperative hindfoot alignment. Foot Ankle Surg 2007;13:41–4.

54. Choi WJ, Yoon HS, Lee JW. Techniques for managing varus and valgus malalignment during total ankle replacement. Clin Podiatr Med Surg 2013;30:35–46.

55. Queen RM, Adams SB Jr, Viens NA, et al. Differences in outcomes following total ankle replacement in patients with neutral alignment compared with tibiotalar joint malalignment. J Bone Joint Surg Am 2013;95:1927–34.

56. Sung KS, Ahn J, Lee KH, et al. Short-term results of total ankle arthroplasty for end-stage ankle arthritis with severe varus deformity. Foot Ankle Int 2014;35: 225–31.

57. Doets HC, Brand R, Nelissen RG. Total ankle arthroplasty in inflammatory joint disease with use of two mobile-bearing designs. J Bone Joint Surg Am 2006; 88:1272–84.

58. Kotnis R, Pasapula C, Anwar F, et al. The management of failed ankle replacement. J Bone Joint Surg Br 2006;88:1039–47.

59. Brigido SA, Wobst GM, Galli MM, et al. Evaluating component migration: comparing two generations of the INBONE(®) total ankle replacement. J Foot Ankle Surg 2015;54:892–5.

60. Jonck JH, Myerson MS. Revision total ankle replacement. Foot Ankle Clin 2012; 17:687–706.

61. Coester LM, Saltzman CL, Leupold J, et al. Long-term results following ankle arthrodesis for post-traumatic arthritis. J Bone Joint Surg Am 2001;83-A:219–28.

62. Fuchs S, Sandmann C, Skwara A, et al. Quality of life 20 years after arthrodesis of the ankle. A study of adjacent joints. J Bone Joint Surg Br 2003;85:994–8.

63. Papa JA, Myerson MS. Pantalar and tibiotalocalcaneal arthrodesis for post-traumatic osteoarthrosis of the ankle and hindfoot. J Bone Joint Surg Am 1992; 74:1042–9.

64. Kile TA, Donnelly RE, Gehrke JC, et al. Tibiotalocalcaneal arthrodesis with an intramedullary device. Foot Ankle Int 1994;15:669–73.

65. Culpan P, Le Strat V, Piriou P, et al. Arthrodesis after failed total ankle replacement. J Bone Joint Surg Br 2007;89:1178–83.

66. Berkowitz MJ, Clare MP, Walling AK, et al. Salvage of failed total ankle arthroplasty with fusion using structural allograft and internal fixation. Foot Ankle Int 2011;32:S493–502.

67. Jeng CL, Campbell JT, Tang EY, et al. Tibiotalocalcaneal arthrodesis with bulk femoral head allograft for salvage of large defects in the ankle. Foot Ankle Int 2013;34:1256–66.

68. Myerson MS, Won HY. Primary and revision total ankle replacement using custom-designed prostheses. Foot Ankle Clin 2008;13:521–38.

69. Doets HC, Zürcher AW. Salvage arthrodesis for failed total ankle arthroplasty. Acta Orthop 2010;81:142–7.
70. Kharwadkar N, Harris NJ. Revision of STAR total ankle replacement to hybrid AES-STAR total ankle replacement-a report of two cases. Foot Ankle Surg 2009;15:101–5.
71. Assal M, Greisberg J, Hansen ST Jr. Revision total ankle arthroplasty: conversion of New Jersey Low Contact Stress to Agility: surgical technique and case report. Foot Ankle Int 2004;25:922–5.
72. Gould JS. Revision total ankle arthroplasty. Am J Orthop (Belle Mead NJ) 2005; 34:361.
73. Hintermann B, Barg A, Knupp M. Revision arthroplasty of the ankle joint. Orthopade 2011;40:1000–7 [in German].
74. Ellington JK, Gupta S, Myerson MS. Management of failures of total ankle replacement with the agility total ankle arthroplasty. J Bone Joint Surg Am 2013;95:2112–8.
75. Ketz J, Myerson M, Sanders R. The salvage of complex hindfoot problems with use of a custom talar total ankle prosthesis. J Bone Joint Surg Am 2012;94: 1194–200.
76. Hanna RS, Haddad SL, Lazarus ML. Evaluation of periprosthetic lucency after total ankle arthroplasty: helical CT versus conventional radiography. Foot Ankle Int 2007;28:921–6.
77. Schuberth JM, Christensen JC, Rialson JA. Metal-reinforced cement augmentation for complex talar subsidence in failed total ankle arthroplasty. J Foot Ankle Surg 2011;50:766–72.

Soft Tissue Reconstruction After Total Ankle Arthroplasty

Yash J. Avashia, MD[a], Ronnie L. Shammas, BS[b],
Suhail K. Mithani, MD[c], Selene G. Parekh, MD, MBA[d],*

KEYWORDS

- Ankle replacement • Soft tissue complications • Wound complications • Flap

KEY POINTS

- Soft tissue management of total ankle replacements begins in the operating room with the use of preventative measures for wound complications.
- Soft tissue and wound complications should be managed with a team approach including the orthopedic surgeon, a plastic surgeon, and perhaps a vascular surgeon or wound care specialist.
- A methodical approach should be taken to managing wound complications following total ankle replacement, with the use of a variety of possible flaps as needed.

INTRODUCTION

End-stage ankle arthrosis is known to cause chronic disability due to its severe impact on pain, health-related quality of life, and function.[1] Although ankle arthrodesis was previously considered the gold standard for treatment, total ankle arthroplasty (TAA) has emerged as a viable alternative treatment. TAA has been performed in selected patients with end-stage ankle arthritis secondary to idiopathic, traumatic, and inflammatory etiologies.

Since the release of the first-generation TAA design in the 1970s to the current day third- and fourth-generation designs, TAAs have seen a reduction in complication profile. However, significant risks still apply. Wound healing problems of the anterior

Disclosure Statement: The authors have nothing to disclose.
[a] Division of Plastic Surgery, Duke University, Room 135, Brown Zone, Duke South, Durham, NC 27710, USA; [b] Division of Plastic Surgery, Duke University, Room 135, Brown Zone, Duke South, Durham, NC 27710, USA; [c] Division of Plastic Surgery, Department of Orthopaedic Surgery, Duke University, 3609 Southwest Durham Drive, Durham, NC 27707, USA; [d] North Carolina Orthopaedic Clinic, Department of Orthopaedic Surgery, Fuqua Business School, Duke University, 3609 Southwest Durham Drive, Durham, NC 27707, USA
* Corresponding author.
E-mail address: selene.parekh@gmail.com

incision can be seen in up to 28% of patients undergoing a TAA.[1,2] Outcomes from a recent meta-analysis showed that the highest risk of TAA failures was with the following complications: deep tissue infection, aseptic loosening of hardware, and implant failure.[3,4] Failures were salvaged with revision of the TAA in the majority of ankles (62%), whereas amputations were rare. Factors that have shown to result in a statistically significant increase in complications include a patient history of diabetes mellitus and smoking, whereas factors that are associated with an increased trend in complications included female sex, history of corticosteroid use, and an underlying inflammatory arthritis.[3,4]

Advancements in soft tissue reconstructive techniques have revolutionized the treatment of traumatic foot and ankle injuries and improved success in limb salvage.[5–7] The collaboration of plastic surgeons and orthopedic surgeons has exponentially improved the treatment of complex foot and ankle problems. A recent retrospective review by Cho and colleagues[8] demonstrated TAA accounting for 22% of all elective orthopedic foot and ankle procedures requiring plastic surgery intervention, with dorsal ankle wounds accounting for 36% of all postoperative referrals for soft tissue management. With the ability to transfer both local and free tissues, salvage of soft tissue complication is often successful and durable.

PREVENTATIVE MEASURES

Although managing soft tissue complications is of importance in patients with TAA, preventative measures have tantamount value. As a preventative strategy, patient selection is critical in minimizing complications. Avoiding higher risk patients with poorly controlled diabetes, peripheral neuropathy, vascular compromise, current smoking, and immunocompromise is advisable, as these have been shown to increase wound complications in foot and ankle surgery.[2] In a retrospective study of 106 TAAs, there was a significant association between inflammatory connective tissue disease, diabetes, and corticosteroid use in patients with wound complications.[9] A patient's medical history must be considered in its entirety before making the judgment as to whether they are a suitable candidate for TAA, and when planning for the proper postoperative care in patients who may be more predisposed to suffer from wound healing complications. Even with attention toward patient selection, the complication rate of TAA still varies between 20% and 28%.[10] Current literature shows revision rates between 14% and 32% at 5 years.[10] While the most common reasons for revision of TAA are aseptic loosening, osteolysis, and talar collapse, deep infection and wound healing problems have also been implicated in failure of TAA.[4]

Meticulous surgical technique in skin closure in conjunction with adjunctive measures designed to minimize wound tension and edema can potentially help reduce the need for postoperative plastic surgery consultation. The authors routinely use a continuous external tissue expander (CETE) in conjunction with negative pressure wound therapy at the time of primary arthroplasty in an attempt to reduce the frequency of wound complications following TAA (**Fig. 1**).

Continuous External Tissue Expander

The goal of this device is to help facilitate wound closure through a more accurate approximation of the skin tissue edge, while also relieving tension from the incision line. A previous study described the use of the Dermaclose CETE (Wound Care Technologies, Incorporated, Chanhassen, Minnesota) as a prophylactic measure to manage surgical incisions of the ankle following TAA.[11] The authors of this study employed the use of CETE in patients who were deemed to be at an increased risk

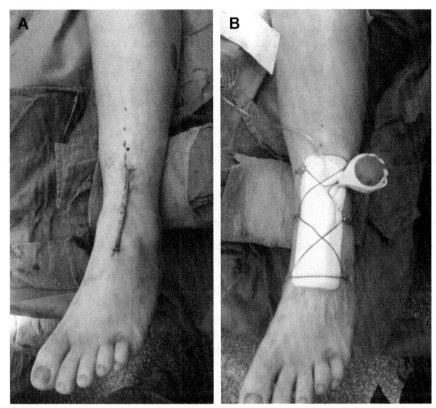

Fig. 1. (A) TAA anterior midline closure. (B) Application of continuous external tissue expander device over negative pressure dressing.

for wound complications. In a series of more than 35 cases utilizing CETE, the authors witnessed a significant decrease in wound-related complications compared with previous patients who underwent standard skin closures. The potential drawbacks of using this device include a theoretically increased risk of skin necrosis secondary to the application of excess tension, and the device's added cost.

Negative Pressure Wound Therapy

Delayed wound healing is one of the most commonly cited complications following TAA, ranging from 4% to 28%.[11] Wound complications following total ankle arthroplasty are multifactorial; however, a general understanding of the current techniques in postoperative wound care may help reduce the occurrence of these complications. There has also been interest in the literature investigating the use of negative pressure wound therapy (NPWT) following TAA as a means to improve patient outcomes following incisional closure.[12] The use of NPWT as a means to improve incisional healing of the foot and ankle has been described, with good patient outcomes and significantly improved rates of wound healing.[12-14]

Postoperative Considerations

Currently, there is no standard for postoperative TAA wound care, with many surgeons choosing to use a combination of dry dressings, casts or splints, and controlled ankle movement boots. Proper postoperative dressing following TAA should focus on reducing tension to the incision pressure and preventative measures for postoperative swelling. For example, immobilization through casting with the foot in dorsiflexion may inadvertently encourage early postoperative edema at the suture line of the ankle. Postoperative swelling may complicate and delay wound healing by decreasing blood flow to the surgical site. Thus, a consideration of how to best address this complication is warranted. Schipper and colleagues[15] described a postoperative compression wrap protocol in TAAs. They reported a significant improvement in wound healing and decreased wound-related complications compared with prior postoperative dressings, which included a padded circumferential cast. In addition, the authors state that an additional advantage of their protocol is the close monitoring of the operative incisions every 2 to 3 days during dressing changes. This allows for prompt action in response to a compromised surgical site.

MANAGEMENT OF WOUND COMPLICATIONS

The standard surgical approach to TAA is through an anterior midline incision extending from the dorsum of the foot to the distal lower portion of the leg. When incisional wound complications occur, there is limited flexibility for conservative management due to the shallow nature of the skin and limited local soft-tissue coverage overlying the arthroplasty. Therefore, an aggressive approach to identifying and treating incisional dehiscence or necrosis is warranted. Management of these complications should be undertaken by a surgeon who is facile in multimodal treatment of wounds, with expertise in vascularized tissue transfer.

Surgical decision making in plastic surgery is complicated by the vast array of procedures suitable for each problem. The reconstructive ladder is a decision-making tool used by plastic surgeons that provides a progressive approach to wound management. This begins with primary wound closure, advancing to grafts, local flaps, and then distant or free tissue transfer.

In the context of the reconstructive ladder, relevant structures requiring coverage in a patient with total ankle arthroplasty include the implant, bone, tendon, muscle, and neurovascular structures. Because these wounds typically occur would some element of edema and resultant vascular compromise of the operative bed, delayed primary closure and primary skin grafting are not typically viable salvage options. Therefore, the true abridged reconstructive ladder for TAA wounds begins with engineered dermal substitutes in combination with skin grafting, followed by local flaps, and ends with free-tissue transfer (**Table 1**). Due to the limited amount of tissue between skin and underlying hardware in total ankle arthroplasty, an aggressive approach to reconstructive management of postoperative wound complications is necessary.

Negative Pressure Wound Therapy, Dermal Regeneration Matrix, and Skin Grafts

NPWT may be employed in limited situations for TAA wound management. This may start during the acute wound management phase when NPWT is used to improve granulation tissue growth on the wound bed to later accommodate the use of skin grafting or dermal substitute. It must be emphasized, however, that the use of negative pressure therapy for total ankle wound complications is limited because of the tenuous wound bed and limited soft-tissue coverage between the skin and the arthroplasty. Its use should be limited to those wounds that are partial thickness through the skin without exposure of underlying structures. In the authors' experience, this is the minority of situations, and thus application of NPWT should be employed sparingly except as a temporary bridge to definitive operative intervention.

Table 1		
Total ankle arthroplasty soft tissue reconstruction options		
Split Thickness Skin Grafting (STSG) Dermal Substitute + STSG	Local Tissue Flaps Reverse Sural Flap Propeller Flap Bipedicle Flap	Free Tissue Transfer Radial Forearm Free Flap (Fasciocutaneous)
• Intact periosteum	• Intact distal run-off	Latissimus Dorsi Free Flap
• Intact peritenon	from AT, PT, or P	(Myocutaneous)
• Uninfected wound	• Prior wound infection	• Poor local soft tissue
• No exposed hardware	• Exposed hardware	options
• Minor dehiscence	• Exposed bone with	• Intact distal run-off
• Small wounds	periosteal stripping	from AT, PT, or P
	• Medium sized wounds	• Prior wound infection
		• Exposed hardware
		• Exposed bone with
		periosteal stripping
		• Large deep wounds

Abbreviations: AT, anterior tibial artery; PT, posterior tibial artery; P, peroneal artery.

In a full-thickness wound with outstanding vascularity, split-thickness skin grafting may be a viable option for reconstruction. Its application in TAA wound complications is also limited because of the same issues, which limit application of NPWT. Often, wounds require more aggressive management with operative debridement employed as an initial intervention for the elimination of avascular tissue or require coverage with vascularized tissue.

In the setting of full-thickness injury with exposure of the underlying tenderness structures with intact peritenon, dermal substitutes have been used to provide better surfacing to the ankle wound and improve the reliability of the wound bed for STSG. The use of dermal substitute also aids in allowing tendons to glide without the negative effects of skin graft contracture and adhesions to underlying tendons. In the authors' experience, this is typically employed in conjunction with an operative debridement to ensure a sterile environment and avoid contamination of the underlying arthroplasty. Office debridements are generally not advisable for wound complications after TAA. The authors apply an occlusive dressing and schedule an operative intervention within 24 hours of recognition of the wound complication.

Integra Dermal regeneration template (Lifesciences, Plainsboro, New Jersey) is a bilayer dermal substitute consisting of a deep dermal layer with a collagen–glycosaminoglycan biodegradable matrix and a superficial layer of semipermeable silicone. The patient's native fibroblasts infiltrate the deep dermal layer and synthesize a neodermis, which is histologically similar in appearance and structure to normal dermis. This outer silicone layer is a temporary layer that prevents dessication of the substitute during its initial phases of incorporation into the patient's wound bed. Four weeks after application, after formation of the neodermis, the silicone layer is removed, and a split-thickness skin grafting may be performed for definitive wound coverage (**Fig. 2**).

Advantages of using dermal substitutes over local flaps are reduced operative time and no significant donor site morbidity. Its use, however, must be limited to settings in which the deeper structures are not exposed. There must be some vascularity to the wound bed. As such, these are applied in an operating room setting with backup plans in place for potential vascularized tissue coverage should the wound bed not appear to be sufficient to enable vascular ingrowth after excisional debridement of compromised tissue. The disadvantage with the 2-staged dermal substitute technique is the requirement for a second operation for skin grafting and its donor site morbidity, but both stages can be performed in an outpatient setting.

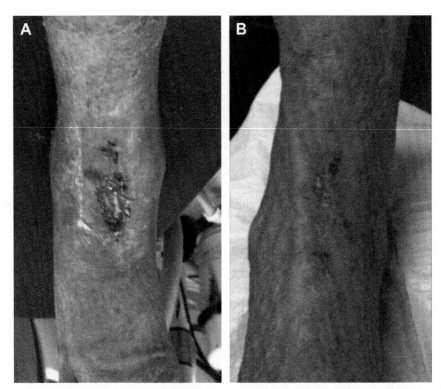

Fig. 2. 69-year-old woman who underwent TAA arthroplasty for persistent right ankle and hindfoot pain secondary to primary osteoarthritis. Postoperative course was complicated by a nonhealing wound of the anterior ankle. Two-staged dermal substitute and skin grafting were elected for reconstruction due to adequate wound bed vascularity and wound size. (A) Wound after application of dermal substitute. (B) Graft/wound site 2 months postoperatively.

Local Flaps

Local tissue flaps are employed when the wound bed is deemed to not have sufficient vascularity to allow for direct grafting or application of a dermal regenerative substitute and if the patient has robust vasculature to allow rotation of adjacent tissue. Selection of local flaps is typically at the discretion of an experienced reconstructive surgeon with expertise in these areas. The technical aspects of elevation and transposition of these types of reconstructive options can be challenging. Various options are available, which are employed in a tailored fashion depending upon individual patient tissue needs.

Reverse sural flap

The fasciocutaneous blood supply of the lower leg consists of septocutaneous and musculocutaneous perforators, fortified by a neuro-venocutaneous plexus.[16]

Championed by Masquelet and colleagues,[17] the distally based reverse sural flap is a skin island flap supplied by the vascular axis of the sural nerve. This was demonstrated by a color latex injection study mapping the vascularity to the skin from arteries accompanying the nerves. The flap is relatively versatile and can be applied to wounds and defects of the anterior ankle, malleoli, and heel (Fig. 3). Further anatomic studies

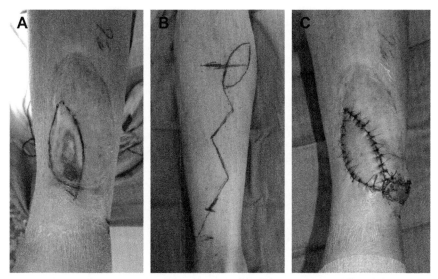

Fig. 3. Patient with an anterior ankle wound managed by reverse sural flap. (*A*) Intraoperative appearance of wound with exposed tibialis anterior tendon. (*B*) Flap markings on posterior aspect of leg. (*C*) Anterior ankle after elevation and inset of reverse sural flap.

have defined that there are 2 longitudinal rows of perforators in the distal sural nerve region from either the posterior tibial or peroneal artery.

Venous drainage in this distally based flap has always been an issue of concern, as it relies on communications between the venae comitantes of the sural nerve and lesser saphenous vein, which do not have valves as the deep venous system of the lower extremity.[18] In a retrospective review of 70 reverse sural flaps, the necrosis rate was 11% in healthy patients, 33% in patients with systemic disease, and 60% when patients had diabetes mellitus, venous insufficiency, or peripheral arterial disease.[19]

Propeller flaps

Making use of peroneal and posterior tibial artery perforators, propeller flaps for distal leg and ankle wounds provide an option for soft tissue reconstruction. The term propeller flap was coined in 1991, an adipocutaneous flap based on a central pedicle may be rotated 90° around its pedicle pivot point.[20] This technique was furthered by Hallock, who reported a similar fasciocutaneous flap that was based on a skeletonized perforator and rotated 180° on an eccentric pivot point.[21] Benefits of the propeller flap are a relatively fast harvest without the need for microsurgery (**Fig. 4**).

Venous congestion is the most frequent complication of propeller flaps, because veins are more prone to torsion than arteries. Common to most flaps of the lower extremity, temporary congestion should be distinguished from true venous insufficiency of the flap. Management of venous congestion for lower extremity fasciocutaneous flaps includes a combination of leech therapy with or without flap dis-insetting and close follow-up and management of secondary wounds. Arterial insufficiency occurs in roughly 5% of cases and is typically limited to necrosis of the skin with preserved underlying subcutaneous tissue. Removal of the eschar normally leaves a well-vascularized subcutaneous wound bed that is amenable for skin grafting or healing by secondary intention.

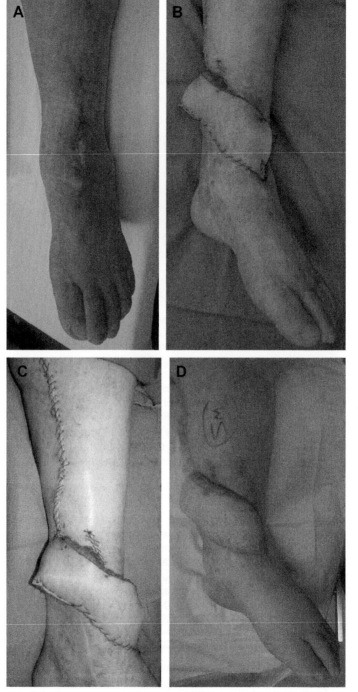

Fig. 4. 69-year-old woman with multiple comorbidities who developed post-traumatic left ankle arthritis. TAA was performed, which was complicated by a nonhealing wound of the anterior ankle with exposed tibialis anterior tendon and limited wound bed vascularity. (*A*) The patient had adequate tissue in the distal third of the lower extremity for a propeller flap. Intraoperatively, Doppler ultrasound aided to identify potential perforators from the posterior tibial artery. (*B*, *C*) Posterior tibial artery pedicled propeller flap inset for wound coverage. (*D*) No wound issues 2 months postoperatively. Subsequent flap debulking and liposuction were performed to improve contour.

Use of these types of flaps is limited to patients who have no distal vascular atherosclerotic disease and typically have strongly palpable pulses.

Bipedicle flaps

Compared with the other anatomic regions, the lower extremity provides the option to raise long longitudinal flaps. The posterior tibial artery provides an advantage to the anterior tibial artery and peroneal artery perforators due its larger caliber perforators.[22] A bipedicle flap receives blood supply from 2 pedicles. Lower extremity bipedicle flaps may be supplied on the posterior tibial, anterior tibial, or peroneal artery perforators. The flaps are based both superiorly and inferiorly with undermining of the flap centrally. These flaps may be advanced over a defect for inset and closure. Donor sites may be closed primarily by undermining or skin grafted. The most distal septocutaneous perforator from the anterior tibial system arises approximately 17 to 22 cm distal to the tibial condyle and runs beneath the extensor digitorum longus muscle. The lateral malleolar artery, a branch off of the anterior tibial artery, serves as the vascular supply for an anteriorly based bipedicle flap. This flap may be used for anterior ankle wounds encountered after TAA.

With limited donor-site morbidity, these flaps provide superior skin color and texture matching due to their adjacent location. Importantly, the harvest and use of a bipedicled flap does not irreversibly distort local vascular anatomy, allowing secondary reconstructive options to remain viable if the bipedicle flap fails. Bipedicled flaps require that the skin and subcutaneous tissue adjacent to the wound are viable to allow for the elevation of a healthy flap and blood supply. Although not substantially reported, the observed complication rate for bipedicle flap may be as high 30%.[23] Application of this type of reconstruction should be undertaken judiciously, and its use is likely limited to small defects.

Free tissue transfer

Free tissue transfer is the most commonly advised reconstructive procedure for defects of the distal third of the leg, including defects of the ankle. This is dictated by a paucity of options for local flaps. The inherent form and function of the foot and ankle also influence types of flap chosen for reconstruction with a goal of matching quantity and quality of tissues. For example, a relatively thick and nonpliable mycocutaneous flap may not be the best option for an anterior ankle wound, as it does not accommodate for range of ankle motion and shoe wearing.

Autologous free tissue transfers for ankle defects rely heavily on arterial anatomy for vascular anastomosis. Although not imperative, obtaining preoperative angiogram provides information to help delineate available vascular sources for flap inflow.[8] Arterial anastomosis can be performed either end-to-end or end-to-side to one of the main lower extremity vessels: anterior tibial, posterior tibial, or peroneal artery. An end-to-side anastomosis may be performed in patients with single-vessel runoff to preserve distal perfusion. A lower extremity Allen test can provide additional information in the patient who does not have vascular imaging.

Free tissue transfer is superior to other forms of soft tissue reconstruction due to its vascularity, tissue quality, and no limitations as far as manipulation of the tissues to accommodate defect size. Although a local fasciocutaneous flap from the lower leg serves predominantly to provide a 2-dimensional reconstructive option for foot and ankle defects, free tissue transfers provide 3-dimensional fill to appropriately circumscribe tendons and exposed bone.[24]

Free tissues available for soft tissue reconstruction may be categorized into free fasciocutaneous flaps or free muscle and/or musculocutaneous flaps. Workhorse flaps for TAA reconstruction include the radial forearm free flap and latissimus dorsi free flap. Although there are several options available for donor sites, the radial forearm free flap provides an appropriate size and tissue volume to address many of the large- and medium-sized defects in TAA patients (**Fig. 5**). This is the authors' preferred method for treatment of deeper wound complications in TAA.

Despite the longer operative time and inpatient admission required for utilization of free tissue transfer, it has proven, in the authors' experience, to be the most reliable method to obtain durable soft tissue coverage in the setting of significant wound complication after TAA.

POSTOPERATIVE MANAGEMENT
Skin Graft or Dermal Substitute Application

Both split-thickness skin grafts and dermal substitutes follow analogous steps for healing. The three phases for skin graft take include plasmatic imbibition, inosculation, and angiogenesis. Skin grafts reach the third phase at around 5 days, and continue to mature over the course of a year. During the initial 5 days, the skin graft is tenuous and requires appropriate dressing.

To avoid complications of fluid collection (seroma or hematoma) and shear forces to the graft until all wound areas have closed, a compression dressing in the form of a bolster should be applied. Vacuum-assisted pressure devices can also be used with a protective interface of petroleum gauze to permit continuous compression on the graft and fluid removal. The first dressing change should take place at 5 days when revascularization has occurred and the graft is well adhered to the wound bed. Split-thickness skin grafts require a moist environment for healing due to the absence of adnexal glands structures that provide this function. Daily moist dressings are applied for up to 2 to 4 weeks, at which point the wound care is transitioned to a topical moisturizer for the remaining year as the graft matures.

Local Adjacent Tissue Transfer

Although local tissue transfers have a relatively reliable vascular source, immediate postoperative care should focus on monitoring the flap for signs of arterial and venous insufficiency. Any arterial insufficiency should be observed throughout the initial weeks. Secondary wounds caused by distal flap ischemia and necrosis may be managed nonoperatively with local wet-to-dry wound care. Venous congestion, however, may threaten the entire flap's survival. For pedicled flaps, troubleshooting a congested flap includes a systematic approach that begins with releasing sutures and often ends with the use of leech therapy. The flap may be delayed if venous congestion is encountered intraoperatively or immediately postoperatively.

Lower extremity elevation is critical in the postoperative period to promote venous blood return. Depending on the local flap and initial postoperative examination, the patient may be allowed to place the lower extremity in a dependent position. Weight-bearing instructions often will be dictated by the stability and hardware concerns related to the TAA. Local flaps do not interfere with the ability to bear weight on a lower extremity.

Free Tissue Transfer

Postoperative care for free tissue transfer is centered on flap monitoring. The microvascular anastomosis is a critical component of the procedure, and complications may arise from thrombosis of the arterial or venous anastomosis. Although the gold standard for flap monitoring is the physical examination, new adjunct technologies

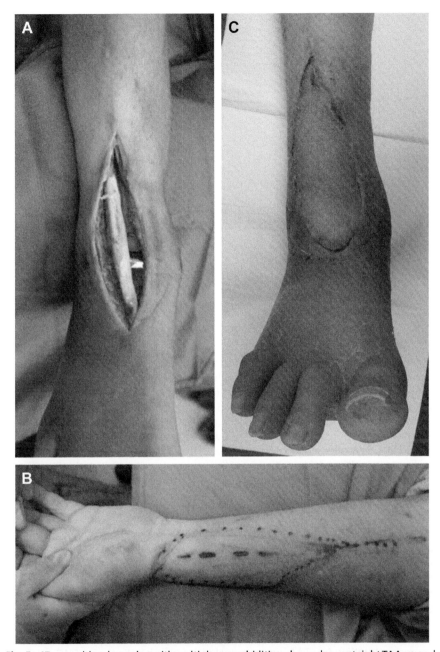

Fig. 5. 47-year-old male smoker with multiple comorbidities who underwent right TAA secondary to significant degenerative joint disease. Five years following the initial surgery, the patient continued to experience stiffness and pain in his right ankle. It was recommended that the patient undergo further arthrodesis with an anterior approach and debridement of the heterotopic ossification around his ankle. (*A*) Following this procedure, the patient suffered from swelling and edema of the lower extremity with wound dehiscence and an exposed tibialis anterior tendon at the wound base. (*B*) A radial forearm free flap from the patient's nondominant hand was planned for wound coverage after poly exchange. (*C*) Appearance of ankle 2 months after procedure with uneventful healing and return to ambulation.

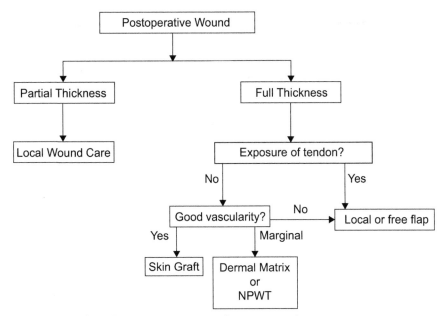

Fig. 6. Options for soft tissue reconstruction for TAA wounds.

have provided plastic surgeons with additional information to better assess the microvascular anastomosis patency and flap viability. Some of these technologies include the implantable microvascular Doppler and transcutaneous tissue oxygenation probe. Typically a patient is admitted for 4 to 5 days after a microvascular procedure. Because of the tenuous nature of the microvascular anastomosis, postoperative lower extremity elevation is required for the first 2 weeks. Transfers from bed to chair may be initiated at 4 days after surgery with leg elevation at all times. After 2 weeks, progressive increase in dependent positioning of the lower extremity is initiated, with weight-bearing instructions dictated by the status of the TAA.

SUMMARY

TAA is an option for patients suffering from end-stage ankle arthrosis. This procedure is associated with wound-healing complications at the ankle. Advancements in soft tissue reconstructive techniques have revolutionized the treatment of traumatic foot and ankle injuries and improved success in limb salvage. In lower limb reconstruction, defects of the lower third of the leg are a challenging problem, due to the paucity of local tissues available for reconstruction. Accurate patient selection, preoperative planning, and careful attention to perioperative and postoperative dressings are mandatory to prevent complications. Options for soft tissue reconstruction for TAA wounds include a combination of NPWT, dermal substitutes and skin grafting, local fasciocutaneous flaps, and free tissue transfer (**Fig. 6**). Prompt recognition of wound-healing complications and aggressive management are of paramount importance in successful salvage. Because of the paucity of tissue, successful salvage necessitates a low threshold for operative debridement and vascularized wound coverage. Postoperative management to address lower extremity venous stasis and swelling aids in improving reconstructive outcomes.

REFERENCES

1. Glazebrook M, Daniels T, Younger A, et al. Comparison of health-related quality of life between patients with end-stage ankle and hip arthrosis. J Bone Joint Surg Am 2008;90(3):499–505.
2. Whalen JL, Spelsberg SC, Murray P. Wound breakdown after total ankle arthroplasty. Foot Ankle Int 2010;31(4):301–5.
3. Gougoulias N, Khanna A, Maffulli N. How successful are current ankle replacements? A systematic review of the literature. Clin Orthop Relat Res 2010; 468(1):199–208.
4. Henricson A, Nilsson JA, Carlsson A. 10-year survival of total ankle arthroplasties: a report on 780 cases from the Swedish Ankle Register. Acta Orthop 2011;82(6): 655–9.
5. Lerman OZ, Kovach SJ, Levin LS. The respective roles of plastic and orthopedic surgery in limb salvage. Plast Reconstr Surg 2011;127(Suppl 1):215s–27s.
6. Levin LS. The reconstructive ladder. An orthoplastic approach. Orthop Clin North Am 1993;24(3):393–409.
7. Levin LS, Condit DP. Combined injuries—soft tissue management. Clin Orthop Relat Res 1996;(327):172–81.
8. Cho EH, Garcia R, Pien I, et al. An algorithmic approach for managing orthopaedic surgical wounds of the foot and ankle. Clin Orthop Relat Res 2014;472(6): 1921–9.
9. Raikin SM, Kane J, Ciminiello ME. Risk factors for incision-healing complications following total ankle arthroplasty. J Bone Joint Surg Am 2010;92(12):2150–5.
10. Noelle S, Egidy CC, Cross MB, et al. Complication rates after total ankle arthroplasty in one hundred consecutive prostheses. Int Orthop 2013;37(9):1789–94.
11. Huh J, Parekh SG. Use of a continuous external tissue expander in total ankle arthroplasty: a novel augment to wound closure. Foot Ankle Spec 2016;9(1):43–7.
12. DeCarbo WT, Hyer CF. Negative-pressure wound therapy applied to high-risk surgical incisions. J Foot Ankle Surg 2010;49(3):299–300.
13. Matsumoto T, Parekh SG. Use of negative pressure wound therapy on closed surgical incision after total ankle arthroplasty. Foot Ankle Int 2015;36(7):787–94.
14. Goldstein JA, Iorio ML, Brown B, et al. The use of negative pressure wound therapy for random local flaps at the ankle region. J Foot Ankle Surg 2010;49(6): 513–6.
15. Schipper ON, Hsu AR, Haddad SL. Reduction in wound complications after total ankle arthroplasty using a compression wrap protocol. Foot Ankle Int 2015; 36(12):1448–54.
16. Follmar KE, Baccarani A, Baumeister SP, et al. The distally based sural flap. Plast Reconstr Surg 2007;119(6):138e–48e.
17. Masquelet AC, Romana MC, Wolf G. Skin island flaps supplied by the vascular axis of the sensitive superficial nerves: anatomic study and clinical experience in the leg. Plast Reconstr Surg 1992;89(6):1115–21.
18. Imanishi N, Nakajima H, Fukuzumi S, et al. Venous drainage of the distally based lesser saphenous-sural veno-neuroadipofascial pedicled fasciocutaneous flap: a radiographic perfusion study. Plast Reconstr Surg 1999;103(2):494–8.
19. Baumeister SP, Spierer R, Erdmann D, et al. A realistic complication analysis of 70 sural artery flaps in a multimorbid patient group. Plast Reconstr Surg 2003; 112(1):129–40 [discussion: 141–2].
20. Hyakusoku H, Yamamoto T, Fumiiri M. The propeller flap method. Br J Plast Surg 1991;44(1):53–4.

21. Hallock GG. The propeller flap version of the adductor muscle perforator flap for coverage of ischial or trochanteric pressure sores. Ann Plast Surg 2006;56(5): 540–2.
22. Hallock GG. Bipedicled fasciocutaneous flaps in the lower extremity. Ann Plast Surg 1992;29(5):397–401.
23. Granzow JW, Li A, Suliman A, et al. Bipedicled flaps in post-traumatic lower-extremity reconstruction. J Plast Reconstr Aesthet Surg 2013;66(10):1415–20.
24. Hallock GG. The role of free flaps for salvage of the exposed total ankle arthroplasty. Microsurgery 2015;37(1):34–7.

How To Diagnose and Treat Infection in Total Ankle Arthroplasty

Yousef Alrashidi, MD, SB-Ortho[a],
Ahmed E. Galhoum, MSc, MRCS (England)[b,c], Martin Wiewiorski, MD[d],
Mario Herrera-Pérez, MD[e], Raymond Y. Hsu, MD[f],
Alexej Barg, MD[f], Victor Valderrabano, MD, PhD[g,*]

KEYWORDS

- Total ankle arthroplasty • Infected total ankle arthroplasty
- Periprosthetic ankle infection • Diagnosis of total ankle arthroplasty infection
- Treatment of total ankle arthroplasty infection

KEY POINTS

- Periprosthetic infection after total ankle arthroplasty (TAA) is a serious complication, often requiring revision surgery, including revision arthroplasty, conversion to ankle arthrodesis, or even amputation.
- Risk factors for periprosthetic ankle infection include prior surgery at the site of infection, low functional preoperative score, diabetes, and wound healing problems more than 14 days postoperatively.
- The clinical presentation of patients with periprosthetic ankle joint infection can be variable and dependent on the infection manifestation: acute versus chronic.
- The initial evaluation in patients with suspected periprosthetic joint infections should include blood tests: C-reactive protein (CRP) and erythrocyte sedimentation rate (ESR).
- Joint aspiration and synovial fluid analysis can help confirm suspected periprosthetic ankle infection.

[a] Orthopaedic Department, College of Medicine, Taibah University, P.O. Box 30001, Almadinah Almunawwarah 41411, Kingdom of Saudi Arabia; [b] Nasser Institute for Research and Treatment, Cairo, Egypt; [c] Department of Orthopaedics and Traumatology, Swiss Ortho Center, Schmerzklinik Basel, Hirschgässlein 15, Basel 4010, Switzerland; [d] Orthopaedic and Trauma Department, Kantonsspital Winterthur, Brauerstrasse 15, 8401 Winterthur, Switzerland; [e] Orthopaedic Department, University Hospital of Canary Islands, La Laguna, Calle El Pilar 50 4 piso, 38002 Tenerife, Spain; [f] Department of Orthopaedics, University of Utah, 590 Wakara Way, Salt Lake City, UT 84108, USA; [g] Orthopaedic Department, Swiss Ortho Center, Schmerzklinik Basel, Swiss Medical Network, Hirschgässlein 15, Basel 4010, Switzerland
* Corresponding author.
E-mail address: vvalderrabano@gsmn.ch

Foot Ankle Clin N Am 22 (2017) 405–423
http://dx.doi.org/10.1016/j.fcl.2017.01.009
1083-7515/17/© 2017 Elsevier Inc. All rights reserved.

INTRODUCTION

Periprosthetic infection after TAA is a serious complication, often requiring revision surgery, including revision arthroplasty, conversion to ankle arthrodesis, or even amputation. There are few studies addressing wound complications and periprosthetic infections in patients who have undergone TAA.

Early diagnosis and treatment of TAA infection is crucial to improving the probability of salvaging the prosthesis. An exact and complete history; careful clinical assessment; standard radiographic assessment including conventional radiographs and possibly advanced imaging (eg, computed tomography [CT]); laboratory work; joint aspiration, and microbiological work-up are necessary for appropriate planning of the therapy. A periprosthetic infection may occur early or later after prosthesis implantation. Patients may present with acute infection or low-grade infection without clinical symptoms.

The primary aims of treatment of infected TAA are eradication of infection; prevention of further complications including avoiding wound issues; and limb salvage. Salvage of the prosthesis is secondary. Data on treatment algorithms for infected TAA are scarce. This article describes diagnostic and treatment algorithms in patients with periprosthetic ankle infections.

EPIDEMIOLOGY AND RISK FACTORS

Unlike for patients with hip or knee arthroplasties, data on periprosthetic ankle infections are limited. Myerson and colleagues[1] performed a retrospective study to describe the demographics and their treatment protocol in patients with periprosthetic ankle infections. In total, 19 patients with infections were described: 14 of 433 cases (3.2%) with the Agility prosthesis (DePuy, Warsaw, IN), 1 of 139 cases (0.7%) with the Salto Talaris prosthesis (Tornier, Saint-Ismier, France), and 4 cases from other institutions. These 19 cases included 15 late chronic infections, 3 early postoperative infections, and 1 acute hematogenous infection.[1] In 2010, Gougoulias and colleagues[2] performed a systematic literature review including 13 level IV studies, with a total of 1105 ankle arthroplasties. Wound healing problems including superficial infections, delayed wound healing, and local skin necrosis, were observed in 66 of 827 cases (8.0%), with a range between 0% and 14.7% in the individual studies. Deep infections were reported in 7 of 827 arthroplasties (0.8%), ranging from 0% to 4.6% in the individual studies.[2] More recently, Zaidi and colleagues[3] performed a systematic review and meta-analysis including 58 clinical publications and 7942 ankle arthroplasties. Postoperative complications were analyzed in 41 articles, with 5579 ankle arthroplasties. Superficial infections were seen in 2.4% of all cases (95% CI, 1.3–3.8). Deep infections occurred in 1.1% of all arthroplasties (95% CI, 0.7–1.7).[3]

Due to the common limitation in the literature addressing TAA — a low number of patients — it is often difficult to draw any clinically meaningful and statistically significant conclusions.[4] Kessler and colleagues[5] performed a matched case-control study that included 26 patients with periprosthetic ankle joint infections and 2 control groups to identify possible risk factors. In this study, the prevalence of periprosthetic joint infection was 4.7%, with the majority of infections (85%) having an exogenous origin. The following statistically significant risk factors were identified: prior surgery at the site of infection (odds ratio [OR] 4.56 in comparison with the age/gender-matched group and OR 4.78 in comparison with the date of surgery–matched group) and low American Orthopaedic Foot and Ankle Society hindfoot score (35.8 vs 49.8 in the age/gender-matched group and 47.6 in the date of surgery–matched group). The mean initial TAA surgical time was significantly longer in the infection group: 119 minutes vs 84 minutes in the age/gender-matched group and 93 minutes in the date of surgery–matched group. Isolated implantation of the ankle prosthesis without a subtalar arthrodesis was also associated with a lower risk of infection. The infection group had a significantly higher number of revision TAA with 23% versus 2% in the age/gender-matched group and 0% in the date of surgery–matched group. Patients with periprosthetic ankle joint infections were most likely to have had poor wound healing (OR 15.38) or for secondary wound drainage (OR 7.00).[5] Patton and colleagues[6] retrospectively reviewed 966 patients with TAA performed between 1995 and 2012. In total, there were 29 cases of infected TAA, resulting in an overall prevalence of 3.2%. The incidence rates of infection in primary TAA and revision ankle arthroplasty were different, 2.4% versus 4%, respectively. The following risk factors were identified as associated with periprosthetic ankle infection: diabetes, prior ankle surgery, and wound healing problems that extend beyond 14 days postoperatively. The percentage of smoking patients, body mass index, and operative time were comparable in groups with and without infection.[6] In a majority of primary ankle arthroplasties, an anterior approach is used for implantation.[7] One of the disadvantages of this approach is possible wound healing issues due to the anatomic vascularity of this region.[8–12] Finally, Young and colleagues[13] presented a case of an infected ankle arthroplasty after a dental procedure treated with a 2-stage revision arthroplasty.

DIAGNOSIS
Definition of Periprosthetic Ankle Infection

Diagnosis of a periprosthetic ankle infection is guided by the definition from the Musculoskeletal Infection Society,[14] which was modified by the International Consensus Group on Periprosthetic Joint Infection in 2014.[15] One major criterion or 3 of 5 minor criteria should be met to diagnose an infection (**Table 1**).[15] Threshold levels for the minor criteria are shown in **Table 2**.[15] In general, the authors recommend the diagnostic algorithm shown in **Fig. 1**.

History and Clinical Examination

A clinical work-up starts with an accurate and complete history. The history often provides important clues that may raise suspicions of a periprosthetic ankle infection.[16] First, the presence of any known risk factors, as discussed previously, should be evaluated. All previous medical and surgical reports and imaging data are collected and carefully analyzed. Special attention should be paid to the data regarding the initial

---

Table 1
Definition criteria of periprosthetic joint infection according to the International Consensus Group on Periprosthetic Joint Infection

Major Criteria	Minor Criteria
• Identification of 2 positive periprosthetic cultures with phenotypically identical microorganisms *OR* • Presence of a sinus tract communicating with the joint	• Elevated serum CRP *AND* elevated ESR • Elevated synovial fluid WBC count *OR* ++ change on leukocyte esterase test strip • Elevated synovial fluid PMN% • Positive histologic analysis of periprosthetic tissue • A single positive culture

Abbreviations: CRP, C-reactive protein; ESR, erythrocyte sedimentation rate; PMN%, polymorphonuclear neutrophil percentage; WBC, white blood cell.

Adapted from Parvizi J, Gehrke T. Definition of periprosthetic joint infection. J Arthroplasty 2014;29(7):1331; with permission.

Table 2
Threshold levels for minor criteria for periprosthetic joint infection

Criterion	Acute Periprosthetic Joint Infection (<90 d)	Chronic Periprosthetic Joint Infection (>90 d)
ESR (mm/h)	Not helpful, no threshold defined	30
CRP (mg/L)	100	10
Synovial WBC count (cells/μl)	10,000	3000
Synovial PMN%	90	80
Leukocyte esterase	+ OR ++	+ OR ++
Histologic analysis of tissue	>5 neutrophils per HPF(×400) in 5 HPF	Same as acute

Abbreviations: CRP, C-reactive protein; ESR, erythrocyte sedimentation rate; HPF, high-power field; PMN%, polymorphonuclear neutrophil percentage; WBC, white blood cell.

index surgery (TAA) and its postoperative course. It is important to analyze all events around the time of the initial surgery, which can be associated with infection development, for example: prolonged operative time, postoperative wound drainage, delayed wound healing, and need for perioperative antibiotic treatment. If antibiotics were used preoperatively, perioperatively, or postoperatively: type and duration of therapy should be noted. Furthermore, any bacteremic events, such as other surgeries or dental work, should be documented.[13,16]

The clinical presentation of patients with periprosthetic ankle joint infections can be variable and dependent on the infection manifestation: acute versus chronic. Patients with acute periprosthetic infections often have severe pain, high fever, toxemia, and/or

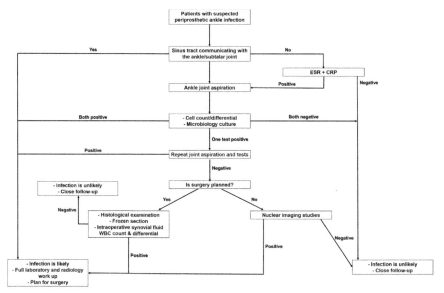

Fig. 1. Diagnostic algorithm in patients with periprosthetic ankle infections. CRP, C-reactive protein; ESR, erythrocyte sedimentation rate; WBC, white blood cell.

local symptoms including increased skin temperature, rubor, joint swelling, and surgical wound drainage. Patients with chronic infections often have nonspecific progressive pain with no systemic signs of infection and minimal if any local findings such as slight perifocal swelling. Formation of skin fistulae and/or drainage of purulent secretions as often seen in patients with periprosthetic hip or knee infections,[16–18] are rare in patients with TAA. Delayed infections may clinically present similarly to patients with aseptic prosthesis failure.[19] Clinical presentation depends on the virulence of the microorganisms, the method of innoculation, and the total duration of the infectious process. Clinical history should elucidate the timeline of all symptoms a patient endorses on presentation. The timing of the onset of a patient's pain and its relation to the index surgery is critical. Specifically, whether or not the pain has been persistent since the index surgery or if there was a pain-free interval postoperatively should be established.

Physical examination starts with a careful inspection of the foot and ankle while walking and standing with special attention given to obvious deformities and the skin and soft tissue condition. The general appearance of the ankle and hindfoot is noted including swelling, joint effusion, erythema, excessive warmth, and wound healing issues. The range of motion of the replaced ankle joint and the subtalar joint should be measured clinically using a goniometer.[20] It should be noted if range of motion is associated with pain. Finally, physical examination should also include a peripheral neurovascular assessment.

Imaging

Radiographic evaluation of affected ankles starts with conventional weight-bearing radiographs including anteroposterior views of the foot and ankle, lateral view of the foot, and the special hindfoot alignment view (Saltzman view).[21] Conventional radiographs may present with nonspecific changes similar to those observed in patients with aseptic loosening. They may be helpful, however, in the differential diagnosis and detection of periprosthetic fracture, osteolysis, or other possible reasons for the pain. In general, computerized tomography (CT) may provide more detail regarding periprosthetic osteolysis in patients with TAA.[22] Single-photon emission (SPECT)-CT has shown to be useful in diagnosis of ankle osteoarthritis and assessment of periprosthetic lucencies in patients with painful TAA[23,24]; however, there is no literature addressing the use of SPECT-CT in patients with suspected periprosthetic ankle infections. In patients with total hip or knee arthroplasties, SPECT-CT with antigranulocyte scintigraphy may help detect a periprosthetic infection and elucidate the foci of the infection.[25] The role of nuclear medicine in the diagnosis of periprosthetic joint infection, however, may be overestimated.[26] MRI can help assess any extraosseous infection involvement including possible abscesses; however, interpretation is often difficult due to implant-associated artifacts.[27,28]

Laboratory Tests

Initial evaluation in patients with suspected periprosthetic joint infections should include blood tests.[16] CRP and ESR are easy to perform and have been shown to be highly sensitive, have a good negative predictive value, and are cost-effective screening tools.[16,29,30] Both markers should be interpreted carefully because they routinely increase postoperatively.[31–33] CRP tends to peak at approximately the second to third postoperative day. ESR tends to peak at the fifth postoperative day. The CRP level is usually back within normal range within 3 weeks but the ESR may remain elevated for longer. Therefore, any second peak in CRP level after the third postoperative day may be a sign of infection.[32,33] As a screening tool, negative results on both tests provide a high negative predictive value for ruling out active periprosthetic joint infection.[34,35] A subset of patients with periprosthetic joint infections however, presents with normal CRP and ESR levels.[36] Specifically, patients with coagulase-negative *Staphylococcus* as well as other low virulent pathogens including *Candida*, *Corynebacterium*, *Mycobacterium*, *Actinomyces*, and *Propionibacterium acnes*, may have seronegative findings.[36,37]

It remains controversial whether serum white blood cell count and differential play an important role in the diagnosis of periprosthetic joint infection.[38,39] In patients with total hip or knee arthroplasties, a serum white blood cell count diagnostic cutoff of 7800 cells/μl has 55% sensitivity and 66% specificity, whereas the neutrophil percentage cutoff of 68% has 52% sensitivity and 75% specificity.[38] Another study demonstrated a weak correlation between joint fluid and blood for white blood cells (R = 0.19), neutrophils (R = 0.31), and lymphocytes (R = −0.22).[39] A serum white blood cell count and differential can be used as additional screening tools; however, these values may not significantly improve the accuracy of diagnosis of a periprosthetic joint infection.

Serum interleukin 6 is a more recently available blood test, which has been described as a more specific marker of acute periprosthetic infection.[40–42] In patients with periprosthetic hip or knee infections, interleukin 6 was shown to have high accuracy, sensitivity, specificity, positive predictive values, and negative predictive values—97%, 100%, 95%, 89%, and 100%, respectively.[40]

Arthrocentesis and Synovial Fluid Analysis

In any patient with an elevated ESR and CRP and clinical symptoms of a periprosthetic ankle infection, joint aspiration and synovial fluid analysis should be performed as the next step. Ankle joint aspiration should be performed under fluoroscopy guidance (**Fig. 2**). Empiric antibiotic therapy before the synovial fluid aspiration should be avoided.[43,44]

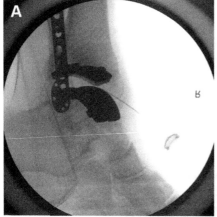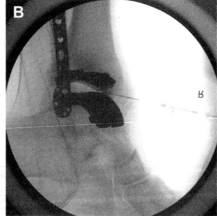

Fig. 2. Ankle joint aspiration. (*A*) A 67-year-old man with a painful total ankle replacement performed 1 year prior. Fluoroscopically guided aspiration of the ankle was performed to rule out a periprosthetic joint infection. Gram stain, crystal analysis, and bacterial and fungal cultures were negative. Cell analysis of synovial fluid demonstrated a white blood cell count of 89/μl, 18% lymphocytes, and 29% mononuclear cells. (*B*) Iodine-based contrast has been used to confirm the intraarticular position of the needle.

The aspirated synovial fluid should be evaluated for a total white blood cell count and a differential with a synovial neutrophil percentage (**Table 3**). In addition, synovial fluid samples should be sent for aerobic, anaerobic, and fungal cultures. In general, synovial fluid white blood cell counts greater than 1700 cells/μl and percentages of neutrophils greater than 60% to 65% are highly suspicious for periprosthetic joint infection.[16,43]

Several synovial fluid biomarkers have been found highly sensitive and specific for periprosthetic joint infections. Alpha-defensin is a naturally occurring antimicrobial peptide and can be used as a synovial fluid biomarker. In patients with total hip or knee arthroplasties, sensitivity and specificity of up to 100% were observed.[55]

Frozen Section and Sonication

The utility of frozen section remains controversial because multiple variables may play a role.[16] Frozen section analysis includes identification of the number of neutrophils per high power field at 400× magnification and the minimum number of fields

Table 3
Available literature on the sensitivity and specificity of synovial fluid white blood cell count in the diagnosis of periprosthetic joint infection

Study	Patients	Synovial Fluid White Cell Count (cells/mm³)			Polymorphonuclear Cells (%)		
		Cutoff	Sensitivity	Specificity	Cutoff	Sensitivity	Specificity
Bedair et al,[45] 2011	146 TKA	>27,800	84%	99%	>89	84%	69%
Della Valle et al,[46] 2007	94 TKA	>3000	100%	98%	NR	NR	NR
Dinneen et al,[47] 2013	27 THA, 28 TKA	>1590	90%	91%	>65	90%	87%
Ghanem et al,[48] 2008	429 TKA	>1100	91%	88%	>64	95%	95%
Mason et al,[14] 2003	86 TKA	>2500	69%	98%	>80	57%	100%
Nilsdotter-Augustinsson et al,[49] 2007	106 THA	>1700	86%	92%	NR	NR	NR
Parvizi et al,[50] 2006	145 TKA	>1760	90%	99%	>73	93%	95%
Schinsky et al,[51] 2008	201 THA	>4200	84%	93%	>80	84%	82%
Shukla et al,[52] 2010	87 THA	>3528	78%	96%	>79	78%	82%
Spangehl et al,[35] 1999	202 THA	>50,000	36%	99%	>80	89%	85%
SURCU,[53] 2012	259 UKA	>6200	90%	96.5%	>60	91%	94%
Trampuz et al,[54] 2004	133 TKA	>1700	94%	88%	>65	97%	98%
Zmistowski et al,[39] 2012	228 TKA	>3000	93%	94%	>75	93%	83%

Abbreviations: NR, not reported; SURCU, Society of Unicondylar Research and Continuing Education; THA, total hip arthroplasty; TKA, total knee arthroplasty; UKA, unicondylar knee arthroplasty.

containing that concentration of inflammatory cells. A general threshold of 5 neutrophils per high-power field is used for screening for periprosthetic joint infection.[16]

Gram stain is not recommended to diagnose periprosthetic joint infections because it has a poor sensitivity between 15% and 27% despite a specificity of 99%.[56,57]

As the current standard, culturing of samples of periprosthetic tissue is performed for the microbiologic diagnosis in patients with periprosthetic joint infections. This method, however, usually demonstrates low sensitivity and specificity. Therefore, sonication is recommended as a novel method for the culturing of the biofilms on the prostheses.[58,59] In a prospective study including 207 total knee prostheses and 124 total hip prostheses, the sensitivities of periprosthetic tissue and sonicate fluid cultures were 60.8% and 78.5%, respectively, and the specificities were 99.2% and 98.8%, respectively.[59] Another study on infected total hip arthroplasties demonstrated that multiple sonicate-fluid cultures increase the sensitivity and specificity of the sonication method to up to 100%.[60]

TREATMENT ALGORITHM

In the current literature, there is little data regarding the optimal treatment of an infected TAA.[7] Most of the available literature has limitations including low numbers of patients and short durations of follow-up. Thus, a treating orthopedic surgeon must apply the basic treatment principles derived from infections of knee and hip arthroplasties.

The 3 ultimate treatment goals of an infected TAA are similar to those of other periprosthetic joint infections: (1) eradication of infection, (2) substantial pain relief, and (3) maintenance/restoration of function. Current treatments include several nonsurgical and surgical options (**Box 1**). The choice of an appropriate treatment depends on several factors including timing (early vs late) and type (superficial vs deep) of infection. A possible treatment algorithm for patients with deep periprosthetic infections is shown in **Fig. 3**. Wound issues in patients with TAA usually require a different approach, discussed later.

TREATMENT OF WOUND ISSUES
Wound Healing Complications

In the current literature, the incidence of wound healing complications after TAA is reportedly up to 40%.[7] Thin dorsal ankle skin, deficient musculature, and limited

---

Box 1
Treatment options in patients with periprosthetic ankle infections

Nonoperative treatment option

- Retention of prosthesis components and antimicrobial therapy

Operative treatment options

- Irrigation and debridement with or without polyethylene exchange with retention of metal prosthesis components
- One-stage or 2-stage revision ankle arthroplasty
- One-stage or 2-stage conversion to ankle arthrodesis
- Prosthesis component removal and implantation of cement spacer as definitive treatment option
- Below-the-knee amputation

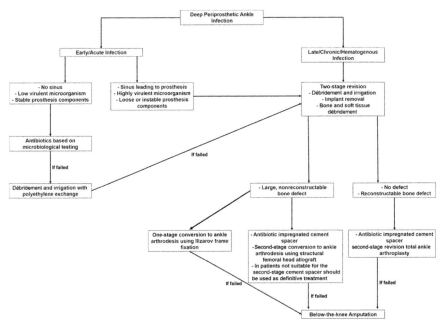

Fig. 3. Treatment algorithm in patients with deep periprosthetic ankle infections.

skin and subcutaneous tissue mobility are factors that underlie the localized trauma and swelling after TAA.[61] The need to involve plastic surgeons in the management of soft tissue problems related to TAA seems more frequent than cases related to other joint arthroplasties.

Postoperative wound complications are defined as the presence of at least 1 of the following: superficial wound dehiscence, severe persistent (more than 96 hours) edema and/or erythema, stitch abscess, and wound drainage.[62,63] Wiewiorski and colleagues[62] analyzed 295 elective foot and ankle operations including 13 total ankle arthroplasties. The overall prevalence of postoperative wound complications was 16.9%. The following statistically significant risk factors have been identified: age greater than or equal to 60 years (OR 8.98), tobacco use (OR 48.77), and tourniquet time greater than or equal to 90 minutes (OR 7.02).[62]

Raikin and colleagues[11] reviewed risk factors and types of wound complications in a retrospective study including 106 Agility ankle arthroplasties. Two different complication groups were observed. The minor complication group included 27 ankles (25%) requiring local wound care or antibiotics without subsequent consequences. The major complication group had 9 ankles (8.5%) requiring surgical irrigation and debridement. Only diabetes was found to have a significant association with the occurrence of minor wound complications. Female gender, inflammatory connective tissue disease, and corticosteroid use were identified as risk factors for major wound complications.[11] Wahlen and colleagues[64] performed a retrospective study including 57 consecutive ankle arthroplasties. Wound breakdown was observed in 16 patients at a median of 17 days after TAA. A significant increase in the rate of wound problems was associated with following risk factors: smoking greater than 12 pack-years, peripheral vascular disease, and cardiovascular disease.[64] Gross and colleagues[65] performed a retrospective analysis of a consecutive series including 1001 primary total ankle arthroplasties; 19 patients had a total of 44 secondary surgical procedures (flap surgeries) to treat wound complications. The most common type of flap performed was a sural pedicle flap followed by a propeller flap. The mean time between initial TAA and flap surgery was 13.1 weeks. There were 4 flap failures with 2 subsequent below-the-knee amputations.[65]

Superficial Wound Necrosis

Superficial wound necrosis can be successfully managed with local wound debridement, daily wound care, and negative pressure wound therapy. Wound necrosis that has failed to heal with daily care or negative pressure wound therapy and/or with exposed tendon (anterior tibial tendon or extensor hallucis longus tendon) requires either rotational or free vascularized flap coverage.[8,65–67] In patients with known risk factors for postoperative wound complications, incisional negative pressure wound therapy should be discussed perioperatively. Matsumoto and Parekh[10] performed a retrospective comparative study on the effect of incisional negative pressure wound therapy on TAA wound healing. Two groups were analyzed, each with 37 patients: a control group and a group with incisional negative pressure wound therapy. There were 9 (24%) wound healing problems in the control group and 1 (3%) in the negative pressure wound therapy group. Incisional negative pressure wound therapy was demonstrated to reduce wound healing issues, with an OR of 0.10.[10]

TREATMENT OF PERIPROSTHETIC INFECTION
Classification of Periprosthetic Joint Infection

Segawa and colleagues[68] introduced a classification of periprosthetic joint infections after total knee arthroplasty. Four different types of deep infection were described (**Table 4**). This classification can be useful to guide appropriate treatment of periprosthetic ankle infections.

Table 4
Four different types of deep periprosthetic joint infection as described by Segawa and colleagues

Type	Description	Treatment Options
I	Positive intraoperative routine cultures in a revision arthroplasty surgery where infection was not expected	Surgical debridement, exchange of components (at least polyethylene), antibiotics (for 4–6 wk)
II	Early postoperative infection (diagnosed within the first 6 postoperative weeks)	Debridement, metal component retention, exchange of polyethylene, antibiotics (for 4–6 wk)
III	Acute hematogenous infection (years after the initial TAA and with documented remote infection source)	• If infection symptoms for less than 2–3 wk: debridement, metal component retention, exchange of polyethylene, antibiotics (for 4–6 wk) • If infection symptoms for more than 2–3 wk: debridement, exchange of all components, antibiotics (for 4–6 wk)
IV	Chronic deep infection	1-stage or 2-stage revision surgery (revision arthroplasty or conversion to ankle arthrodesis), antibiotics

Data from Segawa H, Tsukayama DT, Kyle RF, et al. Infection after total knee arthroplasty. A retrospective study of the treatment of eighty-one infections. J Bone Joint Surg Am 1999;81(10):1434–45.

Early Periprosthetic Infection

Antimicrobial therapy

Retention of prosthesis components and antimicrobial therapy can be considered in cases with the following findings: (1) early postoperative infection with symptom duration less than 4 weeks, (2) absence of sinus tract communicating to any of prosthesis components, (3) pathogen susceptible to antibiotic therapy identified prior to treatment, and (4) presence of adequate periarticular soft tissue envelope.[69] Further indications for this treatment option are the presence of high perioperative risk due to significant comorbidities, low virulence organisms susceptible to a well-tolerated antibiotic therapy, and mechanically stable components without any lucencies at the prosthesis-bone interface.

An infectious disease specialist should be consulted to assist in selecting the most appropriate antimicrobial therapy. This person should be involved at all stages of treatment including ankle joint aspiration, antibiotic therapy, and clinical follow-up.

Irrigation and debridement with or without polyethylene exchange

Irrigation and debridement with component retention remain controversial as a treatment option in patients with periprosthetic ankle infections. In patients with infected hip arthroplasties, irrigation and debridement only resulted in a 20% success rate which increased to 70% when combined with jet lavage and change of all modular components of the hip prosthesis.[69] Similar results were observed in another study including 60 infected total hip arthroplasties.[70] In patients with infected knee arthroplasties, the therapy success rate was 45% and 55.1% in patients with irrigation and debridement without and with polyethylene exchange, respectively.[71] This evidence suggests that if irrigation and debridement are the treatment plan for a periprosthetic ankle infections, it should be done in combination with the exchange of polyethylene. There is limited direct evidence, however, on this surgical option in patients with TAA. Myerson and colleagues[1] reported a cohort of 19 cases of deep periprosthetic ankle infections where irrigation and debridement were performed in 4 patients. All 4 cases failed, however, and patients had recurrent deep infections treated by 2-stage revisions.[1]

Deep Late Chronic Infection/Late Hematogenous Infection

Revision ankle arthroplasty

In patients with deep chronic infections, formation of bacterial biofilms on prosthesis components may result in resistance to both host defense and antibiotic therapy. Therefore, a 2-stage revision surgery including a removal of all components is the most successful surgical treatment in patients with periprosthetic ankle infections **(Fig. 4)**.[72] The most important key points of treatment are the correct identification of the pathogenic organism, the appropriate planning of possibly multiple debridements, and the specific antimicrobial therapy. Revision ankle arthroplasty is a challenging surgical procedure.[73–76] Furthermore, only prostheses with a revision components option should be used.

Surgical steps include the complete removal of all prosthesis components (polyethylene, tibial, and talar) and the temporary insertion of an antibiotic-loaded polymethylmethacrylate [PMMA] cement spacer. After all prosthesis components are removed, the underlying bone including the previous bone-prosthesis interface, should be carefully debrided. Radical debridement is the key to reducing the intraarticular bacterial load. As discussed previously, the removed implants should be sent for sonication analysis.[59] Furthermore, all devitalized and/or infected soft tissues including the ankle joint capsule should be resected as well. Antibiotics used in the PMMA cement must

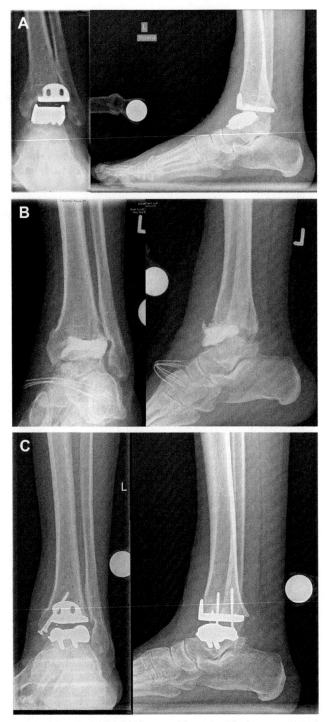

Fig. 4. Two-stage revision TAA. (*A*) A 59-year-old man with deep periprosthetic infection 8 months after initial TAA. Weight-bearing radiographs demonstrated malposition of both prosthesis components. (*B*) Prosthesis removal and implantation of a cement spacer was performed. (*C*) Second-stage procedure, including implantation of revision prosthesis components, was performed 6 weeks later. Left: Anteroposterior view, Right: Lateral view.

be heat stable, available in lyophilized form, and effective against the microorganisms as identified by preoperative microbiologic testing. Intravenous antibiotic therapy guided by microbiologic cultures is recommended for 4 to 6 weeks after spacer implantation.[77] The cement spacer has 2 different functions: (1) prevention of soft tissue contracture by maintaining the ankle joint space and (2) delivery of antibiotics locally to the bone and surrounding soft tissues by elution. The second stage, revision arthroplasty, should only be performed if the eradication of the infection is supported by clinical history and examination, by serologic investigation, and by synovial fluid aspiration.

Cement spacer as a definitive treatment

There is limited literature describing a cement spacer as a definitive treatment option in patients with deep ankle infections. Ferrao and colleagues[78] reported a series of 9 patients with cement spacers as definitive management for postoperative ankle infections. The initial surgeries were TAA and ankle arthrodesis in 6 cases and 3 cases, respectively. The indications for this method of treatment included patients who were asymptomatic after insertion of the cement spacer, patients who did not desire any further revision surgery, and patients with significant comorbidities with increased perioperative risk. In all patients, intravenous antibiotics based on culture sensitivities were delivered for 6 weeks. The average time of cement spacer retention was 20 months, ranging from 6 months to 62 months. At final follow-up, 2 had had subsequent below-the-knee amputations performed as a result of delayed complications. The other 7 patients were all mobile and able to perform basic activities of daily living with minimal discomfort.[78] Lee and colleagues[79] investigated the outcomes of cement arthroplasty as a primary salvage procedure in 16 patients: 9 of these patients had deep ankle infections including 3 patients with previous TAA, 4 patients with previous ankle arthrodesis, 1 patient with open reduction and internal fixation of a talus fracture, and 1 patient with an infected Charcot arthropathy. The cement spacers were retained without breakage for a mean of 39 months ranging from 14 to 100 months. One patient had osteolysis around the spacer. Another patient was diagnosed with subluxation. At

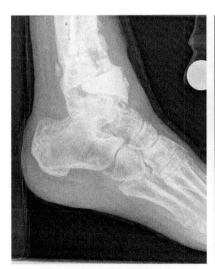
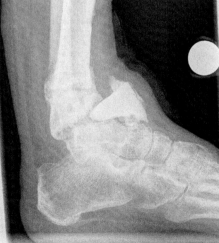

Fig. 5. Cement spacer. Frequent clinical and radiographic follow-ups are necessary for early detection of dislocation of the cement spacer.

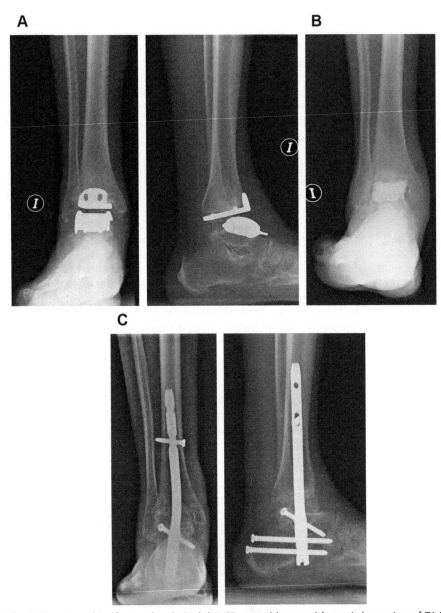

Fig. 6. Two-stage hindfoot arthrodesis. (*A*) A 67-year-old man with septic loosening of TAA 3 years after initial implantation. (*B*) Prosthesis removal and implantation of cement spacer was performed. (*C*) Second-stage procedure, including tibiotalocalcaneal arthrodesis using an intramedullary nail was performed 6 weeks later.

final follow-up, 9 of 16 patients did not require walking aids, 10 used no pain medication, and 9 were able to walk continuously for more than an hour.

Based on the available literature, cement spacers as a definitive treatment can be considered for elderly and less active patients. Regular clinical and radiographic follow-ups are recommended to avoid and identify any associated complications including spacer breakage or subluxation (**Fig. 5**).

Conversion to ankle arthrodesis

Conversion to ankle arthrodesis is the most common salvage procedure for failed TAA.[80–90] Different surgical techniques have been described in the current literature including 1-stage versus 2-stage revision procedures, different fixation types, and tibiotalar versus tibiotalocalcaneal arthrodesis. The specific surgical plan should be based on the preferences of the surgeon and the patient. In patients with significant bone loss after prosthesis removal and bone surface debridement, a second stage involving an intramedullary hindfoot nail and a femoral head allograft may be the best option to compensate for bone loss (**Fig. 6**).

Gross and colleagues[84] performed a systematic review of the literature on ankle arthrodesis after failed TAA including 16 studies and 193 patients. The overall nonunion rate was 10.6%. A blade plate provided the highest union rate of 100% and a tibiotalocalcaneal fusion cage provided the lowest union rate of 50%. The overall complication rate after the revision procedure was 18.2%.[84] Rahm and colleagues[88] demonstrated that salvage ankle arthrodesis after failed TAA resulted in impaired life quality and reduced function combined with significantly higher pain compared to primary ankle arthrodesis.

Below-the-knee amputation

Below-the-knee amputation should be considered an ultimate solution after other limb salvage procedures have failed. Indications include extensive soft tissue deficit that cannot be addressed even with plastic surgery expertise, persistent infection with drainage even after hardware removal and antibiotic spacer insertion, and severe pain.[1,6,91]

REFERENCES

1. Myerson MS, Shariff R, Zonno AJ. The management of infection following total ankle replacement: demographics and treatment. Foot Ankle Int 2014;35(9): 855–62.
2. Gougoulias N, Khanna A, Maffulli N. How successful are current ankle replacements?: a systematic review of the literature. Clin Orthop Relat Res 2010; 468(1):199–208.
3. Zaidi R, Cro S, Gurusamy K, et al. The outcome of total ankle replacement: a systematic review and meta-analysis. Bone Joint J 2013;95(11):1500–7.
4. Barg A, Wimmer MD, Wiewiorski M, et al. Total ankle replacement - indications, implant designs, and results. Dtsch Arztebl Int 2015;112(11):177–84.
5. Kessler B, Sendi P, Graber P, et al. Risk factors for periprosthetic ankle joint infection: a case-control study. J Bone Joint Surg Am 2012;94(20):1871–6.
6. Patton D, Kiewiet N, Brage M. Infected total ankle arthroplasty: risk factors and treatment options. Foot Ankle Int 2015;36(6):626–34.
7. Barg A, Saltzman CL. Ankle replacement. Mann's Surgery of the foot and ankle. Philadelphia: Elsevier Saunders; 2014. p. 1078–162.
8. Hallock GG. The role of free flaps for salvage of the exposed total ankle arthroplasty. Microsurgery 2015;37(1):34–7.
9. Hsu AR, Franceschina D, Haddad SL. A novel method of postoperative wound care following total ankle arthroplasty. Foot Ankle Int 2014;35(7):719–24.
10. Matsumoto T, Parekh SG. Use of negative pressure wound therapy on closed surgical incision after total ankle arthroplasty. Foot Ankle Int 2015;36(7):787–94.

11. Raikin SM, Kane J, Ciminiello ME. Risk factors for incision-healing complications following total ankle arthroplasty. J Bone Joint Surg Am 2010;92(12):2150–5.
12. Schipper ON, Hsu AR, Haddad SL. Reduction in wound complications after total ankle arthroplasty using a compression wrap protocol. Foot Ankle Int 2015; 36(12):1448–54.
13. Young JL, May MM, Haddad SL. Infected total ankle arthroplasty following routine dental procedure. Foot Ankle Int 2009;30(3):252–7.
14. Mason JB, Fehring TK, Odum SM, et al. The value of white blood cell counts before revision total knee arthroplasty. J Arthroplasty 2003;18(8):1038–43.
15. Parvizi J, Gehrke T. Definition of periprosthetic joint infection. J Arthroplasty 2014; 29(7):1331.
16. Springer BD. The diagnosis of periprosthetic joint infection. J Arthroplasty 2015; 30(6):908–11.
17. Kapadia BH, Berg RA, Daley JA, et al. Periprosthetic joint infection. Lancet 2016; 387(10016):386–94.
18. Lima AL, Oliveira PR, Carvalho VC, et al. Periprosthetic joint infections. Interdiscip Perspect Infect Dis 2013;2013:542796.
19. Bauer TW, Parvizi J, Kobayashi N, et al. Diagnosis of periprosthetic infection. J Bone Joint Surg Am 2006;88(4):869–82.
20. Lindsjo U, Danckwardt-Lilliestrom G, Sahlstedt B. Measurement of the motion range in the loaded ankle. Clin Orthop Relat Res 1985;199:68–71.
21. Saltzman CL, El-Khoury GY. The hindfoot alignment view. Foot Ankle Int 1995; 16(9):572–6.
22. Kohonen I, Koivu H, Pudas T, et al. Does computed tomography add information on radiographic analysis in detecting periprosthetic osteolysis after total ankle arthroplasty? Foot Ankle Int 2013;34(2):180–8.
23. Mason LW, Wyatt J, Butcher C, et al. Single-photon-emission computed tomography in painful total ankle replacements. Foot Ankle Int 2015;36(6):635–40.
24. Paul J, Barg A, Kretzschmar M, et al. Increased osseous 99mTc-DPD uptake in end-stage ankle osteoarthritis: Correlation between SPECT-CT imaging and histologic findings. Foot Ankle Int 2015;36(12):1438–47.
25. Yue B, Tang T. The use of nuclear imaging for the diagnosis of periprosthetic infection after knee and hip arthroplasties. Nucl Med Commun 2015;36(4): 305–11.
26. Diaz-Ledezma C, Lamberton C, Lichstein P, et al. Diagnosis of periprosthetic joint infection: The role of nuclear medicine may be overestimated. J Arthroplasty 2015;30(6):1044–9.
27. Cadden AR. Imaging in total ankle replacement. Semin Musculoskelet Radiol 2012;16(3):205–16.
28. Kim DR, Choi YS, Potter HG, et al. Total ankle arthroplasty: an imaging overview. Korean J Radiol 2016;17(3):413–23.
29. Austin MS, Ghanem E, Joshi A, et al. A simple, cost-effective screening protocol to rule out periprosthetic infection. J Arthroplasty 2008;23(1):65–8.
30. Berbari E, Mabry T, Tsaras G, et al. Inflammatory blood laboratory levels as markers of prosthetic joint infection: a systematic review and meta-analysis. J Bone Joint Surg Am 2010;92(11):2102–9.
31. Kim TW, Kim DH, Oh WS, et al. Analysis of the causes of elevated C-reactive protein level in the early postoperative period after primary total knee arthroplasty. J Arthroplasty 2016;31(9):1990–6.
32. Larsson S, Thelander U, Friberg S. C-reactive protein (CRP) levels after elective orthopedic surgery. Clin Orthop Relat Res 1992;275):237–42.

33. White J, Kelly M, Dunsmuir R. C-reactive protein level after total hip and total knee replacement. J Bone Joint Surg Br 1998;80(5):909–11.
34. Greidanus NV, Masri BA, Garbuz DS, et al. Use of erythrocyte sedimentation rate and C-reactive protein level to diagnose infection before revision total knee arthroplasty. A prospective evaluation. J Bone Joint Surg Am 2007;89(7):1409–16.
35. Spangehl MJ, Masri BA, O'connell JX, et al. Prospective analysis of preoperative and intraoperative investigations for the diagnosis of infection at the sites of two hundred and two revision total hip arthroplasties. J Bone Joint Surg Am 1999; 81(5):672–83.
36. Mcarthur BA, Abdel MP, Taunton MJ, et al. Seronegative infections in hip and knee arthroplasty: periprosthetic infections with normal erythrocyte sedimentation rate and C-reactive protein level. Bone Joint J 2015;97(7):939–44.
37. Deirmengian CA, Citrano PA, Gulati S, et al. The C-reactive protein may not detect infections caused by less-virulent organisms. J Arthroplasty 2016;31(9 Suppl):152–5.
38. Toossi N, Adeli B, Rasouli MR, et al. Serum white blood cell count and differential do not have a role in the diagnosis of periprosthetic joint infection. J Arthroplasty 2012;27(8 Suppl):51–4.
39. Zmistowski B, Restrepo C, Huang R, et al. Periprosthetic joint infection diagnosis: a complete understanding of white blood cell count and differential. J Arthroplasty 2012;27(9):1589–93.
40. Di Cesare PE, Chang E, Preston CF, et al. Serum interleukin-6 as a marker of periprosthetic infection following total hip and knee arthroplasty. J Bone Joint Surg Am 2005;87(9):1921–7.
41. Elgeidi A, Elganainy AE, Abou Elkhier N, et al. Interleukin-6 and other inflammatory markers in diagnosis of periprosthetic joint infection. Int Orthop 2014;38(12): 2591–5.
42. Hoell S, Borgers L, Gosheger G, et al. Interleukin-6 in two-stage revision arthroplasty: what is the threshold value to exclude persistent infection before re-implanatation? Bone Joint J 2015;97(1):71–5.
43. Della Valle C, Parvizi J, Bauer TW, et al. Diagnosis of periprosthetic joint infections of the hip and knee. J Am Acad Orthop Surg 2010;18(12):760–70.
44. Parvizi J, Della Valle CJ. AAOS Clinical Practice Guideline: diagnosis and treatment of periprosthetic joint infections of the hip and knee. J Am Acad Orthop Surg 2010;18(12):771–2.
45. Bedair H, Ting N, Jacovides C, et al. The Mark Coventry Award: diagnosis of early postoperative TKA infection using synovial fluid analysis. Clin Orthop Relat Res 2011;469(1):34–40.
46. Della Valle CJ, Sporer SM, Jacobs JJ, et al. Preoperative testing for sepsis before revision total knee arthroplasty. J Arthroplasty 2007;22(6 Suppl 2):90–3.
47. Dinneen A, Guyot A, Clements J, et al. Synovial fluid white cell and differential count in the diagnosis or exclusion of prosthetic joint infection. Bone Joint J 2013;95(4):554–7.
48. Ghanem E, Parvizi J, Burnett RS, et al. Cell count and differential of aspirated fluid in the diagnosis of infection at the site of total knee arthroplasty. J Bone Joint Surg Am 2008;90(8):1637–43.
49. Nilsdotter-Augustinsson A, Briheim G, Herder A, et al. Inflammatory response in 85 patients with loosened hip prostheses: a prospective study comparing inflammatory markers in patients with aseptic and septic prosthetic loosening. Acta Orthop 2007;78(5):629–39.

50. Parvizi J, Ghanem E, Menashe S, et al. Periprosthetic infection: what are the diagnostic challenges? J Bone Joint Surg Am 2006;88(Suppl 4):138–47.

51. Schinsky MF, Della Valle CJ, Sporer SM, et al. Perioperative testing for joint infection in patients undergoing revision total hip arthroplasty. J Bone Joint Surg Am 2008;90(9):1869–75.

52. Shukla SK, Ward JP, Jacofsky MC, et al. Perioperative testing for persistent sepsis following resection arthroplasty of the hip for periprosthetic infection. J Arthroplasty 2010;25(6 Suppl):87–91.

53. Society of Unicondylar Research and Continuing Education. Diagnosis of periprosthetic joint infection after unicompartmental knee arthroplasty. J Arthroplasty 2012;27(8 Suppl):46–50.

54. Trampuz A, Hanssen AD, Osmon DR, et al. Synovial fluid leukocyte count and differential for the diagnosis of prosthetic knee infection. Am J Med 2004;117(8): 556–62.

55. Deirmengian C, Kardos K, Kilmartin P, et al. The alpha-defensin test for periprosthetic joint infection outperforms the leukocyte esterase test strip. Clin Orthop Relat Res 2015;473(1):198–203.

56. Della Valle CJ, Scher DM, Kim YH, et al. The role of intraoperative Gram stain in revision total joint arthroplasty. J Arthroplasty 1999;14(4):500–4.

57. Morgan PM, Sharkey P, Ghanem E, et al. The value of intraoperative Gram stain in revision total knee arthroplasty. J Bone Joint Surg Am 2009;91(9):2124–9.

58. Renz N, Muller M, Perka C, et al. Implant-associated infections - diagnostics. Chirurg 2016;158(15):45–9 [in German].

59. Trampuz A, Piper KE, Jacobson MJ, et al. Sonication of removed hip and knee prostheses for diagnosis of infection. N Engl J Med 2007;357(7):654–63.

60. Janz V, Wassilew GI, Hasart O, et al. Improvement in the detection rate of PJI in total hip arthroplasty through multiple sonicate fluid cultures. J Orthop Res 2013; 31(12):2021–4.

61. Cho EH, Garcia R, Pien I, et al. An algorithmic approach for managing orthopaedic surgical wounds of the foot and ankle. Clin Orthop Relat Res 2014;472(6): 1921–9.

62. Wiewiorski M, Barg A, Hoerterer H, et al. Risk factors for wound complications in patients after elective orthopedic foot and ankle surgery. Foot Ankle Int 2015; 36(5):479–87.

63. Zgonis T, Jolly GP, Garbalosa JC. The efficacy of prophylactic intravenous antibiotics in elective foot and ankle surgery. J Foot Ankle Surg 2004;43(2):97–103.

64. Whalen JL, Spelsberg SC, Murray P. Wound breakdown after total ankle arthroplasty. Foot Ankle Int 2010;31(4):301–5.

65. Gross CE, Garcia R, Adams SB, et al. Soft tissue reconstruction after total ankle arthroplasty. Foot Ankle Int 2016;37(5):522–7.

66. Fukui A, Tanaka Y, Inada Y, et al. Turndown retinacular flap for closure of skin fistula after total ankle replacement. Foot Ankle Int 2008;29(6):624–6.

67. Yamamoto T, Saito T, Ishiura R, et al. Quadruple-component superficial circumflex iliac artery perforator (SCIP) flap: a chimeric SCIP flap for complex ankle reconstruction of an exposed artificial joint after total ankle arthroplasty. J Plast Reconstr Aesthet Surg 2016;69(9):1260–5.

68. Segawa H, Tsukayama DT, Kyle RF, et al. Infection after total knee arthroplasty. A retrospective study of the treatment of eighty-one infections. J Bone Joint Surg Am 1999;81(10):1434–45.

69. Trebse R, Pisot V, Trampuz A. Treatment of infected retained implants. J Bone Joint Surg Br 2005;87(2):249–56.

70. Triantafyllopoulos GK, Poultsides LA, Sakellariou VI, et al. Irrigation and debridement for periprosthetic infections of the hip and factors determining outcome. Int Orthop 2015;39(6):1203–9.
71. Triantafyllopoulos GK, Poultsides LA, Zhang W, et al. Periprosthetic knee infections treated with irrigation and debridement: outcomes and preoperative predictive factors. J Arthroplasty 2015;30(4):649–57.
72. Kessler B, Knupp M, Graber P, et al. The treatment and outcome of periprosthetic infection of the ankle: a single cohort-centre experience of 34 cases. Bone Joint J 2014;96(6):772–7.
73. Hintermann B, Barg A, Knupp M. Revision arthroplasty of the ankle joint. Orthopade 2011;40(11):1000–7 [in German].
74. Hintermann B, Zwicky L, Knupp M, et al. HINTEGRA revision arthroplasty for failed total ankle prostheses. J Bone Joint Surg Am 2013;95(13):1166–74.
75. Hintermann B, Zwicky L, Knupp M, et al. HINTEGRA revision arthroplasty for failed total ankle prostheses. J Bone Joint Surg Am 2013;3(2):e12.
76. Horisberger M, Henninger HB, Valderrabano V, et al. Bone augmentation for revision total ankle arthroplasty with large bone defects. Acta Orthop 2015;86(4):412–4.
77. Joseph TN, Chen AL, Di Cesare PE. Use of antibiotic-impregnated cement in total joint arthroplasty. J Am Acad Orthop Surg 2003;11(1):38–47.
78. Ferrao P, Myerson MS, Schuberth JM, et al. Cement spacer as definitive management for postoperative ankle infection. Foot Ankle Int 2012;33(3):173–8.
79. Lee HS, Ahn JY, Lee JS, et al. Cement arthroplasty for ankle joint destruction. J Bone Joint Surg Am 2014;96(17):1468–75.
80. Culpan P, Le Strat V, Piriou P, et al. Arthrodesis after failed total ankle replacement. J Bone Joint Surg Br 2007;89(9):1178–83.
81. Doets HC, Zurcher AW. Salvage arthrodesis for failed total ankle arthroplasty. Acta Orthop 2010;81(1):142–7.
82. Espinosa N, Wirth SH. Ankle arthrodesis after failed total ankle replacement. Orthopade 2011;40(11):1008, 1010–2, 1014–7. [in German].
83. Espinosa N, Wirth SH. Revision of the aseptic and septic total ankle replacement. Clin Podiatr Med Surg 2013;30(2):171–85.
84. Gross C, Erickson BJ, Adams SB, et al. Ankle arthrodesis after failed total ankle replacement: a systematic review of the literature. Foot Ankle Spec 2015;8(2):143–51.
85. Gross CE, Lewis JS, Adams SB, et al. Secondary arthrodesis after total ankle arthroplasty. Foot Ankle Int 2016;37(7):709–14.
86. Hopgood P, Kumar R, Wood PL. Ankle arthrodesis for failed total ankle replacement. J Bone Joint Surg Br 2006;88(8):1032–8.
87. Kotnis R, Pasapula C, Anwar F, et al. The management of failed ankle replacement. J Bone Joint Surg Br 2006;88(8):1039–47.
88. Rahm S, Klammer G, Benninger E, et al. Inferior results of salvage arthrodesis after failed ankle replacement compared to primary arthrodesis. Foot Ankle Int 2015;36(4):349–59.
89. Sagherian BH, Claridge RJ. Salvage of failed total ankle replacement using tantalum trabecular metal: case series. Foot Ankle Int 2015;36(3):318–24.
90. Zwipp H, Grass R. Ankle arthrodesis after failed joint replacement. Oper Orthop Traumatol 2005;17(4–5):518–33 [in German].
91. Kamrad I, Henricson A, Magnusson H, et al. Outcome after salvage arthrodesis for failed total ankle replacement. Foot Ankle Int 2016;37(3):255–61.

Dealing with the Stiff Ankle

Preoperative and Late Occurrence

Beat Hintermann, MD[a],*, Roxa Ruiz, MD[a], Alexej Barg, MD[b]

KEYWORDS

- Ankle osteoarthritis • Total ankle replacement • Stiffness • Ossifications
- Soft tissue impingement • Revision procedures

KEY POINTS

- Stiffness of the ankle joint can occur preoperatively and postoperatively after total ankle replacement.
- Postoperative formation of proliferative bone and heterotopic ossification is more likely in patients with posttraumatic ankle osteoarthritis and may occur posteriorly and/or anteriorly.
- The radiographic assessment includes bilateral weight-bearing anteroposterior and lateral views of the foot and ankle and hindfoot alignment view.
- Surgical treatment is chosen based on underlying pathology and may include arthroscopic or open debridement.
- All underlying caused should be efficiently addressed, including malpositioning and/or oversized implants, loosening of implants, cyst formation, hindfoot malalignment, soft tissue contractures, and hypertrophic bone formation.

INTRODUCTION

In the past few decades, total ankle replacement (TAR) has become an increasingly recommended and accepted treatment in patients with end-stage ankle osteoarthritis (OA).[1–8] However, controversy still exists with regard to the appropriate indications for TAR,[9] specifically in patients with poor soft tissue conditions and preoperative ankle stiffness.[10,11] These concerns are particularly true for patients with posttraumatic ankle OA, which is the etiology of up to 80% of end-stage ankle degeneration.[12–14] Patients with posttraumatic ankle OA often present with scars resulting from the initial operative treatment of the index injury, limited ankle and subtalar range of motion owing to scarred capsular and periarticular soft tissues, and extra bone formation.[15,16]

ª Orthopaedic Clinic, Kantonsspital Baselland, 4410 Liestal, Switzerland; ᵇ Department of Orthopaedics, University of Utah, 590 Wakara Way, Salt Lake City, UT 84108, USA
* Chairman, Orthopaedic Clinic, Kantonsspital Baselland, 4410 Liestal, Switzerland.
E-mail address: beat.hintermann@ksbl.ch

Foot Ankle Clin N Am 22 (2017) 425–453
http://dx.doi.org/10.1016/j.fcl.2017.01.012

In theory, scarred periarticular structures can be removed or at least reduced during TAR surgery. However, some bony fragments and periarticular scars may elude intraoperative detection and removal. Furthermore, specifically for posterior capsular scaring, resection is often technically demanding and can result in injury of the neurovascular bundle.[17,18]

Postoperative formation of proliferative bone and heterotopic ossifications is more likely in patients with posttraumatic ankle OA and may occur posteriorly[19,20] and/or anteriorly.[21] The proliferative periarticular bony growth in patients with posttraumatic ankle OA may also represent an ongoing inflammatory condition after TAR that predisposes this patient group to gutter disease.[22–25] Most of the currently available implants result in some residual exposure of raw, bleeding cancellous bone after implantation on the tibial and more commonly on the talar side.[26]

Aside from extra bone formation and heterotopic ossifications, a pathologically increased proliferation of periarticular soft tissues may be another underlying cause of ankle stiffness. One reason for this may be compromised periarticular soft tissues owing to the initial injury and surgical treatments, with a loss of elasticity and reduced ankle range of motion.[16,27] Another reason may be overstress of the periarticular soft tissues owing to oversized implants[28] or nonanatomic implants. In particular, this is an issue with the use of cylindrically and not conically shaped talar components, which may overstress the medial ankle ligament structures.[29] Finally, although neglected in the past, a malpositioned talar component in any plane (too medial or lateral, too anterior or posterior, malrotation) may result in overstress of periarticular soft tissues, including ligaments and bony impingement,[30,31] which may cause inferior functional clinical outcomes.[32]

From the current literature, little is known regarding how to address the stiff ankle with arthrofibrosis (**Table 1**) and/or impingement (**Table 2**) in patients who have undergone TAR. This article presents the author's experience in dealing with the preoperatively stiff osteoarthritic ankle, and the stiff ankle after TAR.

PREOPERATIVE STIFF ANKLE

As mentioned, stiffness in an osteoarthritic ankle can originate from extra bone formation that restricts the tibiotalar joint range of motion in the sagittal plane, from soft tissue contracture as a result of previous injuries and possible surgical treatments, and from contracture of muscle–tendon units after scarring of tendons in their sheaths or fibrosis of their muscles. A careful preoperative workup is important to understand fully the underlying pathology, select appropriate treatment modalities, and ensure satisfactory function after TAR.

Indications and Contraindications for Total Ankle Replacement

TAR has become a widely accepted treatment option in patients with end-stage ankle OA. However, the postoperative improvement in ankle range of motion should not be the most expected benefit from this procedure.[68,69] This maxim is particularly true for patients with associated OA of adjacent hindfoot joints and concomitant knee problems, such as painful hyperextension stress and degenerative changes.

The relative contraindications for TAR include a significantly reduced ankle dorsiflexion power owing to neurologic disorders where active dorsiflexion cannot be expected or improved postoperatively.[9] Extended scars around the ankle and atrophy of periarticular soft tissue mantle are also relative contraindications for TAR. The absolute contraindications for TAR include acute or chronic infections with or without

Table 1
Literature review addressing arthrofibrosis in patients who underwent total ankle replacement

Study	Study Type	Patients (Ankles)	TAR Procedure	Prosthesis Type	Follow-up (y)	Arthrofibrosis (%)	Treatment
Barg et al,[33] 2010	PS, SC	8 (10)[a]	Primary (10)	Hintegra (10)	5.6 (2.7–7.6)	1 (10.0)	Open arthrolysis and percutaneous ATL 14 mo after TAR (1)
Barg et al,[34] 2011	RS, SC	16 (21)[b]	Primary (21)	Hintegra (21)	5.3 (3.1–8.6)	2 (9.5)	Open arthrolysis and percutaneous ATL 15 and 18 mo after TAR (2)
Barg et al,[35] 2011	RS, SC	118 (123)[c]	Primary (123)	Hintegra (123)	5.6 (2.4–10.5)	7 (5.7)	Open arthrolysis and percutaneous ATL (7)
Barg et al,[9] 2012	RS, SC	301 (311)	Primary (311)	Hintegra (311)	5.0 (4–9)	2 (0.6)	Open arthrolysis and mobile-bearing inlay exchange (2)
Barg et al,[1] 2013	RS, SC	684 (722)	Primary (722)	Hintegra (722)	6.3 (2–12.2)	5 (0.7)	NR
Barg et al,[36] 2015	PS, MC	18 (18)[d]	Primary (18)	Hintegra (18)	7.5 (2.9–13.2)	1 (5.6)	Open arthrolysis and exchange of mobile-bearing inlay 13 mo after TAR (1)
Brunner et al,[29] 2013	PS, SC	72 (77)	Primary (77)	STAR (77)	12.4 (10.8–14.9)	17 (22.1)	Open arthrolysis and percutaneous ATL at a mean of 3.3 y (0.7–6.3) after TAR (17)
Ellington et al,[37] 2013	RS, SC	53 (53)	Revision (53)	Agility (53)	4.1 (2.2–6.5)	2 (3.8)	Conversion to tibiotalar AD (2)
Giannini et al,[38] 2011	PS, MC	156 (158)	Primary (158)	BOX (158)	1.4 (0.5–4)	3 (1.9)	Open arthrolysis and osteophytes removal medial gutter (3)

(continued on next page)

Table 1
(continued)

Study	Study Type	Patients (Ankles)	TAR Procedure	Prosthesis Type	Follow-up (y)	Arthrofibrosis (%)	Treatment
Haskell and Mann,[39] 2004	RS, SC	189 (189)	Primary (189)	STAR (189)	min 0.3	2 (1.1)	NR
Hintermann et al,[40] 2009	PS, SC	28 (30)	Conversion of ankle AD to TAR (30)	Hintegra (30)	4.6 (3–7.5)	4 (13.3)	NR
Hintermann et al,[41] 2013	RS, SC	116 (117)	Revision (117)	Hintegra (117)	6.2 (2–11.8)	1 (0.9)	Conversion to tibiotalar AD (1)
Horisberger et al,[42] 2015	RS, SC	10 (10)	Revision (10)	Hintegra (10)	4.0 (2.5–6.2)	2 (20)	Conversion to tibiotalar AD (2)
Hsu and Haddad,[4] 2015	RS, SC	59 (59)	Primary (59)	INBONE (59)	2.9 (2–5.4)	9 (15.3)	Open gutter debridement, exostectomy and posterior capsulotomy (9)
Kim et al,[43] 2010	RS, SC	348 (348)	Primary (348)	Hintegra (348)	3.3 (1–6.1)	22 (6.3)	Conversion to tibiotalar AD (2)
Noelle et al,[44] 2013	RS, SC	97 (114)	Primary (114)	STAR (114)	3.0 (min 2)	10 (8.8)	Open arthrolysis, removal of osteophytes, ATL (10)
Rippstein et al,[8] 2011	RS, SC	233 (240)	Primary (240)	Mobility (240)	2.7 (1–3)	1 (0.4)	Open arthrolysis 17 mo after TAR (1)
Saltzman et al,[18] 2003	RS, MC	90 (90)	Primary (90)	Agility (90)	min. 1	1 (1.1)	AS arthrolysis (1)

Abbreviations: AD, arthrodesis; AS, arthroscopic; ATL, Achilles tendon lengthening; BOX, Bologna and Oxford Universities; MC, multicenter; NR, not reported; PS, prospective; RS, retrospective; SC, single center; STAR, Scandinavian Total Ankle Replacement; TAR, total ankle replacement.

a Patients with secondary ankle osteoarthritis owing to hemophilia.
b Patients with secondary ankle osteoarthritis owing to hereditary hemochromatosis.
c Obese patients with end-stage ankle osteoarthritis.
d Patients with secondary ankle osteoarthritis owing to von Willebrand disease.

Table 2
Literature review addressing impingement in patients who underwent TAR

Study	Study Type	Patients (Ankles)	TAR Procedure	Prosthesis Type	Follow-up (y)	Impingement (%)	Treatment
Alvarez-Goenaga,[45] 2008	RS, SC	25 (25)	Primary (25)	Hintegra (25)	2.5 (0.5–5.4)	Anteromedial 2 (8.0)	Open debridement (2)
Barg et al,[46] 2011	PS, SC	26 (52)[a]	Primary (52)	Hintegra (52)	5.0 (2–10)	Medial 2 (3.8)	Open medial debridement (1), local infiltrations (1)
Barg et al,[34] 2011	RS, SC	16 (21)[b]	Primary (21)	Hintegra (21)	5.3 (3.1–8.6)	Subfibular 1 (4.8)	Subfibular debridement and lateral ligament reconstruction (1)
Barg et al,[35] 2011	RS, SC	118 (123)[c]	Primary (123)	Hintegra (123)	5.6 (2.4–10.5)	Medial 3 (2.4), lateral 1 (0.8), dorsal 1 (0.8)	Open debridement (5)
Bolton-Maggs et al,[47] 1985	RS, SC	57 (62)	Primary (62)	ICLH (62)	5.5 (2–11)	Medial/lateral 6 (9.7)	Open debridement (4), conversion to tibiotalar AD (2)
Bonnin et al,[48] 2011	RS, SC	96 (98)	Primary (98)	Salto (98)	8.9 (6.8–11.1)	Subfibular 2 (2.0)	Open debridement (2)
Criswell et al,[49] 2012	RS, SC	64 (65)	Primary (65)	Agility (65)	8 (0.5–11)	Gutter impingement (2)	Open debridement (2)
Freeman et al,[50] 1979	RS, SC	26 (29)	Primary (29)	ICLH (29)	NR	Medial 1 (3.4)	NR
Giannini et al,[51] 2010	PS, MC	51 (51)	Primary (51)	BOX (51)	2.5 (2–4)	lateral 1 (2.0)	Conversion to tibiotalar AD 24 mo after TAR (1)

(continued on next page)

Table 2
(continued)

Study	Study Type	Patients (Ankles)	TAR Procedure	Prosthesis Type	Follow-up (y)	Impingement (%)	Treatment
Jung et al,[21] 2016	RS, SC	54 (54)	Primary (52)	Hintegra (21), Mobility (33)	2.5 (2–5.1)	11 (21.2)	None (9), open debridement (1), AS debridement (1)
Henricson et al,[52] 2010	RS, SC	93 (93)	Primary (93)	AES (93)	3.5 (1.1–6.1)	Medial 7 (7.5), lateral 2 (2.2)	Open debridement (9)
Hintermann et al,[10] 2004	PS, SC	116 (122)	Primary (122)	Hintegra (122)	1.6 (1–3)	Fibulotalar 1 (0.8), anterior 1 (0.8)	Lateral exostectomy (1), anterior capsulotomy and ATL (1)
Hobsen et al,[53] 2009	RS, SC	111 (123)	Primary (123)	STAR (123)	4.0 (2–8)	Fibulotalar 1 (0.8)	Revision of talar component (1)
Karantana et al,[54] 2010	RS, SC	45 (52)	Primary (52)	STAR (52)	6.7 (5–9.2)	Medial 2 (3.8)	AS debridement (2)
Kerkhoff et al,[55] 2015	RS, SC	64 (67)	Primary (67)	Mobility (67)	3.3 (min 1)	Medial/lateral 4 (6.0)	Open debridement (4)
Kim et al,[43] 2010	RS, SC	348 (348)	Primary (348)	Hintegra (348)	3.3 (1–6.1)	16 (4.6)	NR
Knecht et al,[56] 2004	RS, SC	126 (132)	Primary (132)	Agility (132)	4.6 (2–13.5)	Lateral (0.8)	Lateral debridement (1)
Lewis et al,[57] 2015	PS, SC	249 (249)	Primary (249)	INBONE (249)	3.7	Medial/lateral 23 (9.2)	AS debridement (12), open debridement (11)
Muir et al,[58] 2013	RS, SC	123 (129)	Primary (129)	Mobility (129)	4.0 (2–6.3)	Medial 32 (24.8), lateral 35 (27.1)	NR
Murnaghan et al,[59] 2005	RS, SC	22 (22)	Primary (22)	STAR (22)	2.2 (0.7–3.8)	Anterior 1 (4.5)	NR

Study	Type	n		Implant	Follow-up	Location (%)	Treatment (n)
Nodzo et al,[60] 2014	RS, SC	74 (75)	Primary (75)	Salto (75)	3.6 (2–6.1)	Medial/lateral 3 (4.0)	NR
Nunley et al,[61] 2012	RS, SC	82 (82)	Primary (82)	STAR (82)	5.1 (2–9)	Medial/lateral 3 (3.7)	Open debridement (3)
Rippstein et al,[8] 2011	RS, SC	233 (240)	Primary (240)	Mobility (240)	2.7 (1–3)	Anterior 1 (0.4)	Open cheilectomy 22 mo after TAR (1)
Rosello Anon et al,[62] 2015	RS, SC	17 (18)	Primary (18)	Hintegra (18)	3.1 (1–6.1)	Lateral 1 (5.6)	Lateral debridement (1)
Saltzman et al,[63] 2010	RS, MC	37 (37)	Primary (37)	STAR (37)	4.2 (2.2–5.9)	Lateral/posterior 7 (18.9)	Open debridement (7)
Schweitzer et al,[64] 2013	PS, SC	67 (67)	Primary (67)	Salto Talaris (67)	2.8 (2–4.5)	Medial/lateral 4 (6.0)	Open debridement and exostectomy (4)
Staufer,[65] 1977	RS, SC	72 (76)	Primary (76)	Mayo (76)	min 0.5	Talofibular 3 (3.9)	Open debridement (3)
Staufer and Segal,[66] 1981	RS, SC	94 (102)	Primary (102)	Mayo (102)	1.9 (0.5–3.7)	Talofibular 18 (17.6)	None (2), steroid injections (5), open debridement (11)
Valderrabano et al,[67] 2006	PS, SC	147 (152)	Primary (152)	Hintegra (152)	2.8 (2–4)	fibulotalar 1 (0.7)	NR

Abbreviations: AD, arthrodesis; AS, arthroscopic; ATL, Achilles tendon lengthening; BOX, Bologna and Oxford Universities; MC, multicenter; NR, not reported; PS, prospective; RS, retrospective; SC, single center; STAR, Scandinavian Total Ankle Replacement; TAR, total ankle replacement.
[a] Patients with simultaneous bilateral total ankle replacement.
[b] Patients with secondary ankle osteoarthritis owing to hereditary hemochromatosis.
[c] Obese patients with end-stage ankle osteoarthritis.

osteomyelitis, severe hindfoot malalignment and/or instability, and neuromuscular disorders with or without neuroarthropathy.[9,68]

Preoperative Planning

Clinical examination
Preoperative planning starts with the careful assessment of patient history, including a complete review of all available medical records mentioning the previous surgical treatment. The following particular aspects should be addressed in detail: pain, limitations in daily life and recreation activities, and previous and current treatments. All patients should be asked if they had trauma, surgeries, concomitant diseases, or infections in the past. In patient with ankle stiffness and/or equinus contracture, it should be clarified, whether the stiffness and/or contracture progressed in the last months. Patients with any of the aforementioned contraindications should be excluded.

The routine physical examination includes careful inspection of both lower extremities and observation of the patient while walking and standing. The patient's neurovascular status should be evaluated; in particular, the integrity of the tibial nerve function should be proven. Alignment, deformity and foot/ankle/hindfoot position are assessed visually. Muscular functional status and atrophy should be assessed in particular, and special attention should be paid to possible tightness of heel cord and function of plantar flexors, including the posterior tibial muscle and flexor hallucis longus muscle. Next, pain or tenderness to palpation is evaluated. Finally, tibiotalar range of motion is measured in the sagittal plane (plantar flexion/dorsiflexion) and in the coronal plane (eversion/inversion). Ankle range of motion is determined with a goniometer placed along the lateral border of the leg and foot. All goniometer measurements are performed in the weight-bearing position as described by Lindsjö and colleagues.[70] To confirm the range of motion measurement of the tibiotalar joint independent of the midfoot/hindfoot joints, we recommend radiographic measurement of tibiotalar range of motion using weight-bearing lateral radiographs in maximal dorsiflexion and plantar flexion (**Fig. 1**A, B).[8,10,40,71]

Radiographic evaluation
The routine radiographic evaluation includes bilateral weight-bearing anteroposterior and lateral views of the foot and ankle (**Fig. 2**A–C). For appropriate assessment of inframalleolar alignment, a hindfoot alignment view (Saltzman view) should be performed (see **Fig. 2**D)[72,73] Weight-bearing radiographs should be used to identify and quantify degenerative changes, malposition, and deformities of the tibiotalar joint.[74] Furthermore, possible concomitant degenerative changes and/or deformities in the adjacent joints of the hindfoot and midfoot should be identified and assessed. Recently, we started the routine use of weight-bearing computed tomography scans to assess hindfoot alignment and complexity of the degenerative changes of the hindfoot (**Fig. 3**A, B).[75,76] Magnetic resonance imaging (MRI) is not recommended routinely. However, in some cases, MRI may be helpful to evaluate the possible tendon and muscular pathologies.[77] Furthermore, MRI may be used for the detailed quantification of capsular and pericapsular thickening and scarring in patients with arthrofibrosis of the foot and ankle.[78]

Surgical Strategies

Anterior osteophytes
Anterior osteophytes on the tibia and talus are removed before preparation of the ankle for implants (**Fig. 4**A, B). Furthermore, any bone formation in the anteromedial and anterolateral gutters should be removed.

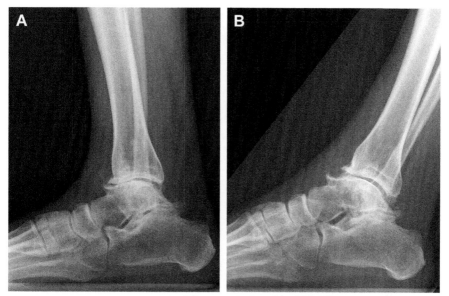

Fig. 1. Weight-bearing lateral radiographs in the maximal dorsiflexion (*A*) and plantar flexion (*B*) are used for measurement of maximal tibiotalar range of motion.

Posterior osteophytes

In general, posterior osteophytes can be removed from an anterior approach, while distracting the ankle after tibial and talar bony cuts for the prosthesis components are performed. Ankle distraction can be achieved using a K-wire based distractor, for example, a Hintermann distractor.

Mild posterior soft tissue contracture

In the most cases, a mild posterior soft tissue contracture can be addressed efficiently by complete resection of the posterior capsule. After insertion of the prosthesis components, manual dorsiflexion stress should be applied to the ankle. The remaining periarticular contracture is then released by gradual mobilization of the ankle. In cases, where a minimum ankle dorsiflexion of 10° cannot be obtained, a percutaneous release of Achilles tendon using a triple hemisection technique[79] should be performed followed by passive ankle mobilization, as described. Here, special attention should be paid to not fully disrupt the released Achilles tendon.

Severe posterior soft tissue contracture (fixed equinus)

In patients with a fixed equinus of more than 5°, a posterior approach is used for extended release of posterior soft tissues. In our experience, a longitudinal approach just along the medial border of the Achilles tendon is the safest approach to expose the posterior capsule of the ankle joint, and, if necessary, to expose the neurovascular bundle safely, including the tibial nerve. The same surgical approach can be used for open lengthening of the Achilles tendon. Special attention should be paid during wound closure to hold the foot in neutral position to avoid any tension across the wound. In markedly fixed equinus feet, we use an external fixator routinely to keep the foot in the neutral position after surgery and to maintain the correction postoperatively.

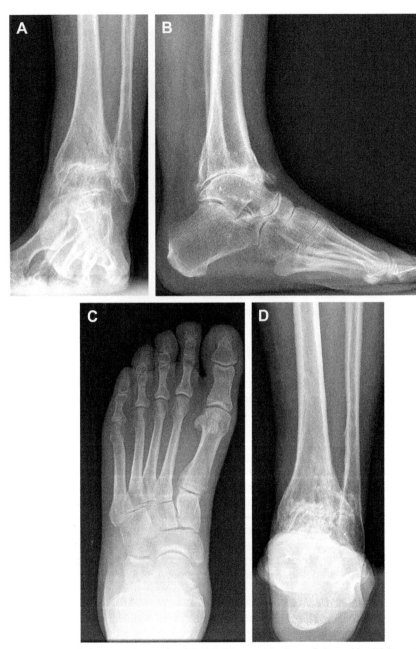

Fig. 2. Weight-bearing radiographs: (*A*) anteroposterior view of the ankle, (*B*) lateral view of the foot and ankle, and (*C*) anteroposterior view of the foot. (*D*) Hindfoot alignment view (Saltzman view). These standard radiographs are taken bilaterally to assess the amount of deviation from contralateral unaffected foot and ankle, and to assess overall deformity.

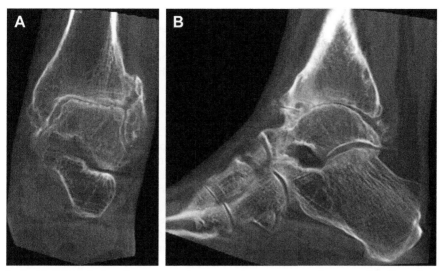

Fig. 3. (A, B) Weight-bearing computed tomography scans are used to assess hindfoot alignment and complexity of the degenerative changes of the hindfoot, such as articular destruction, cyst formation, bone loss, and degenerative disease of peritalar joints.

Tendon contracture

Patients with previous fracture dislocations and/or posteromedial scars after operative fracture treatment often present with a contracture of the posterior tibial tendon. In such cases, the posterior tibial tendon is exposed through an incision of its sheath and explored carefully. In the case of mild scarring, the tendon should

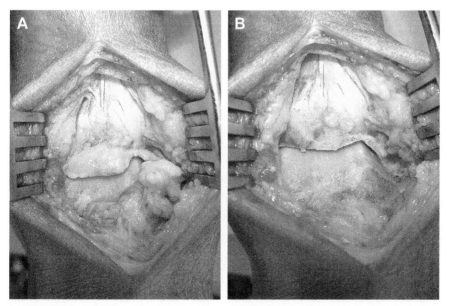

Fig. 4. Exposure of the osteoarthritic ankle through an anterior approach showing osteophyte formation at anterior tibia (A) before and (B) after excision.

be mobilized carefully. However, in the case of extended scarring and/or absent tendon excursion after release, the tendon is excised. In the case of contracture of the flexor hallucis longus tendon (seen preoperatively as a fixed plantar-flexed great toe while dorsiflexing the foot that becomes mobile when the foot is moved into plantar flexion), the tendon is transected through the ankle joint space before inserting the implants.

Surgical Technique

The surgery can be performed under general or regional anesthesia. The patient is placed in a supine position, with an ipsilateral bump until a strictly upward position of the foot is obtained. A pneumatic tourniquet is applied on the ipsilateral thigh.

A standard anterior ankle approach is used between the anterior tibial tendon and extensor hallucis longus tendon. After the tibiotalar joint is exposed, the osteophytes on the tibia and talus are removed, and the medial gutter is cleaned of any bony overgrowth on the talar and medial malleolus sites. Bony resection on the tibia and talus is done using the specific instruments and techniques appropriate for the selected ankle prosthesis. After the medial and lateral gutter debridement is completed and the posterior capsule is resected, the prosthesis components are inserted. The ankle is gradually mobilized into dorsiflexion. In cases, where a minimum dorsiflexion of 10° cannot be obtained, a lengthening of the heel cord is considered. It can be done using different surgical techniques, for example, by a percutaneous release using a triple hemisection technique (Hook procedure)[79] or by a Strayer procedure through a short medial approach.[80] Recently, also a proximal medial gastrocnemius lengthening has been proposed.[81] If there is a substantial posterior tibial tendon contracture (**Fig. 5**A), the tendon is released (see **Fig. 5**B) or excised through an additional posteromedial approach as described.

Patients with a fixed equinus contracture are first positioned prone. The posterior ankle is exposed as described. Special attention is paid not to injure the posteromedial neurovascular bundle, including the tibial nerve. The tibial nerve should be exposed and protected first, before the capsular release and Achilles tendon lengthening is performed. After wound closure, the patient is rolled into a supine position, and the TAR is done. In most patients with a fixed equinus contracture, an external fixator should be

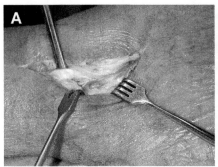
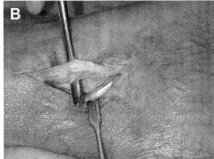

Fig. 5. Scarred posterior tibial tendon causing soft tissue stiffness. (*A*) Exposure of the scarred posterior tibial tendon. (*B*) Tendon after tenolysis showing some preserved excursion; therefore, the tendon was retained.

applied to keep the foot and ankle in a fixed neutral position for 6 weeks postoperatively (**Fig. 6**).

Complications

The main postoperative complications are wound healing problems, in particular in patients with preoperative fixed equinus foot. Therefore, the surgeon may consider a staged procedure, specifically in patients with a large equinus deformity: first, posterior release and application of an external fixator, and second, after wound healing has occurred uneventfully, TAR procedure through an anterior approach. Although not common, a fracture of the malleoli or talus can occur intraoperatively after too extensive a bone resection before implant insertion. In contrast, when hypertrophic bone is not resected sufficiently, the contours of the ankle may be overestimated (**Fig. 7**A, B), potentially leading to the use of oversized implants, which may result in painful overstuffing of the replaced joint. The preoperative clinic and radiographic assessment of the contralateral unaffected ankle may help to reduce this risk. Inappropriate removal of hypertrophic bone may also provoke implantation of components in an incorrect position, which may result in painful dysfunction of the replaced ankle. A careful clinical and fluoroscopic check of trial component position and alignment before the insertion of final components may help to avoid this complication.

Postoperative Management

The postoperative management in this particular patient cohort is identical to the aftercare in patients with uneventful TAR.[9] After 2 to 3 days, the compressive dressing and temporary splint are removed and replaced by a short leg soft cast and a walking boot, respectively. In noncompliant patients, a lower leg scotch cast should be used instead. Early full weight-bearing in the walking boot or cast is allowed as tolerated. At 6 weeks postoperatively, the operated ankle is assessed clinically and radiographically. In patients with appropriate soft tissue status and good prosthesis component integration, free ambulation and a rehabilitation program are initiated. The rehabilitation program includes passive and active mobilization of the ankle, proprioception, coordination, gait improvement, and strength training.

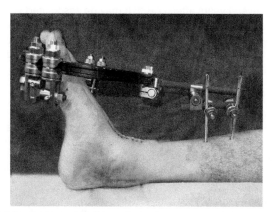

Fig. 6. An external fixator is used in this patient after percutaneous Achilles tendon lengthening for a longstanding equinus foot due to extensive soft tissue damages. The posterior scar is from a previous open procedure to lengthen the Achilles tendon.

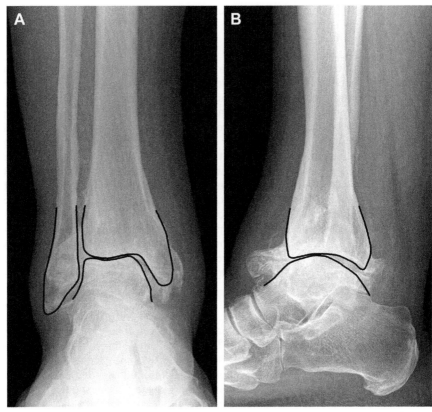

Fig. 7. Hypertrophic bone formation has to be taken into consideration when planning positioning and size of implants. (*A*) Anteroposterior view. (*B*) Lateral view.

THE STIFF ANKLE AFTER TOTAL ANKLE REPLACEMENT

A stiff ankle after TAR can be seen in the early stage of recovery,[82] but also as a progressive process several years after TAR.[29] It may be associated with significant pain and restrictions in daily activities; however, most surprisingly, stiffness could be well-tolerated by many patients, especially if they had limited motion before the TAR. As a general principle, surgical treatment should only be recommended in patients with substantial pain and functional impairment.

Indications and Contraindications for Revision

Isolated scar tissue debridement and hypertrophic bone resection should be performed only in patients with stable and normally aligned prosthesis components without loosening and/or cyst formation. In patients with malalignment of the hindfoot, it should be done in association with realignment surgery. In patients with implant loosening or implant malposition, the debridement should be performed together with revision of components.

Severely compromised periarticular soft tissues around the ankle are a relative contraindication for revision surgery owing to a significantly increased risk for wound healing problems. The absolute contraindications for TAR include acute or chronic infections with or without osteomyelitis.

Preoperative Planning

Clinical examination

Preoperative planning starts with careful assessment of the patient history to learn of any incidental events since the TAR, and to evaluate when and how the stiffness and pain started and how quickly it progressed thereafter. The thorough clinical evaluation includes a careful assessment of periarticular soft tissues, measurement of hindfoot range of motion, and evaluation of muscular function.

Radiographic evaluation

The radiographic assessment includes standard weight-bearing radiographs and hindfoot alignment view (**Fig. 8**A, B). Additionally, functional weight-bearing lateral radiographs in maximal dorsiflexion and plantar flexion should be performed. Alternatively, the true ankle motion in sagittal plan can be assessed using fluoroscopy. A weight-bearing computed tomography scan can help to assess the amount of extra bone formation accurately (**Fig. 9**). The degree of radiographic evidence of bony hypertrophy does not necessarily correlate with symptoms and/or physical examination findings. Single-photon emission computed tomography may help to identify areas of impingement in those patients with equivocal radiographic studies (**Fig. 10**).

Differential diagnosis

The accurate identification of the structures causing ankle pain and/or stiffness may be challenging owing to the proximity of the extrinsic tendons of the foot and ankle. Many of the patients had limited ankle range of motion before replacement surgery, and the resultant motion and excursion can cause pain in these previously dormant tendons. The most commonly affected tendons are the posterior tibial tendon and flexor hallucis longus tendon.

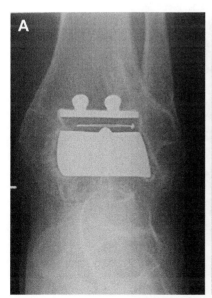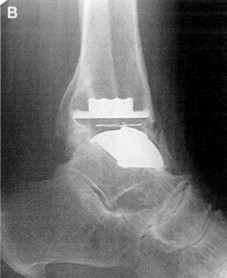

Fig. 8. Standard weight-bearing radiographs in a 52-year-old woman 11 years after total ankle replacement showing extended periarticular bone formation with the ankle fixed in the equinus position. Notice also secondary degenerative disease at the talonavicular joint due to overload. (*A*) Anteroposterior view. (*B*) Lateral view.

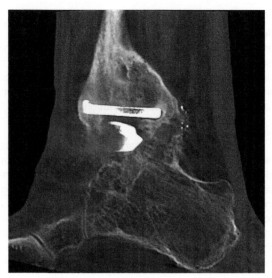

Fig. 9. The computed tomography scan helps to assess extent and localization of ossifications.

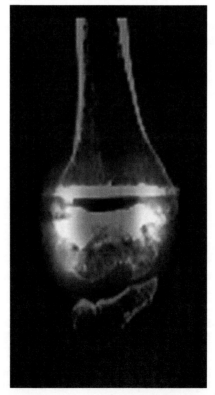

Fig. 10. The single-photon emission computed tomography scan is helpful for assessing activity resulting from bone formation and secondary impingement.

Degenerative changes in the adjacent joints (eg, subtalar and/or talonavicular joint) can be another source for pain around the ankle. Diagnostic injections of local anesthetic directly into the joints can be helpful to confirm the diagnosis.

Surgical Strategies

Arthroscopic surgery
Currently, there is limited literature outlining successful arthroscopic debridement of anterior and gutter impingement after TAR (**Table 3**).[22,83–86] The arthroscopic technique can be used to debride hypertrophic bone on the anterior aspect of the tibia when it overhangs the tibial component (**Fig. 11**). However, arthroscopic debridement is not recommended for posterior overhanging bone structures because of the proximity of the neurovascular bundle. The main disadvantage of arthroscopy after TAR is the potential for damage to the polished surfaces of the implant, which can cause and/or accelerate wear of the polyethylene bearing (**Box 1**). Also, third body wear is possible from residual bone or metallic debris.

Anterior impingement/stiffness
A purely isolated anterior stiffness of the replaced ankle is rare and often presents with an incompetent heel cord. The clinical assessment typically reveals some degree of dorsiflexion, but only very little plantar flexion. Therefore, after debridement of the anterior ankle, including the medial and lateral gutter, the improvement in ankle range of motion should be assessed carefully. If there is no significant improvement in either dorsiflexion or plantar flexion, as a next step the polyethylene insert should be removed and the posterior ankle structures should be debrided. The view of the posterior aspect of the ankle can be substantially improved with manual distraction of the ankle, for example, by using a K-wire–based distractor, such as a Hintermann distractor.

Posterior (and anterior) impingement/stiffness
Despite more advanced imaging modalities, the amount and extent of hypertrophic bone formation cannot always be estimated precisely before the revision surgery (**Fig. 12A, B**). If clinical assessment demonstrates a truly hard stop against dorsiflexion, significant scarring and ossification of the posterior capsule should be expected. In this case, a posteromedial approach is considered for extended open debridement. An additional advantage of this approach is that the posterior tibial tendon can also be explored, evaluated, and released, if necessary.

After complete posterior debridement, the ankle is mobilized manually into maximal dorsiflexion and plantar flexion. If the gained plantar flexion is not satisfactory, an additional anterior debridement through the former anterior approach is performed. Thereafter, if the gained dorsiflexion is not satisfactory, an additional release of the heel cord should be considered.

Component loosening and/or malpositioning
If preoperative clinical and radiographic evaluation revealed loosening of 1 or both components, with or without subsidence, progressive cyst formation or malpositioning, a revision of 1 or both ankle implants is mandatory to achieve appropriate postoperative outcome. Component revision is done according to the type of ankle prosthesis, usually through an anterior approach.[41,88]

Surgical Technique

The surgery can be performed under general or regional anesthesia. The patient is placed in a supine position, with an ipsilateral bump until a strictly upward position

Table 3
Literature review addressing arthroscopic debridement in patients who underwent total ankle replacement

Study	Study Type	Patients (Ankles)	Prosthesis Type	Indication for Arthroscopic Debridement	Surgical Technique	Outcomes
Devos Bevernage et al,[22] 2016	RS, SC	12 (12)	Hintegra (7), Mobility (4), AES (1)	AM imp. (4); AM imp., med. gutter, PTT (1); AM imp., med. gutter (1); ankylosis, ant./post. imp. (1); med. gutter, ankylosis, post. capsular retraction (1); ant. imp., corpus liberum (1); ankylosis, post. HO (1); AM imp., med./lat. gutter (1); med./lat. gutter (1)	Ant. AS (10), ant./post. AS (2)	Mean FU 4.9 ± 2.4 y (2–9.8); AOFAS hindfoot score 64.6 → 73.5; complete pain relief (8); partial pain relief (4); TAR ROM 17°±9° (5°–37°)
Gross et al,[83] 2016	TN	1 (1)	STAR (1)	Med. gutter imp. (1)	Ant. AS using standard AM/AL portals; 2.7-mm arthroscope, 3.5-mm shaver	NR

Richardson et al,[85] 2012	RS, SC	20 (20)	STAR (20)	Med./lat. gutter imp. (20)	Ant. AS using standard AM/AL portals; 2.7-mm arthroscope, 3.5-mm shaver	No wound complications; no postoperative infections; 6 patients developed recurrent symptoms
Shirzad et al,[86] 2011	RS, SC	11 (11)	Salto Talaris (11)	Med./lat. gutter imp. (11)	Ant. AS using standard AM/AL portals; 2.7-mm arthroscope, 3.5-mm shaver	NR

Abbreviations: AES, ankle evolutive system; AL, anterolateral; AM, anteromedial; ant., anterior; AOFAS, American Orthopedic Foot and Ankle Society; AS, arthroscopy; FU, follow-up; HO, heterotopic ossification; imp., impingement; med., medial; NR, not reported; post., posterior; PTT, posterior tibial tendon; ROM, range of motion; RS, retrospective; SC, single center; STAR, Scandinavian Total Ankle Replacement; TAR, total ankle replacement; TN, technical note.

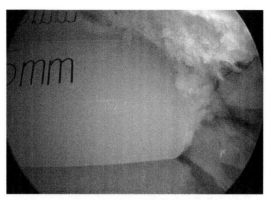

Fig. 11. Arthroscopic debridement of anterior ankle.

of the foot is obtained. It is not necessary to place the patient in a prone position because the entire posterior rim of the distal tibia can be visualized through a posteromedial arthrotomy. A pneumatic tourniquet is applied on the ipsilateral thigh.

In most cases, the previous anterior ankle approach is used between the anterior tibial tendon and extensor hallucis longus tendon (**Fig. 13**A). After the tibiotalar joint is exposed, the scarred anterior capsule is removed, the osteophytes on the tibia and talus are debrided, and the medial and lateral gutters are cleaned of any bone formation (see **Fig. 13**B). Thereafter, the ankle is gradually mobilized into dorsiflexion. If a minimal dorsiflexion of 10° cannot be obtained, the polyethylene insert is removed, and the joint is distracted manually using a K-wire-based distractor, such as a Hintermann distractor. The posterior aspect of the ankle is visualized and the posterior capsule is carefully cut with a large chisel guided first along the flat tibial component and second along the curved talar component. Special attention is paid

---

Box 1
Advantages and disadvantages of using arthroscopic versus open debridement in patients who have undergone total ankle replacement

Advantages

- Less invasive procedure with less postoperative pain[87]
- Shorter recovery[87]
- Lower risk for postoperative complications including wound healing issues
- Faster mobility and weight-bearing after debridement, because there is no need to protect arthrotomy incision
- Outpatient setting possible

Disadvantages

- Technically demanding procedure with technical skills required to bypass scarring tissue
- Scratching/damage of prosthesis component possible
- Difficult to completely visualize medial and lateral gutters
- Longer surgery time if using radiofrequency ablation, shaver or burr
- Posteromedial debridement associated with injury risk of neurovascular bundle

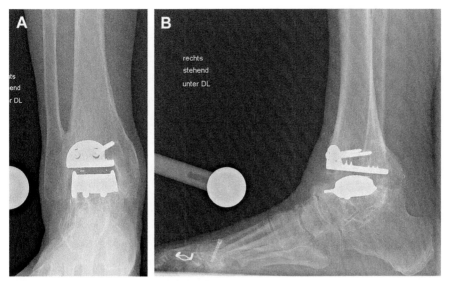

Fig. 12. Extended periarticular ossification with stiffness of the ankle in a 59-year-old woman 11 years after total ankle replacement because of a severe posttraumatic osteoarthritis. The patient had sustained a complex ankle fracture with subsequent infection. (*A*) Anteroposterior view. (*B*) Lateral view.

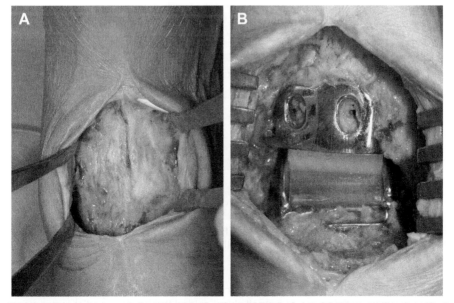

Fig. 13. Anterior approach (same patient as **Fig. 11**). (*A*) Exposure of the scarred and ossified anterior capsule. (*B*) After resection of the capsule, the medial and lateral gutters are also debrided.

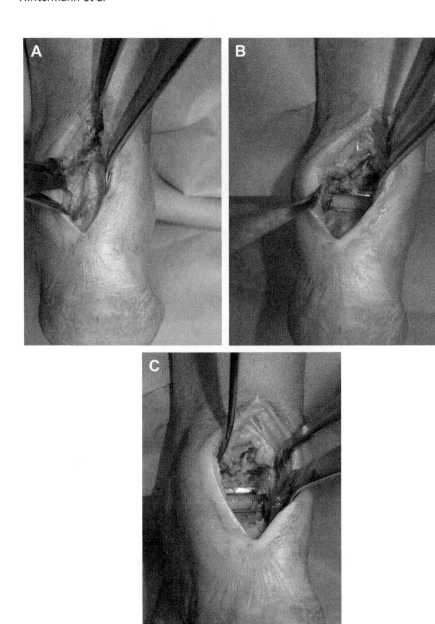

Fig. 14. Posterior approach (same patient as **Fig. 11**). (*A*) Exposure of scarred and ossified posterior capsule along medial border of Achilles tendon. The medial (*B*) and lateral (*C*) gutters are also debrided.

posteromedially not to injure the neurovascular bundle. The medial and lateral edges are cut vertically with the use of a small chisel guided through the medial gutter along the medial malleolus and through the lateral gutter along the fibula, respectively. The posterior capsule and the ossification can usually be removed using a rongeur until posterior fat and flexor hallucis longus tendon can be visualized. If a dorsiflexion of 10° can still not be obtained, a lengthening of heel cord is considered.

In patients with significant posterior bony overhang, the incision is placed along the course of posterior tibial tendon. The incision should be long enough to reflect the entire posterior medial soft tissues off the posterior aspect of the distal tibia. A bladed retractor is placed across the entire exposed posterior tibia to the syndesmosis to provide adequate exposure. On the medial side, a small Hohmann retractor is placed on the posteromedial talus. Ossifications and scarred capsular structures are removed and posterior ankle is debrided. If a minimum dorsiflexion of 10° can still not be obtained, a lengthening of the heel cord should be performed.

In patients with extended bone formation on the posterior aspect of the ankle, including a bony bridge between the tibia and talus, a posterior approach along the medial aspect of the Achilles tendon should be performed, as described in detail (**Fig. 14**A). Ossifications and scarred capsular structures are removed and posterior ankle is debrided (See **Fig. 14**B, C). If afterward a minimum dorsiflexion of 10° can still not be obtained, a lengthening of the heel cord should be performed (**Fig. 15**A, B). **Fig. 16** shows the situation after combined anterior and posterior resection.

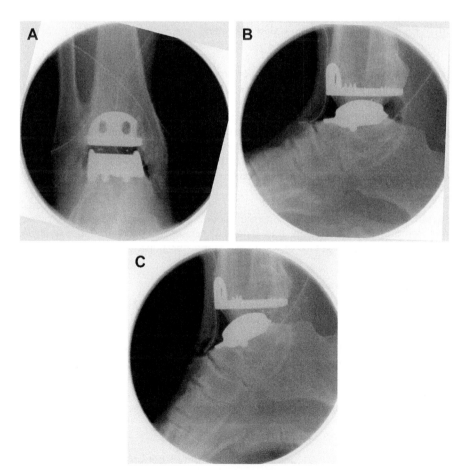

Fig. 15. Intraoperative fluoroscopic check. (*A*) Anteroposterior view. (*B*) Lateral view of the foot in maximal dorsiflexion; and (*C*) foot in maximal plantar flexion.

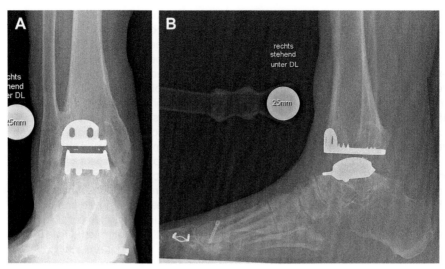

Fig. 16. Weight-bearing radiographs showing the ankle 1 year after debridement (same patient as **Fig. 11**). (*A*) Anteroposterior view. (*B*) Lateral view.

In patients with component loosening or progressive periprosthetic cyst formation, 1 or both components are removed. The entire ankle is debrided, including resection of scarred capsular structures. Hypertrophic bone is also removed while special attention is paid not to weaken the remaining bone stock. The cysts are completely debrided and the bone stock is prepared to receive a new component.

Localized bone defects are filled by autograft or allograft, and bone matrix can also be used to obtain an appropriate bone–prosthesis interface. If available, special revision prosthesis components should be used.

Complications

The main postoperative complications are wound healing problems caused by preexisting compromised soft tissue and extensive tissue resection around the ankle. Although uncommon, fracture of the malleoli and component migration can occur postoperatively.

Postoperative Management

After 2 to 3 days, the compressive dressing and temporary splint are removed and replaced by a short leg soft cast and a walking boot, respectively. In noncompliant patients, a lower leg fiberglass cast should be used instead. Early full weight-bearing is allowed in the walking boot or cast as tolerated. At 6 weeks postoperatively, the ankle is assessed clinically and radiographically. In patients with appropriate soft tissue status and good prosthesis components integration, free ambulation and rehabilitation are initiated. The rehabilitation program includes passive and active mobilization of the ankle, proprioception, coordination, gait improvement, and strength training.

RESULTS

In a collective review of 501 primary TAR performed between January 2008 and December 2013, 92 ankles (18.4%) showed a limited dorsiflexion (<3°) preoperatively. Extended bony and capsular resection was done in all patients, and in 34 ankles

(6.8%), an additional Achilles tendon lengthening was performed. The American Orthopedic Foot and Ankle Society score increased from 47 preoperatively to 72 at the last follow-up (minimum of 2 years).

Revision of the ankle replacement because of painful stiffness was performed in 43 ankles (6.8%). An anterior approach was used in all but 3 ankles, a posteromedial approach was used in 16 ankles, and a posterior approach was used in 8 ankles. The Achilles tendon was lengthened in 7 ankles (1.4%), and the posterior tibial tendon was revised in 5 ankles (1.0%). With the revision surgery, the American Orthopedic Foot and Ankle Society score improved from 61 to 70; overall range of motion increased from 26° to 30°. Delayed wound healing was seen in 2 patients, but it healed uneventfully without additional surgery.

SUMMARY

In patients with a stiff ankle replacement, appropriate resection of scarred capsular structures, hypertrophic bone formation debridement, and careful release of tendons should be performed to achieve good postoperative outcomes. However, appropriately sized and correctly implanted components are required to restore the ankle function to as normal as possible. Although not proven, based on our experience, the better a TAR is balanced, the less likely scar and heterotopic bone formation will occur postoperatively.[89,90] In patients with a stiff and painful ankle replacement, a detailed preoperative diagnostic workup is mandatory to fully understand the underlying pathologic process and to plan the best appropriate treatment. As a principle, all underlying causes should be addressed appropriately, including malpositioning and/or oversized implants, loosening of implants, cyst formation, hindfoot malalignment, soft tissue contractures, and hypertrophic bone formation.

ACKNOWLEDGMENTS

The authors thank Christine Schweizer for her help in preparing the article and the figures. The authors also thank Joshua R. Harmer and Raymond Y. Hsu, MD for their help in correcting this article.

REFERENCES

1. Barg A, Zwicky L, Knupp M, et al. HINTEGRA total ankle replacement: survivorship analysis in 684 patients. J Bone Joint Surg Am 2013;95(13):1175–83.

2. Daniels TR, Mayich DJ, Penner MJ. Intermediate to long-term outcomes of total ankle replacement with the Scandinavian Total Ankle Replacement (STAR). J Bone Joint Surg Am 2015;97(11):895–903.

3. Daniels TR, Younger AS, Penner M, et al. Intermediate-term results of total ankle replacement and ankle arthrodesis: a COFAS multicenter study. J Bone Joint Surg Am 2014;96(2):135–42.

4. Hsu AR, Haddad SL. Early clinical and radiographic outcomes of intramedullary-fixation total ankle arthroplasty. J Bone Joint Surg Am 2015;97(3):194–200.

5. Nwachukwu BU, Mclawhorn AS, Simon MS, et al. Management of end-Stage ankle arthritis: cost-utility analysis using direct and indirect costs. J Bone Joint Surg Am 2015;97(14):1159–72.

6. Queen RM, Sparling TL, Butler RJ, et al. Patient-reported outcomes, function, and gait mechanics after fixed and mobile-bearing total ankle replacement. J Bone Joint Surg Am 2014;96(12):987–93.

7. Ramaskandhan JR, Kakwani R, Kometa S, et al. Two-year outcomes of MOBILITY total ankle replacement. J Bone Joint Surg Am 2014;96(7):e53.
8. Rippstein PF, Huber M, Coetzee JC, et al. Total ankle replacement with use of a new three-component implant. J Bone Joint Surg Am 2011;93(15):1426–35.
9. Barg A, Knupp M, Henninger HB, et al. Total ankle replacement using HINTE-GRA, an unconstrained, three-component system: surgical technique and pit-falls. Foot Ankle Clin 2012;17(4):607–35.
10. Hintermann B, Valderrabano V, Dereymaeker G, et al. The HINTEGRA ankle: rationale and short-term results of 122 consecutive ankles. Clin Orthop Relat Res 2004;(424):57–68.
11. Shi GG, Huh J, Gross CE, et al. Total ankle arthroplasty following prior infection about the ankle. Foot Ankle Int 2015;36(12):1425–9.
12. Barg A, Pagenstert GI, Hugle T, et al. Ankle osteoarthritis: etiology, diagnostics, and classification. Foot Ankle Clin 2013;18(3):411–26.
13. Saltzman CL, Salamon ML, Blanchard GM, et al. Epidemiology of ankle arthritis: report of a consecutive series of 639 patients from a tertiary orthopaedic center. Iowa Orthop J 2005;25(1):44–6.
14. Valderrabano V, Horisberger M, Russell I, et al. Etiology of ankle osteoarthritis. Clin Orthop Relat Res 2009;467(7):1800–6.
15. Holzer N, Salvo D, Marijnissen AC, et al. Radiographic evaluation of posttrau-matic osteoarthritis of the ankle: the Kellgren-Lawrence scale is reliable and cor-relates with clinical symptoms. Osteoarthritis Cartilage 2014;23(3):363–9.
16. Horisberger M, Valderrabano V, Hintermann B. Posttraumatic ankle osteoarthritis after ankle-related fractures. J Orthop Trauma 2009;23(1):60–7.
17. Myerson MS, Mroczek K. Perioperative complications of total ankle arthroplasty. Foot Ankle Int 2003;24(1):17–21.
18. Saltzman CL, Amendola A, Anderson R, et al. Surgeon training and complications in total ankle arthroplasty. Foot Ankle Int 2003;24(6):514–8.
19. Choi WJ, Lee JW. Heterotopic ossification after total ankle arthroplasty. J Bone Joint Surg Br 2011;93(11):1508–12.
20. Lee KB, Cho YJ, Park JK, et al. Heterotopic ossification after primary total ankle arthroplasty. J Bone Joint Surg Am 2011;93(8):751–8.
21. Jung HG, Lee SH, Shin MH, et al. Anterior heterotopic ossification at the talar neck after total ankle arthroplasty. Foot Ankle Int 2016;37(7):703–8.
22. Devos Bevernage B, Deleu PA, Birch I, et al. Arthroscopic debridement after total ankle arthroplasty. Foot Ankle Int 2016;37(2):142–9.
23. Kim BS, Choi WJ, Kim J, et al. Residual pain due to soft-tissue impingement after uncomplicated total ankle replacement. Bone Joint J 2013;95(3):378–83.
24. Schuberth JM, Babu NS, Richey JM, et al. Gutter impingement after total ankle arthroplasty. Foot Ankle Int 2013;34(3):329–37.
25. Schuberth JM, Wood DA, Christensen JC. Gutter impingement in total ankle ar-throplasty. Foot Ankle Spec 2016;9(2):145–58.
26. Barg A, Saltzman CL. Ankle replacement. Mann's surgery of the foot and ankle. Philadelphia: Elsevier Saunders; 2014. p. 1078–162.
27. Valderrabano V, Hintermann B, Horisberger M, et al. Ligamentous posttraumatic ankle osteoarthritis. Am J Sports Med 2006;34(4):612–20.
28. Hintermann B. Total ankle arthroplasty: historical overview, current concepts and future perspectives. Vienna (Austria): Springer; 2005.
29. Brunner S, Barg A, Knupp M, et al. The Scandinavian Total Ankle Replacement: long-term, eleven to fifteen-year, survivorship analysis of the prosthesis in seventy-two consecutive patients. J Bone Joint Surg Am 2013;95(8):711–8.

30. Saltzman CL, Tochigi Y, Rudert MJ, et al. The effect of agility ankle prosthesis misalignment on the peri-ankle ligaments. Clin Orthop Relat Res 2004;424(1): 137–42.

31. Tochigi Y, Rudert MJ, Brown TD, et al. The effect of accuracy of implantation on range of movement of the Scandinavian total ankle replacement. J Bone Joint Surg Br 2005;87(5):736–40.

32. Barg A, Elsner A, Anderson AE, et al. The effect of three-component total ankle replacement malalignment on clinical outcome: pain relief and functional outcome in 317 consecutive patients. J Bone Joint Surg Am 2011;93(21): 1969–78.

33. Barg A, Elsner A, Hefti D, et al. Haemophilic arthropathy of the ankle treated by total ankle replacement: a case series. Haemophilia 2010;16(4):647–55.

34. Barg A, Elsner A, Hefti D, et al. Total ankle arthroplasty in patients with hereditary hemochromatosis. Clin Orthop Relat Res 2011;469(5):1427–35.

35. Barg A, Knupp M, Anderson AE, et al. Total ankle replacement in obese patients: component stability, weight change, and functional outcome in 118 consecutive patients. Foot Ankle Int 2011;32(10):925–32.

36. Barg K, Wiewiorski M, Anderson AE, et al. Total ankle replacement in patients with von Willebrand disease: mid-term results of 18 procedures. Haemophilia 2015; 21(5):e389–401.

37. Ellington JK, Gupta S, Myerson MS. Management of failures of total ankle replacement with the agility total ankle arthroplasty. J Bone Joint Surg Am 2013;95(23):2112–8.

38. Giannini S, Romagnoli M, O'connor JJ, et al. Early clinical results of the BOX ankle replacement are satisfactory: a multicenter feasibility study of 158 ankles. J Foot Ankle Surg 2011;50(6):641–7.

39. Haskell A, Mann RA. Perioperative complication rate of total ankle replacement is reduced by surgeon experience. Foot Ankle Int 2004;25(5):283–9.

40. Hintermann B, Barg A, Knupp M, et al. Conversion of painful ankle arthrodesis to total ankle arthroplasty. J Bone Joint Surg Am 2009;91(4):850–8.

41. Hintermann B, Zwicky L, Knupp M, et al. HINTEGRA revision arthroplasty for failed total ankle prostheses. J Bone Joint Surg Am 2013;95(13):1166–74.

42. Horisberger M, Henninger HB, Valderrabano V, et al. Bone augmentation for revision total ankle arthroplasty with large bone defects. Acta Orthop 2015;86(4): 412–4.

43. Kim BS, Knupp M, Zwicky L, et al. Total ankle replacement in association with hindfoot fusion: outcome and complications. J Bone Joint Surg Br 2010;92(11): 1540–7.

44. Noelle S, Egidy CC, Cross MB, et al. Complication rates after total ankle arthroplasty in one hundred consecutive prostheses. Int Orthop 2013;37(9):1789–94.

45. Alvarez-Goenaga F. Total ankle replacement. First 25 cases. Rev Esp Cir Ortop Traumatol 2008;52(3):224–32.

46. Barg A, Henninger HB, Knupp M, et al. Simultaneous bilateral total ankle replacement using a 3-component prosthesis: outcome in 26 patients followed for 2-10 years. Acta Orthop 2011;82(6):704–10.

47. Bolton-Maggs BG, Sudlow RA, Freeman MA. Total ankle arthroplasty. A long-term review of the London Hospital experience. J Bone Joint Surg Br 1985;67(5): 785–90.

48. Bonnin M, Gaudot F, Laurent JR, et al. The Salto total ankle arthroplasty: survivorship and analysis of failures at 7 to 11 years. Clin Orthop Relat Res 2011;469(1): 225–36.

49. Criswell BJ, Douglas K, Naik R, et al. High revision and reoperation rates using the agility total ankle system. Clin Orthop Relat Res 2012;470(7):1980–6.
50. Freeman MaR, Kempson GE, Tuke MA, et al. Total replacement of the ankle with the ICLH prosthesis. Int Orthop 1979;2(3):327–31.
51. Giannini S, Romagnoli M, O'connor JJ, et al. Total ankle replacement compatible with ligament function produces mobility, good clinical scores, and low complication rates: an early clinical assessment. Clin Orthop Relat Res 2010;468(10): 2746–53.
52. Henricson A, Knutson K, Lindahl J, et al. The AES total ankle replacement: a mid-term analysis of 93 cases. Foot Ankle Surg 2010;16(2):61–4.
53. Hobson SA, Karantana A, Dhar S. Total ankle replacement in patients with significant pre-operative deformity of the hindfoot. J Bone Joint Surg Br 2009;91(4): 481–6.
54. Karantana A, Hobson S, Dhar S. The Scandinavian Total Ankle Replacement: survivorship at 5 and 8 years comparable to other series. Clin Orthop Relat Res 2010;468(4):951–7.
55. Kerkhoff YRA, Kosse NM, Louwerens JW. Short term results of the mobility total ankle system: clinical and radiographic outcome. Foot Ankle Surg 2016;22(3): 152–7.
56. Knecht SI, Estin M, Callaghan JJ, et al. The Agility total ankle arthroplasty. Seven to sixteen-year follow-up. J Bone Joint Surg Am 2004;86-A(6):1161–71.
57. Lewis JS Jr, Green CL, Adams SB Jr, et al. Comparison of first- and second-generation fixed-bearing total ankle arthroplasty using a modular intramedullary tibial component. Foot Ankle Int 2015;36(8):881–90.
58. Muir D, Aoina J, Hong T, et al. The outcome of the mobility total ankle replacement at a mean of four years: can poor outcomes be predicted from pre- and postoperative analysis? Bone Joint J 2013;95(10):1366–71.
59. Murnaghan JM, Warnock DS, Henderson SA. Total ankle replacement. Early experiences with STAR prosthesis. Ulster Med J 2005;74(1):9–13.
60. Nodzo SR, Miladore MP, Kaplan NB, et al. Short to midterm clinical and radiographic outcomes of the Salto total ankle prosthesis. Foot Ankle Int 2014;35(1): 22–9.
61. Nunley JA, Caputo AM, Easley ME, et al. Intermediate to long-term outcomes of the STAR total ankle replacement: the patient perspective. J Bone Joint Surg Am 2012;94(1):43–8.
62. Rosello Anon A, Martinez Garrido I, Cervera Deval J, et al. Total ankle replacement in patients with end-stage ankle osteoarthritis: clinical results and kinetic gait analysis. Foot Ankle Surg 2014;20(3):195–200.
63. Saltzman CL, Kadoko RG, Suh JS. Treatment of isolated ankle osteoarthritis with arthrodesis or the total ankle replacement: a comparison of early outcomes. Clin Orthop Surg 2010;2(1):1–7.
64. Schweitzer KM, Adams SB, Viens NA, et al. Early prospective clinical results of a modern fixed-bearing total ankle arthroplasty. J Bone Joint Surg Am 2013;95(11): 1002–11.
65. Stauffer RN. Total ankle joint replacement. Arch Surg 1977;112(9):1105–9.
66. Stauffer RN, Segal NM. Total ankle arthroplasty: four years' experience. Clin Orthop Relat Res 1981;(160):217–21.
67. Valderrabano V, Pagenstert G, Horisberger M, et al. Sports and recreation activity of ankle arthritis patients before and after total ankle replacement. Am J Sports Med 2006;34(6):993–9.

68. Barg A, Wimmer MD, Wiewiorski M, et al. Total ankle replacement - indications, implant designs, and results. Dtsch Arztebl Int 2015;112(11):177–84.
69. Gougoulias N, Khanna A, Maffulli N. How successful are current ankle replacements? A systematic review of the literature. Clin Orthop Relat Res 2010; 468(1):199–208.
70. Lindsjö U, Danckwardt-Lilliestrom G, Sahlstedt B. Measurement of the motion range in the loaded ankle. Clin Orthop Relat Res 1985;(199):68–71.
71. Coetzee JC, Castro MD. Accurate measurement of ankle range of motion after total ankle arthroplasty. Clin Orthop Relat Res 2004;(424):27–31.
72. Barg A, Amendola RL, Henninger HB, et al. Measurement of supramalleolar alignment on the anteroposterior and hindfoot alignment views: influence of ankle position and radiographic projection angle. Foot Ankle Int 2015;36(11):1352–61.
73. Saltzman CL, El-Khoury GY. The hindfoot alignment view. Foot Ankle Int 1995; 16(9):572–6.
74. Linklater JM, Read JW, Hayter CL. Ch 3 imaging of the foot and ankle. In: Coughlin M, Saltzman CL, Anderson RB, editors. Mann's surgery of the foot and ankle. 9th edition. Philadelphia: Elsevier Saunders; 2014. p. 61–120.
75. Colin F, Horn Lang T, Zwicky L, et al. Subtalar joint configuration on weightbearing CT scan. Foot Ankle Int 2014;35(10):1057–62.
76. Krahenbuhl N, Tschuck M, Bolliger L, et al. Orientation of the subtalar joint: measurement and reliability using weightbearing CT scans. Foot Ankle Int 2016;37(1): 109–14.
77. Hintermann B. What the orthopaedic foot and ankle surgeon wants to know from MR imaging. Semin Musculoskelet Radiol 2005;9(3):260–71.
78. Linklater JM, Fessa CK. Imaging findings in arthrofibrosis of the ankle and foot. Semin Musculoskelet Radiol 2012;16(3):185–91.
79. Salamon ML, Pinney SJ, Van Bergeyk A, et al. Surgical anatomy and accuracy of percutaneous Achilles tendon lengthening. Foot Ankle Int 2006;27(6):411–3.
80. Pinney SJ, Sangeorzan BJ, Hansen ST Jr. Surgical anatomy of the gastrocnemius recession (Strayer procedure). Foot Ankle Int 2004;25(4):247–50.
81. Barouk P. Technique, indications, and results of proximal medial gastrocnemius lengthening. Foot Ankle Clin 2014;19(4):795–806.
82. Hintermann B, Valderrabano V, Knupp M, et al. The HINTEGRA ankle: short- and mid-term results. Orthopade 2006;35(5):533–45 [in German].
83. Gross CE, Neumann JA, Godin JA, et al. Technique of arthroscopic treatment of impingement after total ankle arthroplasty. Arthrosc Tech 2016;5(1):e1–5.
84. Lui TH, Roukis TS. Arthroscopic management of complications following total ankle replacement. Clin Podiatr Med Surg 2015;32(4):495–508.
85. Richardson AB, Deorio JK, Parekh SG. Arthroscopic debridement: effective treatment for impingement after total ankle arthroplasty. Curr Rev Musculoskelet Med 2012;5(2):171–5.
86. Shirzad K, Viens NA, Deorio JK. Arthroscopic treatment of impingement after total ankle arthroplasty: technique tip. Foot Ankle Int 2011;32(7):727–9.
87. Scranton PE Jr, Mcdermott JE. Anterior tibiotalar spurs: a comparison of open versus arthroscopic debridement. Foot Ankle 1992;13(3):125–9.
88. Hintermann B, Zwicky L, Knupp M, et al. HINTEGRA revision arthroplasty for failed total ankle prostheses. J Bone Joint Surg Am 2013;95(13):1166–74.
89. Barg A, Suter T, Zwicky L, et al. Medial pain syndrome in patients with total ankle replacement. Orthopade 2011;40(11):991–2, 994–9. [in German].
90. Hintermann B. Ankle joint prosthetics in Switzerland. Orthopade 2011;40(11):963 [in German].

Experience with Navigation in Total Ankle Arthroplasty. Is It Worth the Cost?

Christopher W. Reb, DO[a], Gregory C. Berlet, MD[b],*

KEYWORDS

• Accuracy • Technique • Outcomes • Value

KEY POINTS

- Emergence of a navigation-assisted total ankle replacement (TAR) system approved by the Food and Drug Administration raises the question of whether or not the technology is worth the additional cost.
- TAR implant malalignment has negative mechanical and kinematic effects.
- Reliance on 2-dimensional radiographs appears to be a confounder to accurate TAR placement.
- Navigation provides 3-dimensional preoperative templating and patient-specific cut guides.
- Compared with conventional systems, navigation offers comparable, if not improved, tibial component accuracy but the highest reported accuracy for the talus component.

In recent history, the market for total ankle arthroplasty (TAR) has expanded. This was driven by increasing demand from an educated population for an alternative surgical option to ankle fusion as a treatment of end-stage ankle arthritis. Commensurate with this demand, the number of surgeons skillful at TAR has grown, thereby increasing its availability. Other important factors contributing to this trend of improved access include improvements in surgeon training through fellowships, training courses, and skills laboratories[1]; improvements in technique, including the use of intraoperative imaging, alignment guides,[2] and captured cut guides; improvements in implant materials and designs; and an expanding literature base.

For the surgeon, both cognitive and psychomotor skills improve as experience is acquired, leading to better preoperative planning and technical execution of the

---

Disclosure: Dr G.C. Berlet is a paid consultant for Wright Medical Technology, Inc. Dr C.W. Reb has nothing to disclose.
[a] Division of Foot and Ankle Surgery, Department of Orthopaedics and Rehabilitation, University of Florida College of Medicine, 3450 Hull Road, Gainesville, FL 32607, USA; [b] Orthopedic Foot and Ankle Center, 300 Polaris Parkway, Suite 2000, Westerville, OH 43082, USA
* Corresponding author.
E-mail address: ofacresearch@orthofootankle.com

operation. With the emergence of a navigation-assisted TAR system approved by the Food and Drug Administration, the question raised is whether or not a computer-assisted strategy aimed at improving surgical precision in achieving an individualized predefined target is worth the additional cost of both surgeon and engineering time, as well as the cost of the advanced imaging.

Of the factors under the surgeon's control, when performing TAR, optimal placement of correctly sized implants is elemental to prolonging the working life of the implant. Component position and alignment affect the distribution of forces within the system. The relevant forces include the distribution of contact stress at the bearing surface, the strains born by associated ligaments,[3] and the forces at the interfaces between bone and prosthetic materials.[4]

The mechanical effects of implant malalignment are well characterized for TAR. For example, the ankle joint bears forces up to 5 times the body's weight during ambulation.[5] As a result, even slight joint incongruity secondary to component malalignment results in unevenly distributed contact stresses leading to potentially destructive focal contact pressures.

Espinosa and colleagues[6] reported a validated finite element analysis model used to compare the effect of talar component malalignment on bearing surface contact stresses between the fixed-bearing Agility (DePuy Synthes Companies, Warsaw, IN) and the mobile-bearing Mobility (DePuy Synthes Companies, Warsaw, IN) prostheses. As for the Agility, the average contact pressures exceeded the 10 MPa thresholds for polyethylene delamination, even when optimally aligned. These magnitudes became substantially higher and more narrowly distributed from edge loading by the talar component when the components were coronally malaligned. Agility pressure distributions were similar for neutral and axial rotation malalignment, with malalignment creating potentially damaging contact pressures; whereas, the average contact pressures with Mobility prostheses were less than 10 MPa when optimally aligned, but exceeded this threshold through edge loading with as little as 2° of coronal malalignment. Rotational malalignment did not elevate pressure magnitudes nor alter their distributions, presumably due to accommodation by the mobile bearing. This study shows that coronal malalignment is not tolerated, regardless of mobile or fixed-bearing design.

Corroborating these findings, Fukuda and colleagues[4] used a human cadaveric model to assess loaded static and dynamic pressure distributions in response to talar component rotation for the Agility prosthesis. They demonstrated a decrease in contact area and substantial focal increase in contact stresses with talar component axial malalignment, particularly in internal rotation. Additionally, they demonstrated increased rotational torques at the bone-implant interface below the talar component in axially malaligned positions.

Additionally, variations in TAR component positioning will affect ankle kinematics. Saltzman and colleagues[3] used a cadaveric model of simulated gait to demonstrate relative changes in ankle ligament lengths in response to variations in Agility tibial component position. Subsequently, Tochigi and colleagues[7] used a similar methodology to demonstrate diminished loaded ankle range of motion when the talus component of the mobile-bearing Scandinavian TAR (STAR) prosthesis (Small Bone Innovations, Inc, Morrisville, PA) was implanted in nonanatomic sagittal plane positions and when the polyethylene bearing was considered to be too thick or too thin.

Cenni and colleagues[8] reported a retrospective case series of 14 mobile-bearing Box total ankles (Finsbury Orthopaedics Limited, Leatherhead, UK), which were assessed clinically and with radiographs preoperatively and at approximately 7 and 13 months postoperatively. Overall, they found acceptable ankle range of motion for all prostheses. However, they did note small but statistically significant increases in range of motion in instances in which there was larger sagittal plane polyethylene-to-tibial-component motion, where the talar component was located more anteriorly than the tibial component, and among talus components with more anterior inclination, respectively.

However, limited outcomes data support the importance of accurate implant positioning on clinical outcomes. Barg and colleagues[9] observed a consistent trend among 317 mobile-bearing Hintegra prostheses (Integra LifeSciences Corporation (France), Plainsboro, NJ) in which better short-term to intermediate-term clinical outcomes occurred in patients with the talar component in ideal sagittal alignment with the tibial component. The investigators concluded that the small but statistically significant magnitudes of difference observed for visual analog scale pain, ankle range of motion, and American Orthopaedic Society Ankle hindfoot score were clinically important indicators of the need for accurate implant positioning.

Whereas the ideal in situ parameters for each implant system are specific to its unique design features, the ability to select the correct prosthesis for the patient and to skillfully implant it are acquired skills. In this way, the outcomes of TAR are operator dependent to an important extent. The learning curve for a surgeon new to performing TAR appears to level off at approximately 25.[10] However, this phenomenon really reflects gross improvements in minimizing the negative effects of subjectivity and technical error early in one's experience with TAR. The learning curve for achieving outcome consistency across the nuanced breadth of challenges potentially facing an ankle arthroplasty surgeon is not well characterized.

An important confounder to accurate TAR implantation lies in the reliance on 2-dimensional imaging. Adams and colleagues[2] retrospectively compared tibial component alignment accuracy when using either intramedullary or extramedullary alignment guides. There were 153 INBONE II prostheses (Wright Medical Technology, Inc, Arlington, TN) implanted using intramedullary alignment, and 83 Salto Talaris prostheses (Integra LifeSciences Corporation) implanted using extramedullary alignment. Both radiographic tibial implant alignment and observer measurements were highly precise. However, when corrected for the specific surgeon-intended alignment, intramedullary alignment was significantly more accurate in the sagittal plane.

Prissel and colleagues[11] used weight-bearing ankle radiographs to evaluate observer reliability among 13 candidate coronal and sagittal plane parameters for possible use with the INBONE II prosthesis. Intraclass correlation (ICC) of 0.75 or greater was chosen to indicate sufficient reproducibility for clinical use. Overall, only 2 parameters showed sufficient reproducibility for both intraobserver and interobserver reliability. One was preoperative distal tibial articular surface alignment relative to the tibial anatomic axis on the coronal view; the other was the height of the posterior aspect of the talus component relative to a line between the superior aspects of the talonavicular joint and the calcaneus tuberosity on the lateral view. For both measurements, ICC values indicated excellent to near perfect (ICC >0.90) intraobserver and interobserver reliability.

Tochigi and colleagues[12,13] evaluated radiographic methods for assessing sagittal plane tibiotalar alignment. They accurately noted that intraarticular landmarks are often obscured in ankle osteoarthritis (OA) and are absent following TAR. Therefore, they proposed using extra-articular radiographic landmarks. The tibial-axis–to-talus ratio (T-T ratio) was defined as the ratio into which the mid-longitudinal axis of the tibial shaft divides the longitudinal talar length. The posterior-tibia-axis–to-talus ratio (P-T ratio) was defined as the same ratio but using the posterior tibial diaphyseal line instead. They found measurement errors ranging between 2% and 6% for these parameters, despite variations in limb rotation between 10° internal to 10° external and despite changes in ankle joint flexion angles. Moreover, they demonstrated excellent observer reliability for both parameters when using clinical radiographs from patients with and without ankle OA.

Braito and colleagues[14] demonstrated wide variation in radiographic measurements about the Hintegra total ankle prosthesis with limb positioning varying within 3 planes of freedom. They corroborated these findings by demonstrating comparable variances in the same measurements when obtained from a retrospective case series of TAR patients.

In addition to their heterogeneous methodology and results, it is important to note that none of these radiographic studies used a gold standard of comparison, such as standing full-length lower limb films or computed tomography (CT) scans, for assessing radiographic measurement accuracy. Further, no studies have addressed observer consistency in relation to characteristics of preoperative deformity.

Taken as a body of knowledge, we interpret these data to guide us toward a TAR implantation technique that is based on reliable and reproducible landmarks, and using implantation techniques that have the proposed benefit of accuracy and reproducibility of implantation.

In the context of joint replacement surgery, the term "navigation" refers to computer software–assisted surgical planning and execution based on a digital model of the patient's anatomy. The primary goal of navigation is process improvement (**Box 1**). Whereas Leardini and colleagues[15] developed a system to covert preoperative radiographs into a navigation system, there is one FDA-approved navigated TAR system (PROPHECY INBONE II and PROPHECY INFINITY Preoperative Navigation System, Wright Medical Technology, Inc, Arlington, TN). This system uses a preoperative ankle and hindfoot CT scan to generate patient-specific captured cut guides for intraoperative use.

As in other forms of navigation-assisted surgery, proprietary software generates a highly accurate rendering of the patient's bony anatomy (**Fig. 1**). Based thereupon, the software then allows the surgeon to interact with the computer model. The surgical strategy is developed through stepwise consideration of the elements of the surgery. This process identifies loose bodies for removal; the location, size, and shape of osteophytes; the presence of bone deficits; the 3-plane nature of any preexisting deformity; and the desired features, position, and sizes of the final implants (**Fig. 2**). Once the virtual surgery is completed, the final plan is used to generate patient-specific bone models and captured cut guides for the tibia and talus (**Fig. 3**).

Presently, outcomes data related to navigated TAR are limited. In a cadaveric model, Adams and colleagues[16] compared radiographic alignment of the STAR

Box 1
Goals of navigation for total ankle replacement

1. Accuracy: patient-specific plan with final implant positions as intended.

2. Precision: reproducible result of the process.

3. Efficiency: shorter time to goal.

4. Value: long-term lower total cost per case from fewer complications/revisions from technical errors.

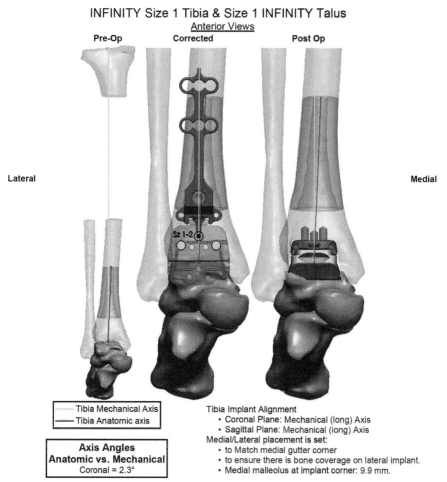

INFINITY Size 1 Tibia & Size 1 INFINITY Talus
Anterior Views

Pre-Op   Corrected   Post Op

Lateral   Medial

| Tibia Mechanical Axis |
| Tibia Anatomic axis |

Axis Angles
Anatomic vs. Mechanical
Coronal = 2.3°

Tibia Implant Alignment
 • Coronal Plane: Mechanical (long) Axis
 • Sagittal Plane: Mechanical (long) Axis
Medial/Lateral placement is set:
 • to Match medial gutter corner
 • to ensure there is bone coverage on lateral implant.
 • Medial malleolus at implant corner: 9.9 mm.

Fig. 1. Prophecy assessment of mechanical and anatomic alignment with proposed position of tibial cut guide and final tibial prosthesis position (Infinity implant).

prosthesis tibial component following use of either the standard extramedullary alignment jig and cut block or a computer-navigated system designed for use in total knee arthroplasty (VectorVision, BrainLAB, Munich, Germany). They found that tibial component alignment was highly accurate when using the jig and this was not significantly improved by computer navigation assistance. The investigators did not address the talar component.

Berlet and colleagues[17] assessed the accuracy and precision of the PROPHECY INBONE system by using live intraoperative navigation technology (Optotrak Certus, First Principles software; Northern Digital Inc, Waterloo, Ontario, Canada) as the gold standard of comparison. The primary outcome was the accuracy of surgeon placement of both the CT-derived patient-specific cut guides and the final implants. Overall, the guides were placed within 1° of rotational goal with less than 1 mm of translation. The implant rotational alignments were within 2° and 2 mm of target.

CASE18714 - Bone Void Appendix

Any bone voids are shown below relative to the implant and resection plane. Please refer to the patient's CT scan for more details.

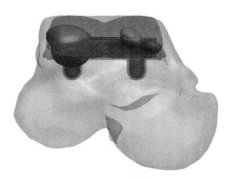

Anterior view of talus with implant.

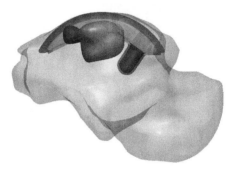

Sagittal view of talus with implant.

Fig. 2. Talus implant and effect of bone voids in local anatomy (Infinity talus).

Hsu and colleagues[18] compared 3-month postoperative plain-film radiographic coronal and sagittal plane tibial component alignment to the preoperative plan. All postoperative measurements were within 3° of the plan, but the average was less than 1°; however, observer reliability was not reported. Additionally, neutral alignment was achieved regardless of preoperative deformity. Tibial component size prediction was highly accurate and talar component size prediction was 75% accurate. The investigators' impression was that this variability was likely due to intraoperative surgeon preferences.

Clinical outcomes data are limited to a single case report. Hanselman and colleagues[19] reported acceptable radiographic and clinical outcome at 8 months in a 54-year-old male patient with preoperative varus ankle deformity of 29°.

Taken as a whole, the TAR literature appears to show that in the present era, implant positions are reproducibly falling within relatively narrow tolerances across the spectrum of prosthetic designs and instrumentation systems. However, it also suggests a clinically significant threshold for implant malpositioning lies within a few millimeters or degrees of target.

Given the current evidence, the value of adopting navigation for TAR can be estimated only based on benefits other than a proven clinical outcomes improvement

Post Op

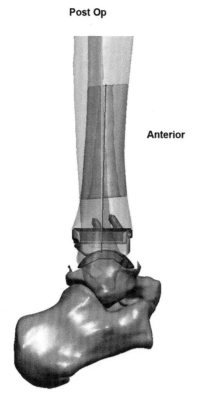

Anterior

Fig. 3. Final position of the tibia and talus components as seen on the lateral view (Infinity tibia and talus).

directly attributable to its use. To that end, preoperatively, the navigation processes assists the surgeon in customizing the surgical strategy to the patient through unique 3-dimensional templating and virtual surgery. Intraoperatively, the patient-specific cut guides reduce instrumentation (**Box 2**), steps, and obviate reliance on jig-based estimation of the appropriate mechanical alignment of the implants. Compared with conventional systems, navigation offers comparable, if not improved, tibial component accuracy, but the highest reported accuracy for the talus component.

To better inform this conversation, well-observed longitudinal outcomes studies are warranted. The potential advantages to surgeons include a flattening of the learning curve, enhanced accuracy, and reproducibility across a wide variety of clinical challenges.

Box 2
Benefits of reduced instrumentation with navigation for total ankle replacement

1. Quicker set up
2. Fewer trays through processing
3. Fewer intraoperative steps
4. Fewer posteriorly directed steps

REFERENCES

1. Saltzman CL, Amendola A, Anderson R, et al. Surgeon training and complications in total ankle arthroplasty. Foot Ankle Int 2003;24(6):514–8.
2. Adams SB Jr, Demetracopoulos CA, Viens NA, et al. Comparison of extramedullary versus intramedullary referencing for tibial component alignment in total ankle arthroplasty. Foot Ankle Int 2013;34(12):1624–8.
3. Saltzman CL, Tochigi Y, Rudert MJ, et al. The effect of agility ankle prosthesis misalignment on the peri-ankle ligaments. Clin Orthop Relat Res 2004;424: 137–42.
4. Fukuda T, Haddad SL, Ren Y, et al. Impact of talar component rotation on contact pressure after total ankle arthroplasty: a cadaveric study. Foot Ankle Int 2010; 31(5):404–11.
5. Fischer AG, Wolf A. Assessment of the effects of body weight unloading on overground gait biomechanical parameters. Clin Biomech 2015;30(5):454–61.
6. Espinosa N, Walti M, Favre P, et al. Misalignment of total ankle components can induce high joint contact pressures. J Bone Joint Surg Am 2010;92(5):1179–87.
7. Tochigi Y, Rudert MJ, Brown TD, et al. The effect of accuracy of implantation on range of movement of the Scandinavian total ankle replacement. J Bone Joint Surg Br 2005;87(5):736–40.
8. Cenni F, Leardini A, Cheli A, et al. Position of the prosthesis components in total ankle replacement and the effect on motion at the replaced joint. Int Orthop 2012; 36(3):571–8.
9. Barg A, Elsner A, Anderson AE, et al. The effect of three-component total ankle replacement malalignment on clinical outcome: pain relief and functional outcome in 317 consecutive patients. J Bone Joint Surg Am 2011;93(21): 1969–78.
10. Simonson DC, Roukis TS. Incidence of complications during the surgeon learning curve period for primary total ankle replacement: a systematic review. Clin podiatr Med Surg 2015;32(4):473–82.
11. Prissel MA, Berlet GC, Scott RT, et al. Radiographic assessment of a medullary total ankle prosthesis: a test of agreement and reliability. Foot Ankle Spec 2016. [Epub ahead of print].
12. Tochigi Y, Suh JS, Amendola A, et al. Ankle alignment on lateral radiographs. Part 1: sensitivity of measures to perturbations of ankle positioning. Foot Ankle Int 2006;27(2):82–7.
13. Tochigi Y, Suh JS, Amendola A, et al. Ankle alignment on lateral radiographs. Part 2: reliability and validity of measures. Foot Ankle Int 2006;27(2):88–92.
14. Braito M, Liebensteiner M, Dammerer D, et al. Poor accuracy of plain radiographic measurements of prosthetic migration and alignment in total ankle replacement. J Orthop Surg Res 2015;10:71.
15. Leardini A, Rapagna L, Ensini A, et al. Computer-assisted preoperative planning of a novel design of total ankle replacement. Comput Methods Programs Biomed 2002;67(3):231–43.
16. Adams SB Jr, Spritzer CE, Hofstaetter SG, et al. Computer-assisted tibia preparation for total ankle arthroplasty: a cadaveric study. Int J Med Robot 2007;3(4): 336–40.
17. Berlet GC, Penner MJ, Lancianese S, et al. Total ankle arthroplasty accuracy and reproducibility using preoperative CT scan-derived, patient-specific guides. Foot Ankle Int 2014;35(7):665–76.

18. Hsu AR, Davis WH, Cohen BE, et al. Radiographic outcomes of preoperative CT scan-derived patient-specific total ankle arthroplasty. Foot Ankle Int 2015;36(10): 1163–9.
19. Hanselman AE, Powell BD, Santrock RD. Total ankle arthroplasty with severe pre-operative varus deformity. Orthopedics 2015;38(4):e343–6.

Is There Anything to Learn from a National Joint Registry?

Dawson Muir, FRACS

KEYWORDS

- Ankle arthroplasty • National joint registry • Outcome • Big data • Compliance
- Data integration • Elimination of bias • Implant surveillance

KEY POINTS

- National Joint Registries (NJRs) eliminate potential bias due to the historic dominance of developer series.
- Concerns relate to over interpretation of data, compliance with revision reporting and the potential for mandatory publication of surgeon's specific data.
- Surgeon- and institution-based outcomes provide close to real-time feedback that can alter practice.
- NJRs have potential to independently monitor introduction of new implants and provide early warning of those performing poorly.
- Registries must be integrated with other robust data sets and adequately funded to audit compliance.

INTRODUCTION

National joint registries (NJRs) have been established in Northern Europe for over 20 years. Since then, many other countries have begun collecting and reporting national data for total ankle arthroplasty (TAA).

With relatively small numbers implanted, a large variety of available designs, and with any long-term reports dominated by designer groups, TAA is ideally placed to benefit from large national or even pooled national registries.

The existing registry-based literature has been reviewed with respect to what is already known. The potential positives and down sides of registry data are highlighted.

DEMOGRAPHICS OF NATIONAL REGISTRIES

National arthroplasty registries were first established in Sweden. Their knee register was founded in 1976 and hip register in 1979.[1] Since then, numerous countries

The author has nothing to disclose.
Grace Orthopaedic Centre, 335 Cheyne Road, Tauranga 31125, New Zealand
E-mail address: dawson.muir@orthocentre.co.nz

have created national registries. Ankle replacements were added to the Swedish, Norwegian, and Finnish registries in the early 1990s.[2–4] They were followed by New Zealand in 2000,[5] Australia in 2007,[6] and England and Wales in 2009.[7] These registries are all embedded in their multi-implant national arthroplasty registries with an established culture of reporting.

National ankle registries have more recently been established in France, Denmark, Belgium, The Netherlands, and Germany. To date, these young registries are yet to get close to the greater than 85% coverage recommended for national registries.[1,8]

In the United States, big data repositories such as Medicare have been used to identify trends in TAA,[9] but incomplete coverage and lack of specific information erode their value. A national registry was launched in 2010 but does not currently include TAA,[10] and it remains to be seen whether it will achieve wide acceptance.

The European Foot and Ankle Society, in cooperation with the European Arthroplasty Register, is setting up an umbrella registry based on implant tracking.[11] This has potential to provide more robust audit of national registry compliance.

This article is restricted largely to established national registries with extensive coverage and current annual reports in English.

WHY HAVE A REGISTRY?

The aim of a national registry is to decrease the socioeconomic burden associated with failure and morbidity. This is achieved through several mechanisms (**Box 1**).

The Generalizability Cascade

Across all arthroplasty, designer groups or those affiliated with implant companies report better results when compared with registries.[12] There are many potential reasons for this, including surgeon experience, the designer's better appreciation of the nuances of the device, and several potential sources for bias. This is certainly true in TAA. About 50% of cases in outcome reports come from designer groups,[13] with an average 9- to 10-year survival of 84% to 95%.[14–17] Equivalent data from registries are more sobering (**Table 1**).

Expressed another way, the annual failure rate of surgeon designers is 1.1% compared with nondesigner series 1.7% and finally national joint registries of 3.2%. This hierarchy of survival data represents the generalizability cascade.[20]

Often overlooked as an alternative explanation for inferior registry survivorship is the inclusion of an array of devices with proven inferior survival.

Box 1
Benefits of registries

   i. Generalizable outcome data—all surgeons, no exclusions, no conflict of interest

   ii. Timely feedback to individual surgeons and institutions

   iii. Monitoring the performance of types of TAA and surgical techniques close to real time

   iv. Provide a warning system for early failure

   v. Allow easy identification of patients for recall or more in-depth research

   vi. Potential to expand data collection with (a) patient-reported outcome measures and/or (b) groups such as fusion or supramalleolar osteotomy

---

Table 1 Survival rates from established national registries								
Years	3	4	5	6	7	8	9	10
Sweden	—	—	81	—	—	—	—	69
Finland	—	—	83	—	78	—	—	—
Norway	—	—	89	—	—	—	—	76[a]
New Zealand	94.2	—	90.2	—	—	—	83.1[c]	—
Australia	91.7	89.9	—	—	87.6[b]	—	—	—
England/Wales	97.2	—	—	—	—	—	—	—

[a] Small numbers (confidence interval 71–85).
[b] Excludes rheumatoid arthritis patients who had slightly better survival.
[c] Updated in 2014 with addition of missed revisions.
Data from Refs.[6,7,9,18,19]

Monitoring the Performance of Implants

Following the explosion of availability of different designs and implantation techniques, robust monitoring of the introduction and ultimately long-term outcome is imperative. This has been dramatically demonstrated in total hip arthroplasty. The Australian registry first identified higher than expected revision rates in young women with large metal-on-metal hip resurfacing when compared with conventional implants in 2005.[6] A specific hip implant was implicated soon afterward. Similarly, the Swedish registry identified high failure of a Sulzer hip when only 30 had been implanted, whereas in the United States 17,500 of these replacements had been implanted, and an estimated 3000 have required revision.[1]

In TAA, the impact of registries has been more modest. The Ramses ankle was highlighted by the New Zealand Joint Registry (NZJR) in 2006 after very few had been implanted.[18] The NZJR, which has been collecting postoperative patient-reported outcome scores since its inception, found that the 6-month scores correlated with early requirement for revision[21] and could potentially function as an early warning sign for poor performance in the future. Data from the Swedish registry have shown poor results for the single-coat Scandinavian Total Ankle Replacement (STAR, LINK Orthopaedics Hamburg, Germany).[22,23] This device has a single layer of hydroxyapatite sprayed on the smooth metal and has a 14-year survival of 47% versus a 64% 12-year survival for the later version with a Titanium plasma spray plus calcium phosphate later. The role of the implant bone interface is further supported by the failure mechanism (59% of the failures for the single layer device were caused by aseptic loosening compared with 42% in the double-layer device). Most recently, the double-layer STAR (LINK Orthopaedics, Hamburg, Germany) was flagged by the Australian registry in 2015 with higher early failure after only 40 had been implanted.[6] Potential confounders such as learning curve and patient selection make it difficult to draw conclusions from these highlighted examples. However, despite good long-term reports for the STAR from designer and nondesigner groups,[24,25] the registry results, as well as the widespread abandonment of this device in countries with registries, should provide caution to users.

As the quality of registry data improves with larger numbers of universally popular designs that have better medium- and long-term survivorship, there will be a superior generalizable benchmark to compare newer designs. Ultimately, in countries with registries, one can learn in a timely fashion of the risks and results of large-scale experimentation with new implant technology[1]

Monitoring Trends

Overall

National registries provide useful retrospective insights into the patient population and implant usage. The most compelling trend is the reducing numbers of TAA. Total numbers peaked in Sweden[26] and Norway[2] in 2009, New Zealand[19] in 2010, and Australia[6] in 2011. No data have been published for the United States since 2014, when an increasing trend was reported up until the end of 2011 in the Medicare population.[9] In Sweden, there has also been a reduction in the number of institutions and surgeons performing TAA.[22] Similarly, in New Zealand there are now only 3 surgeons performing greater than 10 TAAs per annum. This is likely to be, at least in part, because of the registry. No one wants to be an outlier at the wrong end of the bell curve. Diminished enthusiasm for TAA may also come from unflattering comparison with hip and knee outcomes. For example, the rate of revision per 100 component years of 2.13 for ankles looks unpleasant when compared with total knee rates of 0.49.[19]

Registry specific

By the end of 2014 the NJR in the United Kingdom had 2554 primary ankles registered with a mean age of 68 years and 58% male. Following withdrawal of the mobility, other devices are becoming more popular, especially fixed bearing implants.[7]

Also by the end of 2014, there were 1504 primaries registered in Australia with mean age 66 years and 61% male. The most common implants in 2014 were Salto followed by Hintegra. 274 ankles were implanted in 2011 compared with 146 in 2015.[6] This represents the most dramatic decline in all registries.

In New Zealand, as of February 2016, there were 1275 primaries in the NZJR with mean age 65.5 years and 62% male.

At the end of 2014 there were 958 ankles in the Norwegian registry,[27] and 1130 in the Swedish version.[26] These 2 registries, and the Finnish registry, have higher percentages of patients with rheumatoid disease (up to one-third vs 10% in New Zealand and even less in Australia). This may reflect genetic differences, better treatment of rheumatoid arthritis in recent years, or that New Zealand and Australian surgeons are more aggressive at recommending replacement for isolated osteoarthritis. The latter may be true given the higher per capita usage in New Zealand and Australia.

Implant specific

Pooled registry data demonstrate dominance of 3 component mobile bearing designs, representing 97% of all prostheses used from 2000 to 2011 **(Table 2)**.[10] The STAR, Buechel Pappas (Endotec Orange, New Jersey), Ankle Evolution System (Transysteme-JMT, Nimes, France), Agility (DePuy, Warsaw, Indiana), and more recently the Mobility (DePuy International, Leeds, United Kingdom) have declined and/or been withdrawn.

Salto, Hintegra and Zenith are currently popular designs, with small numbers of Trabecular Metal Zimmer and Infinity appearing in 2014 to 2015.[7,19]

What Registries Can Tell About Revision

Preoperative demographics

New Zealand, Sweden, and Australia have demonstrated higher revision rates for younger and post-trauma patients.[6,19,26] In Sweden, this elevated risk was statistically significant in females.[22] All registries show similar or better survivorship for rheumatoid patients.

Table 2
Implant usage in registries

	Australia	NJR (England/Wales)	New Zealand	Norway	Sweden	Total
Mobility	565	1111	450	100	269	2495
STAR	40	166	47	615	324	1192
Salto	346	185	513	100	0	1144
Zenith	8	584	0	0	0	592
Hintegra	353	174	15	11	36	589
CC1	4	0	0	149	78	232
Rebalance	36	0	0	15	130	181
Fusion	—	—	—	—	1667	—
Supra-Malleolar Osteotomy	—	—	—	—	31	—

Total numbers of common implants in registries (as at end of 2014 from 2015 annual reports).

Failure mode

Standardization of reporting revision or reoperation is essential to extracting useful data. Defining reasons for reoperation are more complex than for hip and knee arthroplasty. A Canadian group found 572 unique terms used to describe adverse events in 117 studies.[28] A guideline developed by this group provides a useful framework to draft a revision/reoperation registry document to minimize confusion and hopefully harmonize better with registry forms from other countries (**Fig. 1**). Henricson and colleagues[29] also defined revision as removal of any component apart from incidental polyethylene exchange. This has been adopted by the Swedish registry and the NJR.

A meta-analysis of failure mode used published results from the Norwegian, Swedish, and New Zealand registries from 1997 to 2007. Sadoghi and colleagues[30] found revision for aseptic loosening at 38%, technical errors in 15%, pain without other cause in 12%, infection in 9.8%, instability in 8.5%, implant breakage in 5.3%, and periprosthetic fracture in 2%. Whether failure is assigned to technical error is subjective, requires insight, and depends on whether it is offered as an option on the form. Many revisions for malalignment, instability, periprosthetic fracture, or early subsidence could potentially be characterized as surgeon error. Apart from identifying technical error as a potential reason for failure, registries do not provide any superior data with respect to failure mode than other series.

Failure of specific implants

Given that there is only 1 randomized-controlled trial in the literature[31] and no standardized outcome reporting and clinical series, registries are the only means of obtaining some measure of direct comparison between implants using revision as an endpoint. Only the New Zealand and Swedish registries use patient-reported outcome measures. When comparing implant survival, variable lengths of follow-up must be accounted for. The best way to do this is to report the failure rate per 100 component years. This is derived by dividing the number of prostheses revised by the observed component years multiplied by 100. The observed component years is the number of registered primaries multiplied by the number of years each component has been in place (**Table 3**).

NEW ZEALAND JOINT REGISTRY   **FREE PHONE 0800 274-989**

RE-OPERATION / REVISION ANKLE JOINT REPLACEMENT

Date:	
BMI:	
Side: **	Patient Label [89 x 28 mm]
Town / City:	
Hospital:	
Theatre No:	

Date of Primary Arthroplasty:............................   **Date of Prior Revision / Re-operation:**...................

REASON FOR THIS REVISION/REOPERATION (more than one may apply)

☐ Access   ☐ Impingement

☐ Osteolysis: Talus ☐   Tibia ☐   ☐ Periprosthetic #

☐ Pain ? Cause   ☐ Deep infection (confirmed ☐   suspected ☐)

☐ Subjacent arthritis   ☐ Pain due to malalignment

☐ Bearing Failure (wear ☐   fracture ☐)   ☐ Failure to osseointergrate

☐ Subsidence Talus ☐   Tibia ☐   ☐ Other...

REVISION PROCEDURE	
☐ Bearing exchange for wear or fracture	☐ Extraction +/- cement spacer
☐ Tibia: standard ☐ revision ☐ custom ☐ allograft composite ☐	☐ Amputation
☐ Talus: standard ☐ revision ☐ custom ☐ allograft composite ☐	☐ Additional Procedures ....
☐ Fusion: TT ☐ TTC ☐	
CEMENT: **Tibia** ☐	**Talus** ☐

OR _RE-OPERATION_ PROCEDURE	
☐ Osteotomy	☐ Tendon surgery
☐ Debridement for infection (bearing exchange for access ☐)	☐ Subjacent Fusions
☐ Debridement for impingement: open ☐ arthroscopic ☐	☐ Lateral ligament repair
☐ Grafting of cysts: with bearing exchange ☐	☐ ORIF Peri prosthetic #
☐ Other:	

PRIMARY SURGEON: Consultant ☐   Fellow Unsuperv. ☐   Registrar Unsuperv. ☐
                                              Fellow Superv. ☐   Registrar Superv. ☐

OPERATION TIME: Start Skin Time........   Finish Skin Time.......

Fig. 1. Proposed reoperation and revision form for NZJR to improve accurate indication and classification of the surgical episode.

This method of comparison can identify poor performing implants. Unfortunately, at this time, even in registries, small numbers of patients with a long enough follow-up of designs currently in use limit the utility of this data.

Evaluation of revisions

The New Zealand and Swedish registries have continued to analyze patients after revision or fusion. The NZJR reported generally poor outcomes for its revision cohort.[19]

Table 3
Comparison of 3 implants from New Zealand Joint Registry (2015 annual report)

	Number	Observed Component Years	Number Revised	Rate/100 Component Years
Mobility	450	2320	52	2.24
Salto	513	1716	19	1.11
Ramses	513	78	5	6.43

Using the revision rate/100 component years allows direct comparison between designs with variable follow-up length.

The Swedish group has published similarly unflattering results of revision[32] and salvage fusion.[33] This group reported on 69 revisions with 24 failing again after a median 25 months. Of 33 with the revision still in situ, 29 completed their validated self-reported foot and ankle score (SEFAS). For salvage fusions, despite 90% primary union, the outcome scores were equivalent to the revision cohort. Only 47% were satisfied or very satisfied. These complete, unselected national cohorts are an important addition to the body of literature on this challenging problem.

Provision of surgeon's specific data

Being able to compare results to the national average can influence practice.[34] Outlier committees have been set up in several registries to review surgeon, institution, and implant performance. The process must be confidential at least initially and conducted with sensitivity.

PROBLEMS WITH REGISTRIES

Several issues have already been raised. The difficulties faced by national registries can be summarized by defining what they require to function well.

Requirements for an effective registry include

I. A culture of open and diligent reporting
II. Stable long-term funding (ideally independent of data ownership)
III. Strong governance to protect data, robust mechanisms to interact with industry, and strategies to address outliers
IV. Internationally standardized reporting
V. Publication that avoids overinterpretation of observational data
VI. Good coverage, ideally greater than 90% of primary procedures
VII. Even better compliance with revision
VIII. Timely feedback to surgeons to support best practice

Culture

Countries with existing hip and knee registries have an established culture of reporting and pre-existing mechanisms to collect, analyze, and audit data. Without this, it takes more than a few dedicated individuals to develop an effective registry.

The Funding and Control

Most national registries are government funded. Without adequate funding, it is likely that the quality of reporting and audit will suffer first. Independent ownership should prevent dissemination of surgeon's specific data. This is of particular concern in the United Kingdom, where the data are owned by the government.[34]

Overinterpretation

National registries fall into the category of big data.[35] Although they are repositories of more specific information than most databases, they share problems such as misclassification, lumping, confounders, and potentially meaningless significance of statistical power.

For example, lumping all STAR implants together could lead to erroneous conclusions regarding outcome of a more recent design. Without knowledge of confounders, which local surgeons may be aware of, a true effect cannot be quantified. Fundamentally, registries are hypothesis-generating tools rather than replacements for well-designed studies.[35,36] Misclassification is a possible explanation for an unexpected finding from the NZJR. Hooper and colleagues[37] found higher infection rates for hip and knee replacement in Laminar flow theaters as opposed to conventional theaters, despite having no definition of what constitutes Laminar flow in the registry documentation.

Incomplete coding can make validation difficult. If big national health data sets are not side specific or fail to record the implant removal aspect of a fusion, they cannot be reliably used to audit revision compliance.

When interpreting registry information the reader must be aware of what is missing and the methods of quality control and audit within the database.[35] Work is being done to standardize reporting guidelines for publishing big data, including registries.[35]

Revision Compliance—Can the data be trusted?

This is the greatest problem facing ankle registries (**Fig. 2**). Without integration with an accurate external independent data base, one cannot guarantee revision compliance. In no joint is this more problematic than the ankle.[38] When validating the Norwegian registry, poor compliance was found with conversion to fusion.[38] As yet unpublished data from the NZJR from 2013 (Puna and colleagues) found similar results. Of 887 primary ankles, the registry had documented 65 revision procedures in 58 ankles.

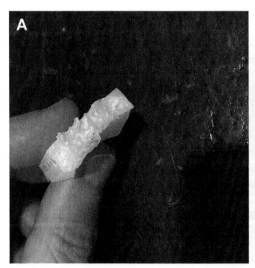
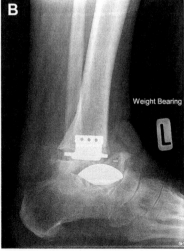

Fig. 2. (*A*) Exchanged bearing at 9 years. (*B*) Mobile bearing Salto with talar fracture and collapse immediately prior to conversion to fusion. Both cases were overlooked as revisions by the operating theater staff.

Following phone interview with patients and contact with all the treating surgeons to provide additional information on those who volunteered further surgery or who could not be traced, an additional 59 revisions were uncovered. Importantly, all 3 amputation cases and 35 fusions had been overlooked. In ankle arthroplasty, missing extraction fusions markedly diminish revision accuracy. Having highlighted these omissions, one can be confident that capture will improve, but short of repeating the process, there is no way to be sure in New Zealand. The British Orthopaedic Foot and Ankle Society reports its revision rate may be under-reported. This registry currently contains only 12 conversion to fusion.[7] The Australian registry has only 5 documented fusions.[6]

Better comprehensive national health data sets that are side specific and reliably capture extraction without reimplantation are operating in most countries with full International Society of Arthroplasty Registry Membership. In countries where a significant proportion of TAAs are performed in private hospitals, there must be the same standard of reporting from those hospitals to cross-check compliance.

Other strategies to audit capture include implant retrieval registries.[39] The planned European implant registry will serve this purpose also. Linking payment with submission of a registry form would be a powerful tool to get close to universal coverage of primary surgery but may not be as effective for revision or reoperation in ankle arthroplasties.

Documentation of validation of revision compliance with high capture rates should be mandatory for publication in quality peer-reviewed journals.

SUMMARY

Currently, interpretation of registry data is fraught with confounders and potential data capture problems. To date, registry publications largely support the level IV evidence from case series but with inferior results, which probably more closely approximate general usage. However, there is plenty to be optimistic about. As registries accumulate increasing numbers of better performing devices with longer follow-up, this will allow more rapid comparison with new designs and continue to inform and influence surgical decision making.

REFERENCES

1. Von Knoch F, Malchau H. Why do we need a national joint replacement registry in the United States? Am J Orthop 2009;38(10):500–3.
2. Henricson A, Skoog A, Carlsson A. The Swedish ankle arthroplasty register: an analysis of 531 arthroplasties between 1993 and 2005. Acta Orthop 2007; 78(5):569–74.
3. Skytta E, Koivu H, Eskelinen A, et al. Total ankle replacement a population based study of 515 cases from the Finnish Arthoplasty Register. Acta Orthop 2010; 81(1):114–8.
4. Fevang B-T, Lie S, Havelin L, et al. 257 ankle arthroplasties performed in Norway between 1994 and 2005. Acta Orthop 2007;78(5):575–83.
5. Tomlinson M, Harrison M. The New Zealand joint registry report of 11 year data for ankle arthroplasty. Foot Ankle Clin N Am 2012;17:719–23.
6. The Australian Orthopaedic Association Joint Replacement Registry Annual Report 2015. Available at: https://aoanjrr.sahmri.com. Accessed October 1, 2016.
7. National Joint Registry for England, Wales, Northern Ireland and the Isle of Man 2015 Annual Report. Available at: www.njrcentre.org.uk. Accessed October 1, 2016.

8. International Society of Arthroplasty Registers. Bylaws (revised March 2013). Available at: http://www.isarhome.org/statements. Accessed October 1, 2016.

9. Pugely A, Lu X, Amendola A, et al. Trends in the use of total ankle replacements and ankle arthrodesis in the united states Medicare population. Foot Ankle Int 2014;35(3):207–15.

10. Roukis T, Prissel M. Registry data trends of total ankle replacement use. J Foot Ankle Surg 2013;52:728–35.

11. Kofoed H, Kostuj T, Goldberg A. European registers for total ankle replacement. Foot Ankle Surg 2013;19:1.

12. Bedair H, Lawless B, Malchau H. Are implant designer series believable? Comparison of survivorship between designer series and national registries. J Arthroplasty 2013;28:728–31.

13. Labek G, Klaus H, Schlichtherle R, et al. Revision rates after total ankle arthroplasty in sample based clinical studies and national registries. Foot Ankle Int 2011;32(8):740–5.

14. Barg A, Zwicky L, Knupp M, et al. Hintegra total ankle replacement: survivorship analysis in 684 patients. J Bone Joint Surg Am 2013;95:1175–83.

15. Bonnin M, Gaudot F, Laurent J-R, et al. The Salto total ankle arthroplasty. Survivorship and analysis of failures at 7 to 11 years. Clin Orthop Relat Res 2011; 469:225–36.

16. Kofoed H. Scandinavian Total Ankle Replacement (STAR). Clin Orthop Relat Res 2004;424:73–9.

17. Knect S, Estin M, Callaghan J, et al. The agility total ankle arthroplasty : seven to sixteen year follow up. J Bone Joint Surg Am 2004;86(6):1161–71.

18. Labek G, Todorov S, Iovanescu L, et al. Outcome after total ankle arthroplasty – results and findings from worldwide arthroplasty registers. Int Orthop 2013;37: 1677–82.

19. The New Zealand Joint Registry: six year report 2015. Available at: www.nzoa. org.nz/new-joint-registry. Accessed October 1, 2016.

20. Zaidi R, Cro S, Gurusamy K, et al. The outcome of total ankle replacement. A systematic review and meta-analysis. Bone Joint J 2013;95-B:1500–7.

21. Hosman A, Mason R, Hobbs T, et al. A New Zealand national joint registry review of 202 total ankle replacements followed for up to 6 years. Acta Orthop 2007; 78(5):584–91.

22. Henricson A, Nilsson J-A, Carlsson A. 10 year survival of total ankle arthroplasties. A report on 780 cases from the Swedish Ankle Register. Acta Orthop 2011;82(6):655–9.

23. Henricson A, Carlsson A. Survival Analysis of the Single and Double-Coated STAR Ankle up to 20 years: long term follow up of 324 cases from the Swedish Ankle Registry. Foot Ankle Int 2015;36(10):1156–60.

24. Mann J, Mann R, Horton E. STAR ankle: long term results. Foot Ankle Int 2011;32: 473–84.

25. Nunley J, Caputo A, Easley M, et al. Intermediate to long term outcomes of the STAR total ankle replacement: the patient perspective. J Bone Joint Surg Am 2012;94:43–8.

26. The Swedish Ankle Registry Annual Report for 2014. Available at: www. swedankle.se. Accessed October 1, 2016.

27. The Norwegian Hip Register annual report 2015. Report 2015 – English. Available at: nrlweb.ihelse.net. Accessed October 1, 2016.

28. Mercer J, Penner M, Wing K, et al. Inconsistency in the report of adverse events in total ankle arthroplasty: a systematic review of the literature. Foot Ankle Int 2016;37(2):127–36.

29. Henricson A, Carlsson A, Rydholm U. What is a revision of total ankle replacement? Foot Ankle Surg 2011;17(3):99–102.

30. Sadoghi P, Liebensteiner M, Agreiter M. Revision surgery after total joint arthroplasty: a complication - based analysis using worldwide arthroplasty registers. J Arthroplasty 2013;28:1329–32.

31. Wood P, Sutton C, Mishra, et al. A randomised controlled trial of two mobile bearing total ankle replacements. J Bone Joint Surg Br 2009;91:69–74.

32. Kamrad A, Henricson A, Karlsson M, et al. Poor prosthesis survival and function after component exchange of total ankle prosthesis. Acta Orthop 2015;86(4):407–11.

33. Kamrad I, Henricson A, Magnusson H, et al. Outcome after salvage arthrodesis for failed total ankle replacement. Foot Ankle Int 2015;37(3):255–61.

34. Haddad F, Manktelow A, Skinner J. Publication of surgeon level data from registers: who benefits? Bone Joint J 2016;98-B:1–2.

35. Perry D, Parsons N, Costa M. 'Big data' reporting guidelines. Bone Joint J 2014;96-B:1575–7.

36. Konan S, Haddad F. Joint registries: a Ptolemaic model of data interpretation? Bone Joint J 2013;95-B:1585–6.

37. Hooper GJ, Rothwell AG, Frampton C, et al. Does the use of laminar flow and space suits reduce early deep infection after total hip and knee replacement?: the ten-year results of the New Zealand Joint Registry. J Bone Joint Surg Br. 2011;93(1):85–90.

38. Espehaug B, Furnes O, Havelin L, et al. Registration completeness in the Norwegian Arthroplasty Register. Acta Orthop 2006;77(1):49–56.

39. Sabah S, Henckel J, Koutsouris S, et al. Are all metal on metal hip revision operations contributing to the National Joint Registry implant survival curves? A study comparing the London Implant Retrieval Centre and National Joint Registry datasets. Bone Joint J 2016;98-B:33–9.

Pearls and Pitfalls for a Surgeon New to Ankle Replacements

Federico Giuseppe Usuelli, MD[a],*, Camilla Maccario, MD[a,b]

KEYWORDS

- Total ankle replacement • Ankle arthritis • TAR • Prosthesis • Mobile bearing
- Fix bearing • Pitfalls

KEY POINTS

- Surgeon learning curve, patient selection, and implant choice are the key elements for a successful total ankle replacement (TAR).
- High-volume reference-center should play a role in the training of new surgeons.
- Bone-stock loss, deformity, and patient's age are not absolute contraindications for TAR, but they are the main parameters in the decision-making process.
- The most common approach is the anterior and it provides the best exposure of the ankle joint. Lateral approach can be more demanding, but provides a direct exposure of the center of rotation of the ankle joint.
- Mobile-bearing TAR has accommodative movement, but it requires perfect balance with soft tissues and bony procedures.

INTRODUCTION

The first total ankle replacement (TAR) was similar to an inverted total hip replacement and was performed by Lord and Marotte in 1970.[1] However, first-generation TAR designs had unacceptably high complication and failure rates.[2,3]

After 3 implant generations, numerous modifications in their design, and different surgical approaches, TAR now represents a reliable alternative to fusion.[4,5] TAR long-term results compared with those of ankle fusion continue to be one of the most debated topics in foot and ankle surgery.[6,7] A recent systematic review of intermediate and long-term outcomes comparing TAR with arthrodesis showed comparable risks of early complications and long-term failure for both procedures.[8,9] Newer

Disclosures: F.G. Usuelli is a consultant for Zimmer-Biomet, Integra, Geistlich. C. Maccario has no disclosures.
ᵃ C.A.S.C.O. Foot and Ankle Unit- IRCCS Galeazzi, via Riccardo Galeazzi 4, Milano 20161, Italy;
ᵇ Universita' degli Studi di Milano, via Festa del Perdono, 7, Milano 20122, Italy
* Correspondent author.
E-mail address: fusuelli@gmail.com

studies reported implant survival rates from 70% to 95% for follow-up from 2 to 12 years.[10–13]

These encouraging recent data are supported by gait analysis findings. For instance, it has been proved that a mobile-bearing TAR more closely resembled normal gait when compared with gait patterns of patients with arthrodesis.[14] The principle behind both joint-preserving surgeries and TAR is that restoring the joint to a near-normal state, may improve ankle function, but also delay the onset of peritalar complex arthritis.[15] Three main factors play a role in the final outcome: the surgeon, the patient and the implant itself.

DISCUSSION
The Surgeon

In the past decade, there is an ongoing debate between surgeons supporting ankle fusion, and surgeons supporting TAR. Many comparison studies between fusion and TAR have been designed and published, but it is extremely difficult to find a clear definitive answer from these studies.[16,17] In fact it is very challenging, if not impossible to design and perform a true prospective randomized fusion versus TAR study.

A proper approach is to accept that there are patients eligible for TAR and others are candidates for ankle fusion, with a limited mismatch area between the 2 groups. New studies are needed to clarify these boundaries.

Nonetheless, the enthusiasm toward TAR is tempered with caution, as a comparison of international registry data with clinical study results has found that implant designers reported significantly lower revision rates compared with those data reported in the registries.[18]

On the other side, nondesigner studies, reporting less encouraging results, are often affected by low-volume issues, and surgeon learning curve.[19–21]

The role of the operative learning curve in TAR has been investigated by various scholars and has produced contradictory results. Some findings did not show any evidence of a learning curve in TAR,[22,23] and others showed a reduction in perioperative complications and revisions with the increase of expertise.[19,20,24–26] Most of the studies have compared consecutive series of TAR cases to determine if a learning curve was present from the initial to more recent procedures.[27,28]

The practice of a young surgeon approaching TAR may be more affected by studies designing an ideal cutoff around which clinical and radiological outcomes can be considered stable and reliable.[29] Further studies are needed to determine how to structure surgical training to limit complications and optimize final results.

The epidemiologic features of ankle arthritis may suggest identifying reference centers both for the treatment of this pathology and for specific training for the surgeons involved in its treatment.[30] It is a principle that had inspired health policy in many other medical specialties (obstetrics, for instance), successfully reducing risks and complications for patients.[31]

In particular, the role of high-volume reference centers in the training process is not only limited to the surgical-technique learning curve, but is also extended to the chance for a young surgeon to be exposed and deal with minor and major complications that may occur after TAR implantations.

Minor complications are those that are manageable without further surgery and risk-system failure, whereas major complications are those that require additional surgery and lead to implant failure.[16,32] According to this classification, medial impingement, articular stiffness, delay in wound healing, and intraoperative fractures can be counted among minor complications. Aseptic loosening, deep infection, implant mobilization, severe malalignment, implant failure, and talar avascular necrosis (AVN) are included as major complications.

THE PATIENT
Patient Expectations

Ankle arthritis is commonly of posttraumatic origin.[16,33] Therefore, it is likely to affect young patients with high-level expectations.[16,33,34] Furthermore, a posttraumatic patient usually has a healthy contralateral ankle to compare with. This is the most important challenge for a surgeon: patients must be aware that a replaced ankle would never be as good as the healthy one. Every patient should be well informed on the expected outcomes to avoid illusions and unrealistic expectations.

One of the most important focus for the patients is to achieve a complete restoration of the range of motion, but this should not be the most important goal for the surgeon. Previous studies stated that the stiffness of a replaced joint may be a reason for patient complaints, but it is not strictly related to any poor functional outcomes.[8,35,36] This topic should be preoperatively discussed.

One of the most annoying minor complications is referred medial pain.[8,34] It may be linked to a thigh triceps surae or to a bone medial impingement.[37,38] In the first case, stretching activities should be recommended. Only in a few selected cases of clear bone medial impingement, arthroscopic medial debridement may be considered.

Last, during the short-term and long-term follow-up, patients can develop foot symptoms that may be not related to the previous TAR procedure. The surgeon should be very careful to plan a revision TAR, before the exclusion of any other independent foot pathologies.

Patient Selection

Every patient's individual combination of criteria has to be assessed and balanced thoroughly before surgery (**Fig. 1**).

"The ideal indication for TAR is a nonobese individual with a body mass index (BMI) ranging from 20 to 25 kg/m^2, low demand, severe pain secondary to ankle arthritis, well-aligned and stable hindfoot, reasonable mobility, a good bone-stock and has no significant comorbidities."[16]

There are probably no patients for TAR if we look for candidates without any relative contraindications.

Posttraumatic end-stage ankle arthritis, for instance, often presents at least moderate deformities.[16,33] Biomechanics understanding, surgical technique development, and design evolution may explain a recent trend toward extended indications.

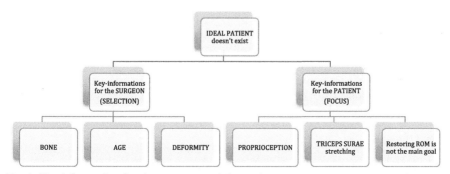

Fig. 1. Key information for the surgeon and the patient.

According to these principles, previous studies assessed that BMI greater than 25 kg/m^2, coronal deformity greater than 15°, partial areas of avascular bone, traumatic bone loss, or a history of previous infections represent relative rather than absolute contraindications.[16,33,34]

Acute or chronic infections, AVN of more than one-third of the talus, neuromuscular disorders, neuro-arthropathy (Charcot arthropathy of the midfoot or hindfoot), and diabetic syndrome with polyneuropathy are still absolute contraindications.[16,33,34]

Any preoperative assessment should be planned on weight-bearing radiographs. In most cases, additional computed tomography scans may be required to understand bone-stock quality and to identify preexisting bone cysts. With this proper imaging planning, the surgeon should be able to assess the feasibility of a TAR, according 3 main factors: bone, age, and deformity.[33,34]

Bone

Idiopathic and posttraumatic AVN more frequently affects the talar bone. In case of a subtotal AVN, talus will eventually develop subchondral collapse and secondary arthritis. This can occur at the ankle or at the subtalar joint or simultaneously in both joints.[16]

Fusion of the involved joints has been the only treatment of choice in similar cases for decades.[39] Nowadays, new TAR designs have allowed extended indications, especially with new talar component resurfacing designs.[40] These implants require a limited bearing surface and reduce the need of residual healthy bone. Furthermore, TAR and simultaneous subtalar joint fusion has been shown to be a safe and reliable procedure, at the end of the learning curve process of the surgeon.[41] Therefore, a combined procedure can be planned in case of arthritis developing in both joints (TAR and subtalar joint fusion), reducing the postoperative stiffness of a combined fusion of both ankle and subtalar joint (tibiotalocalcaneal fusion).

Age

Young patients are generally more demanding in terms of postoperative function of their ankle joint, return to sports, and recreational activities.

Age is an important consideration in TAR, but there is no hard evidence that age substantially affects the final outcome of TAR. The one concern with doing ankle replacements in younger patients is the longevity of the components, and salvage options once it fails.

Previous studies has suggested that clinical outcomes and implant survivorship of TAR are inferior in younger patients.[8,23,24,42] This is in contrast to studies on total hip and total knee arthroplasty.[43,44]

Recent studies have shown that TAR is a reliable alternative to ankle fusion also in young patients. Kofoed and Lundberg-Jensen[45] reported equivalent survivorship TAR in patients younger and older than 50 years. Rodrigues-Pinto et al[46] found a greater increase in the American Orthopaedic Foot and Ankle Society score and similar rates of complication and survivorship in patients younger than 50 compared with patients older than 50. Dermetracopoulus and colleagues[47] stated that the outcomes of TAR in younger patients were comparable to those of older patients at early follow-up. In addition, the incidences of complications, reoperation, and revision were similar between age groups.

Deformity

Posttraumatic arthritis accounts for 75% to 80% and rheumatoid disease for 12% to 15% of end-stage ankle arthritis.[48–50] In posttraumatic cases, patients are likely to develop deformities, bone-stock loss, and severe ankylosis. Between 30% and

40% of end-stage ankle arthritis cases present severe malalignment (higher than 10° in any planes).[51] In severe deformities, hindfoot osteotomies or arthrodesis and supramalleolar osteotomies in combination with TAR procedures are recommended (**Figs. 2 and 3**).[51,52]

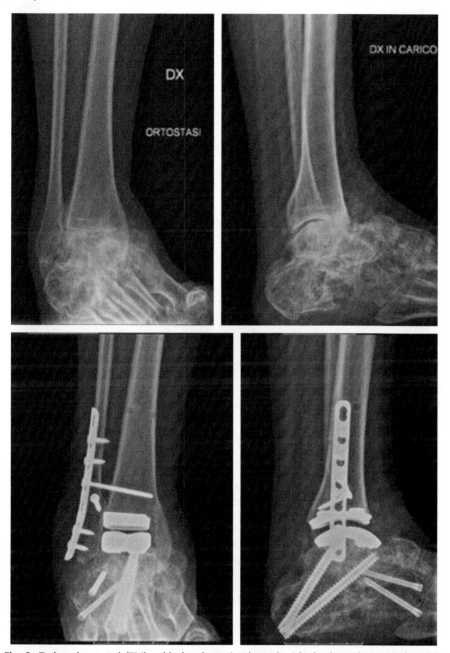

Fig. 2. Trabecular metal (TM) ankle has been implanted with the lateral approach. Additional procedures were fibular shortening osteotomy, subtalar joint fusion, and shortening of the lateral column with calcaneus-cuboid joint fusion.

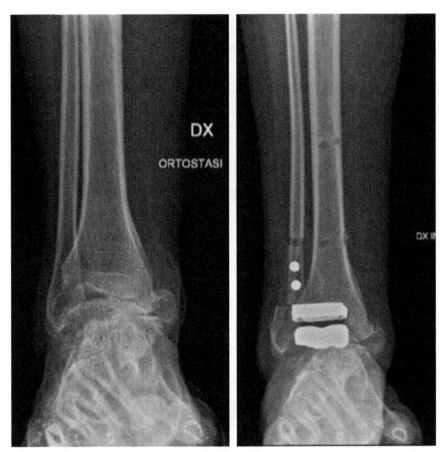

Fig. 3. TM ankle has been implanted with the lateral approach. The additional procedure was Z-shape lengthening abduction fibular osteotomy.

Minor deformities at the level of the ankle can be corrected with bone cuts during the operation (**Fig. 4**).

Doets and colleagues[53] reported an increased failure rate was encountered in ankles with a preoperative deformity of greater than 10° in the frontal plane.

Hobson and colleagues[54] compared patients with a preoperative hindfoot deformity less than 10° with a group with greater deformity (11°–30°) and found no difference in range of motion, complication, and survival rate.

Several studies reported good results in younger patients and in cases with preoperative malalignment.[46,53,54] In this population, TAR can be planned and successfully performed only by experienced surgeons at the end of their learning curve. Inexperienced surgeons should be tutored when dealing with these cases.

ANKLE REPLACEMENT
Anterior Approach

The anterior approach is the most common approach for total ankle arthroplasty (**Fig. 5**).[55] Passing between the anterior tibial and extensor hallucis longus tendons, it allows excellent visualization of anterior ankle joint including the distal tibia, tibiotalar

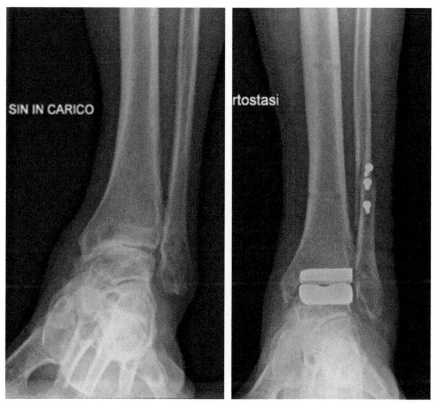

Fig. 4. TM ankle has been implanted with the lateral approach and standard technique for minor deformity.

joint, and talar dome. The downside for this surgical approach may be the risk of wound complications, especially in case of a previously violated soft tissue envelope.[25,56] Although wound-healing problems are not considered as major complications, surgeons should be mindful because of the related risk of implant exposure and consequent deep-infection risk.

Lateral Approach

The most important hypothetical advantage described for this approach is a reduced risk of healing complications of superficial wounds.[40] In our personal series that covers more than 120 cases, this does not appear to be a significant advantage compared with the anterior approach. The one advantage of the lateral approach is that if wound problems develop, there is no direct exposure of the ankle implant. However, the lateral plate would be exposed. For this reason, the investigator suggests performing a long oblique osteotomy to be able to fix it with 2 free 3.5 cortex screws and avoid any plate exposure in case of wound-healing issues (**Fig. 6**).

Furthermore, the transfibular approach may represent a significant challenge in terms of deformities corrections for a young surgeon, but it allows a direct visualization of the center of rotation of the ankle, with an advantage in terms of joint restoration.

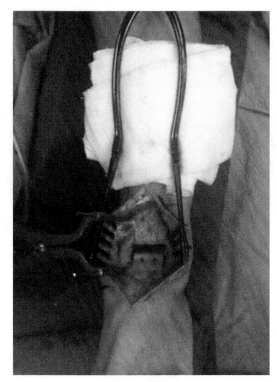

Fig. 5. Anterior approach.

Mobile and Fix Bearing

TAR implants are available with either fixed or mobile polyethylene (PE) bearings, and there is little consensus on the benefits and drawbacks of each type. The performance and complications of fix-bearing (FB) and mobile-bearing (MB) implants are well documented in the literature.[57,58] MB and FB have both advantages and disadvantages. The surgeon's choice may be related to training, with surgeons in Europe and Asia more likely exposed to MB-TAR and surgeons in the United States more likely exposed to FB-TAR.

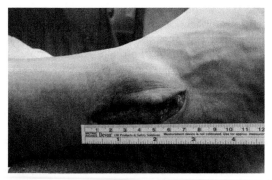

Fig. 6. Lateral approach.

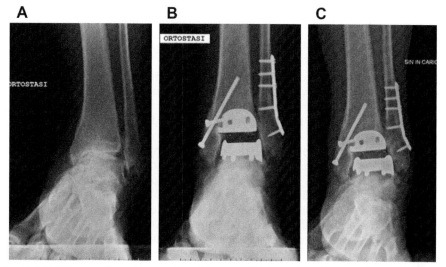

Fig. 7. MB-TAR needs to be balanced. In this case, MB Hintegra has been implanted with the anterior approach. Medial malleolus lengthening osteotomy to balance the deltoid ligament tension, fibular shortening osteotomy, and peroneus longus pro brevis transfer were simultaneously performed. (*A*) Preoperative; (*B*) 2-year follow-up; (*C*) 5-year follow-up.

Mobile bearing

MB design allows more flexible articulation with lower shear forces at the bone-implant interface but are susceptible to anteroposterior or lateral subluxation of the PE bearing, which may lead to tibial component overhang or malleolar impingement.[59,60]

One hypothetical advantage of the MB is the posterior talar shifting on the sagittal plane that has been shown by some independent investigators.[61–63] In fact, sagittal plane malalignment frequently occurs in ankle osteoarthritis, and the talus is often anteriorly translated. A compensatory movement may help the surgeon to deal with this deformity.[61–63] However, the exact mechanism of postoperative translation of the talus relative to the tibia after TAA remains unclear. It suggests that the surgeon should be mindful that the position of the components may change from their initial position during the immediate postoperative period as the surrounding soft tissues adjust to the new alignment and motion of the ankle. To benefit from this compensative movement, the prosthesis must be well balanced (**Fig. 7**).

Fix bearing

FB design provides a stable joint without the risk of subluxation of the PE bearing but is theoretically susceptible to loosening of the tibial component due to high shear forces at the bone-implant interface.[57,64] FB-TAR has been the only alternative in the United States for many years and it is recently gaining popularity in Europe.

FB aims to improve the talar centering, allowing for a reduction of malleolar impingement, and reducing particulate debris that may be responsible for subchondral bone cyst formation. FB does not allow any postoperative adaptive shifting; therefore, the correct center of rotation must be intraoperatively achieved.

SUMMARY

TAR is a reliable treatment for ankle osteoarthritis, but a new surgeon should be aware of the learning curve. Reference centers should be identified and involved in the training process. Proper selection of the patient and a comprehensive discussion of expectations are the keys for a successful treatment.

REFERENCES

1. Lord G, Marotte JH. Prothese totale de cheville: technique et premiers resultants: a propos de 12 observations. Rev Chir Orthop Reparatrice Appar Mot 1973;59: 139–51.
2. Hamblen DL. Editorial. Can the ankle be replaced? J Bone Joint Surg Br 1985;67: 689.
3. Kopp FJ, Patel MM, Deland JT, et al. Total ankle arthroplasty with the Agility prosthesis: clinical and radiographic evaluation. Foot Ankle Int 2006;27:97–103.
4. Kitaoka HB, Patzer GL. Clinical results of the Mayo total ankle arthroplasty. J Bone Joint Surg Am 1996;78:1658–64.
5. Knecht SI, Estin M, Callaghan JJ, et al. The Agility total ankle arthroplasty. Seven to sixteen-year followup. J Bone Joint Surg Am 2004;86-A:1161–71.
6. Brunner S, Barg A, Knupp M, et al. The Scandinavian total ankle replacement: long-term, eleven to fifteen-year, survivorship analysis of the prosthesis in seventy-two consecutive patients. J Bone Joint Surg Am 2013;95(8):711–8.
7. Nunley JA, Caputo AM, Easley ME, et al. Intermediate to long-term outcomes of the STAR Total Ankle Replacement: the patient perspective. J Bone Joint Surg Am 2012;94(1):43–8.
8. Haddad SL, Coetzee JC, Estok R, et al. Intermediate and long-term outcomes of total ankle arthroplasty and ankle arthrodesis: a systematic review of the literature. J Bone Joint Surg Am 2007;89(9):1899–905.
9. Saltzman CL, Mann RA, Ahrens JE, et al. Prospective controlled trial of STAR total ankle replacement versus ankle fusion: initial results. Foot Ankle Int 2009;30(7): 579–96.
10. Anderson T, Montgomery F, Carlsson A. Uncemented STAR total ankle prostheses. Three to eight-year follow-up of fifty-one consecutive ankles. J Bone Joint Surg Am 2003;85(7):1321–9.
11. Bonnin M, Judet T, Colombier JA, et al. Midterm results of the Salto total ankle prosthesis. Clin Orthop Relat Res 2004;424:6–18.
12. Buechel FF Sr, Buechel FF Jr, Pappas MJ. Twenty-year evaluation of cementless mobile-bearing total ankle replacements. Clin Orthop Relat Res 2004;424:19–26.
13. Schutte BG, Louwerens JW. Short-term results of our first 49 Scandinavian total ankle replacements (STAR). Foot Ankle Int 2008;29(2):124–7.
14. Singer S, Klejman S, Pinsker E, et al. Ankle arthroplasty and ankle arthrodesis: gait analysis compared with normal controls. J Bone Joint Surg Am 2013; 95(24). e191(1–10).
15. Hintermann B, Knupp M, Barg A. Joint-preserving surgery of asymmetric ankle osteoarthritis with peritalar instability. Foot Ankle Clin 2013;18(3):503–16. Review.
16. Krause FG, Schmid T. Ankle arthrodesis versus total ankle replacement: how do I decide? Foot Ankle Clin 2012;17(4):529–43.
17. Espinosa N, Klammer G. Treatment of ankle osteoarthritis: arthrodesis versus total ankle replacement. Eur J Trauma Emerg Surg 2010;36(6):525–35.
18. Labek G, Klaus H, Schlichtherle R, et al. Revision rates after total ankle arthroplasty in sample-based clinical studies and national registries. Foot Ankle Int 2011;32(8):740–5.
19. Haskell A, Mann RA. Perioperative complication rate of total ankle replacement is reduced by surgeon experience. Foot Ankle Int 2004;25(5):283–9.

20. San Giovanni TP, Keblish DJ, Thomas WH, et al. Eight-year results of a minimally constrained total ankle arthroplasty. Foot Ankle Int 2006;27(6):418–26.

21. Clement RC, Krynetskiy E, Parekh SG. The total ankle arthroplasty learning curve with third-generation implants: a single surgeon's experience. Foot Ankle Spec 2013;6(4):263–70.

22. Hosman AH, Mason RB, Hobbs T, et al. A New Zealand national joint registry review of 202 total ankle replacements followed for up to 6 years. Acta Orthop 2007;78:584–91.

23. Spirt AA, Assal M, Hansen ST Jr. Complications and failure after total ankle arthroplasty. J Bone Joint Surg Am 2004;86-A:1172–8.

24. Henricson A, Skoog A, Carlsson A. The Swedish Ankle Arthroplasty Register: an analysis of 531 arthroplasties between 1993 and 2005. Acta Orthop 2007;78: 569–74.

25. Myerson MS, Mroczek K. Perioperative complications of total ankle arthroplasty. Foot Ankle Int 2003;24:17–21.

26. Schuberth JM, Patel S, Zarutsky E. Perioperative complications of the Agility total ankle replacement in 50 initial, consecutive cases. J Foot Ankle Surg 2006;45: 139–46.

27. Schimmel JJ, Walschot LH, Louwerens JW. Comparison of the short-term results of the first and last 50 Scandinavian total ankle replacements: assessment of the learning curve in a consecutive series. Foot Ankle Int 2014;35(4):326–33.

28. Lee KB, Cho SG, Hur CI, et al. Perioperative complications of HINTEGRA total ankle replacement: our initial 50 cases. Foot Ankle Int 2008;29(10):978–84.

29. Usuelli FG, Maccario C, Pantalone A, et al. Identifying the learning curve for total ankle replacement using a mobile bearing prosthesis. Foot Ankle Surg, in press.

30. Reuver JM, Dayerizadeh N, Burger B, et al. Total ankle replacement outcome in low volume centers: short-term followup. Foot Ankle Int 2010;31(12):1064–8.

31. Zeitlin J, Blondel B, Ananth CV. Characteristics of childbearing women, obstetrical interventions and preterm delivery: a comparison of the US and France. Matern Child Health J 2015;19(5):1107–14.

32. Rodrigues-Pinto R, Muras J, Martín Oliva X, et al. Functional results and complication analysis after total ankle replacement: early to medium-term results from a Portuguese and Spanish prospective multicentric study. Foot Ankle Surg 2013; 19(4):222–8.

33. Barg A, Knupp M, Henninger HB, et al. Total ankle replacement using HINTEGRA, an unconstrained, three-component system: surgical technique and pitfalls. Foot Ankle Clin 2012;17(4):607–35.

34. Colombier JA, Judet T, Bonnin M, et al. Techniques and pitfalls with the Salto prosthesis: our experience of the first 15 years. Foot Ankle Clin 2012;17(4): 587–605.

35. Wood PL, Deakin S. Total ankle replacement. The results in 200 ankles. J Bone Joint Surg Br 2003;85:334–41.

36. Stengel D, Bauwens K, Ekkernkamp A, et al. Efficacy of total ankle replacement with meniscal-bearing devices: a systematic review and meta-analysis. Arch Orthop Trauma Surg 2005;125:109–19.

37. Valderrabano V, von Tscharner V, Nigg BM, et al. Lower leg muscle atrophy in ankle osteoarthritis. J Orthop Res 2006;24(12):2159–69.

38. Valderrabano V, Nigg BM, von Tscharner V, et al. J. Leonard Goldner Award 2006. Total ankle replacement in ankle osteoarthritis: an analysis of muscle rehabilitation. Foot Ankle Int 2007;28(2):281–91.

39. Myerson M, Christensen JC, Steck JK, et al. Avascular necrosis of the foot and ankle. Foot Ankle Spec 2012;5(2):128–36.

40. Tan EW, Maccario C, Talusan PG, et al. Early complications and secondary procedures in transfibular total ankle replacement. Foot Ankle Int 2016;37(8):835–41.

41. Usuelli FG, Maccario C, Manzi L, et al. Clinical outcome and fusion rate following simultaneous subtalar fusion and total ankle arthroplasty. Foot Ankle Int 2016; 37(7):696–702.

42. Fevang BT, Lie S, Havelin LI, et al. 257 ankle arthroplasties performed in Norway between 1994 and 2005. Acta Orthop 2007;78(5):575–83.

43. Long WJ, Bryce CD, Hollenbeak CS, et al. Total knee replacement in young, active patients: long-term follow-up and functional outcome: a concise follow-up of a previous report. J Bone Joint Surg Am 2014;96(18):e159.

44. Bisschop R, Brouwer RW, Van Raay JJAM. Total knee arthroplasty in younger patients: a 13-year follow-up study. Orthopedics 2010;33(12):876.

45. Kofoed H, Lundberg-Jensen A. Ankle arthroplasty in patients younger and older than 50 years: a prospective series with long-term follow-up. Foot Ankle Int 1999; 20(8):501–6.

46. Rodrigues-Pinto R, Muras J, Martín Oliva X, et al. Total ankle replacement in patients under the age of 50. Should the indications be revised? Foot Ankle Surg 2013;19(4):229–33.

47. Demetracopoulos CA, Adams SB Jr, Queen RM, et al. Effect of age on outcomes in total ankle arthroplasty. Foot Ankle Int 2015;36(8):871–80.

48. Saltzman CL, Zimmerman MB, O'Rourke M, et al. Impact of comorbidities on the measurement of health in patients with ankle osteoarthritis. J Bone Joint Surg Am 2006;88:2366–72.

49. Chou LB, Coughlin MT, Hansen S Jr, et al. Osteoarthritis of the ankle: the role of arthroplasty. J Am Acad Orthop Surg 2008;16:249–59.

50. Rippstein PF, Huber M, Coetzee JC, et al. Total ankle replacement with use of a new three-component implant. J Bone Joint Surg Am 2011;93:1426–35.

51. Wood PL, Sutton C, Mishra V, et al. A randomised, controlled trial of two mobile-bearing total ankle replacements. J Bone Joint Surg Br 2009;91:69–74.

52. Thomas R, Daniels TR, Parker K. Gait analysis and functional outcome following ankle arthrodesis for isolated ankle arthritis. J Bone Joint Surg Am 2006;88: 526–35.

53. Doets HC, Brand R, Nelissen RG. Total ankle arthroplasty in inflammatory joint disease with use of two mobile-bearing designs. J Bone Joint Surg Am 2006; 88:1272–84.

54. Hobson SA, Karantana A, Dhar S. Total ankle replacement in patients with significant pre-operative deformity of the hind-foot. J Bone Joint Surg Br 2009;91: 481–6.

55. Hintermann B, Barg A. The HINTEGRA total ankle arthroplasty. In: Wiesel SW, editor. Operative techniques in orthopaedic surgery. 1st edition. Philadelphia: Lippincott Williams & Wilkins; 2010. p. 4022–31.

56. Pyevich MT, Saltzman CL, Callaghan JJ, et al. Total ankle arthroplasty: a unique design. Two- to twelve-year follow-up. J Bone Joint Surg Am 1998;80:1410–20.

57. Valderrabano V, Pagenstert GI, Müller AM, et al. Mobile- and fixed-bearing total ankle prostheses: is there really a difference? Foot Ankle Clin 2012;17(4):565–85.

58. Gaudot F, Colombier JA, Bonnin M, et al. A controlled, comparative study of a fixed-bearing versus mobile-bearing ankle arthroplasty. Foot Ankle Int 2014; 35(2):131–40.

59. Lewis G. Biomechanics of and research challenges in uncemented total ankle replacement. Clin Orthop Relat Res 2004;424:89–97.
60. Conti SF, Wong YS. Complications of total ankle replacement. Clin Orthop Relat Res 2001;391:105–14.
61. Lee KB, Kim MS, Park KS, et al. Effect of anterior translation of the talus on outcomes of three-component total ankle arthroplasty. BMC Musculoskelet Disord 2013;14:260.
62. Usuelli FG, Maccario C, Manzi L, et al. Posterior talar shifting in mobile-bearing total ankle replacement. Foot Ankle Int 2016;37(3):281–7.
63. Wood PL, Prem H, Sutton C. Total ankle replacement: medium-term results in 200 Scandinavian total ankle replacements. J Bone Joint Surg Br 2008;90(5):605–9.
64. Mehta S, Donley B, Jockel J, et al. The Salto Talaris total ankle arthroplasty system: a review and report of early results. Semin Arthroplasty 2010;21(4):282–7.

Index

Note: Page numbers of article titles are in **boldface** type.

A

Accuracy, of total ankle arthroplasty using navigation assistance system, **455–463**

Agility implants, stemmed, revision of, **341–360**
    background, 342–347
    outcomes, 355–359
    surgical technique, 347–355

Alignment correction, of lower limb before, during, and after total ankle arthroplasty, **311–339**
    avoiding postoperative disaster, 336–338
    clinical evaluation, 313–315
    considerations for adjunctive procedures, 322–324
    deformity of foot distal to ankle, 318–322
    deformity proximal to ankle joint, 316–318
    intraoperative considerations, 324–336
        multiplanar, 334–336
        procurvatum, 332–334
        recurvatum, 331–332
        valgus ankle, 327–331
        varus ankle, 324–327
    treatment and consideration of deformity, 315

Ankle arthrodesis. *See* Arthrodesis, ankle.

Ankle arthroplasty, total. *See* Total ankle arthroplasty.

Ankle, stiff. *See* Stiff ankle.

Arthritis, end-stage ankle, total ankle arthroplasty for, 251–489
    ankle arthrodesis *versus* total ankle arthroplasty, **251–266**
    kinematics and function with total ankle replacements *versus* normal ankles, **241–249**
    osteolysis mechanism in, **267–275**
    in presence of talar varus or valgus deformities, **277–300**

Arthrocentesis, and synovial fluid analysis, in diagnosis of periprosthetic infection, 410–411

Arthrodesis, ankle, 252–256
    contraindications, 252
    outcomes, 256
    technique, 252–256
    versus total ankle arthroplasty, 260–262

Arthroplasty, total ankle. *See* Total ankle arthroplasty.

Arthroscopic surgery, for stiff ankle after total ankle arthroplasty, 441

B

Biomechanics, of total ankle replacements *versus* normal ankles, 242

Foot Ankle Clin N Am 22 (2017) 491–502
http://dx.doi.org/10.1016/S1083-7515(17)30041-4
1083-7515/17

foot.theclinics.com

Moving?

Make sure your subscription moves with you!

To notify us of your new address, find your **Clinics Account Number** (located on your mailing label above your name), and contact customer service at:

Email: journalscustomerservice-usa@elsevier.com

800-654-2452 (subscribers in the U.S. & Canada)
314-447-8871 (subscribers outside of the U.S. & Canada)

Fax number: 314-447-8029

Elsevier Health Sciences Division
Subscription Customer Service
3251 Riverport Lane
Maryland Heights, MO 63043

ELSEVIER

Printed and bound by CPI Group (UK) Ltd, Croydon, CR0 4YY

08/05/2025

01864699-0004